R0061494779

01/2012

D1238699

# OPEN HEART

# OPEN HEART

## The Radical Surgeons
## Who Revolutionized Medicine

### DAVID K.C. COOPER, MD

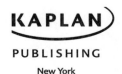

PUBLISHING

New York

© 2010 David Cooper

Published by Kaplan Publishing, a division of Kaplan, Inc.
1 Liberty Plaza, 24th Floor
New York, NY 10006

Printed in the United States of America

10 9 8 7 6 5 4 3 2 1

Library of Congress Cataloging-in-Publication Data

Cooper, D. K. C. (David K. C.), 1939–
    Open heart : the personal stories of the daring young men who pioneered heart surgery/ by David Cooper.
        p. ; cm.
    Other title: Personal stories of the daring young men who pioneered heart surgery
    Includes bibliographical references and index.
    ISBN 978-1-60714-490-8 (alk. paper)
    1. Heart—Surgery—History. 2. Thoracic surgeons—Biography. I. Title.
II. Title: Personal stories of the daring young men who pioneered heart surgery.
    [DNLM: 1. Thoracic Surgery—Biography. 2. Cardiac Surgical Procedures—history. 3. History, 20th Century. 4. Thoracic Surgery—history.
WZ 112.5.C2 C776o 2010]
    RD598.C6635 2010
    617.4'12092'2—dc22

2010011389

Kaplan Publishing books are available at special quantity discounts to use for sales promotions, employee premiums, or educational purposes. For more information or to purchase books, please call the Simon & Schuster special sales department at 866-506-1949.

*"It is not the critic who counts; not the man who points out how the strong man stumbled, or whether the doer of deeds could have done them better. The credit belongs to the man who is actually in the arena, whose face is marred by dust and sweat and blood; who strives valiantly, who errs and comes short again and again; who knows the great enthusiasms, the great devotions; who spends himself in a worthy cause; who, at the best, knows in the end the triumph of high achievement, and who, at the worst, if he fails, at least fails while daring greatly, so that his place shall never be with those timid souls who know neither victory nor defeat."*

— THEODORE ROOSEVELT

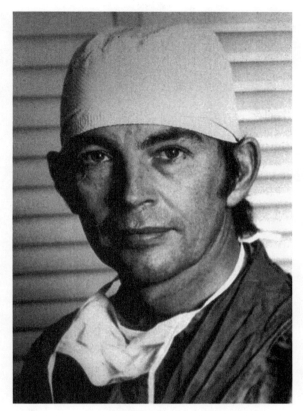

*Chris Barnard, the South African heart transplant surgeon, who epitomizes the daring young men who pioneered heart surgery.*

# CONTENTS

# Men Who Dared to Fail

*"Only those who dare to fail greatly*
*Can ever achieve greatly."*
— Robert Kennedy

PERFORMING HEART SURGERY has never been for the faint of heart. In no other specialty is a surgeon more likely to take a living patient into the operating room in the morning only to wheel out a dead one in the afternoon. In breaking the ultimate bad news to waiting relatives, the heart surgeon must confront the suspicion — and sometimes the reality — that death has resulted directly from his or her own error in technique or judgment. Yet even when the surgeon is beyond reproach, and even when death remains only one among many potential outcomes, the pressure takes a toll, and it requires a healthy self-regard to carry on despite it.

For more than 50 years — since my time as a medical student at London's renowned Guy's Hospital, where I came under the influence of Russell Brock and Donald Ross, two of the heart surgeons featured in this book — I have observed the world of the heart surgeon from a distinct vantage point — as a member of the profession. Heart surgery was the "cutting edge" of medicine at that time, and I can still feel the thrill of the very thought of operating on the heart itself — the source of life.

"The heart is the chief mansion of the soul," wrote the 16th-century surgeon Ambroise Paré, "the organ of vital faculty, the beginning of life...the first to live and the last to die." How bold and courageous must be the men who did this work, I thought. It excited me like nothing before or since.

While I was carrying out postgraduate research, Christiaan Barnard performed his dramatic first human heart transplant, electrifying this field once more. I was present at the first heart transplant performed in the United Kingdom by Donald Ross at the National Heart Hospital in 1968, the 11th such operation in the world.

I then completed my training in general surgery and cardiothoracic surgery in the United Kingdom, after which I had the pleasure and privilege of working with Chris Barnard for a number of years in South Africa. I was impressed by his surgical knowledge and intelligence, and came under the influence of his charm and sense of humor—his obvious charisma. I came to know him well, and we maintained close contact until his sudden death in 2001. Indeed, it was through Barnard's auspices that I found myself in 1987 taking up an appointment at the Oklahoma Transplantation Institute in Oklahoma City, where Chris was scientist-in-residence after retiring from his position in Cape Town.

It was in Oklahoma City that the director of the Institute, Nazih Zuhdi, suggested to me that I write the story of the development of heart surgery. The subject had never been approached through the point of view of the surgeons who had actually contributed. Zuhdi, himself a pioneer in this field, suggested that I visit these men and learn their stories firsthand. Indeed, he facilitated my introduction and visits to several of them. A few, of course, had already died, but from 1987 onward, I managed to personally interview many of the great pioneers and even more of their colleagues and trainees. I was able to speak to others at length by telephone and, by the time I came to put this book together, I had recorded the detailed personal experiences of more than 60 of these surgeons and their associates. They are a memorable bunch, lacking neither audacity nor eccentricity.

In a letter to Robert Hooke, Isaac Newton wrote, "If I have seen further, it is by standing on the shoulders of giants." In our own time, in the process of interviewing test pilots and astronauts, Tom Wolfe picked up the phrase "the right stuff" to describe the "giants" of early space exploration. Tom Starzl, the great pioneer of organ transplantation, attributed the same, ineffable quality — "the right stuff" — to the leaders in the development of heart surgery.

It is now almost 60 years since the first open heart operation was performed under hypothermia in 1952, since a heart-lung machine was first used successfully in 1953, and since the first successful series of open heart operations using these machines was begun in 1955. It is more than 40 years since the first heart transplant hit the headlines.

Today, probably well over a million heart operations are performed worldwide each year. Heart surgery has now moved from the exotic to the routine, and yet, for the individual undergoing such an intervention, there is nothing at all commonplace about having one's chest cracked open and one's heart tinkered with. Well-known patients such as Dick Cheney, Larry King, David Letterman, Charlie Rose, Arnold Schwarzenegger, Robin Williams, and former President Bill Clinton can attest to the dramatic impact of such a personal crisis.

Because the men I profile in this book pursued and achieved their goals, the lives of all of us today — young and old, rich and poor — have been changed for the better. Without them, blue babies would continue to die in childhood, young adults would continue to die miserable deaths from valve disease, and older people would not be given a "second chance" through coronary artery surgery or heart transplantation. These men have affected our everyday lives much more than the early astronauts who, like these pioneering surgeons, had "the right stuff."

Two points that we shall discuss later are worthy of brief mention here. First, the drive and enthusiasm of the surgeons not only established heart surgery but also stimulated advances in cardiology, which progressed significantly on the coattails of cardiac surgery. Indeed, the work of the surgeons was a stimulus to the whole of medicine.

For example, the concept of intensive care came directly from experience with heart surgery. Second, the medicolegal climate was quite different from today. Experimentation on both animals and patients was far less regulated than it is today—almost unregulated—greatly facilitating exploration of innovative surgical techniques, at a speed that would be impossible today.

This book probes the questions "Who were these men?" and "What drove them to do what they did?" My aim in writing this book is to acquaint the reader not only with what these men achieved, but with who they were—their personalities, strengths, and weaknesses—and how life subsequently treated them. Having recorded my interviews with these pioneers, whenever possible I allow them to use their own voices in describing their thoughts and recollections. In some respects, therefore, this book can be considered an oral history of heart surgery—that is, the achievements of these men "in their own words."

It is an account of astounding scientific progress, interwoven with unique insights into the personalities, flaws, and foibles of the figures who made it possible. These young men—who were often only in their 30s when they made their breakthroughs—all shared a technical flair, and they all took bold and innovative steps to treat their desperately ill patients, but they were or are as different from one another as chalk from cheese. Some were solid establishment figures, others outsiders or mavericks; some staid conservatives, others flamboyant and charismatic. Some were rash to the point of recklessness, whereas others made cautious progress in little increments over many years. Those in the early years of "closed" heart surgery (not involving use of a heart-lung machine) tended to be individualists; those who came along later needed to be team leaders. But whether they were extroverts or reclusive, whether they wore their ego on their sleeve or kept it close to the vest, they all had an extraordinary singleness of mind and a courage that allowed them to do what they did.

To quote Thomas Carlyle, "A well-written life is almost as rare as a well-spent one." The lives of the surgeons about whom I have written were certainly well spent. I greatly enjoyed learning something about them as people, about their varied, often fascinating lives, and in particular, their awesome surgical achievements. I hope you, the reader, will equally enjoy reading about them.

*David Cooper*
*2010*

## CHAPTER 1

# The Long and Rugged Road: The First 2,500 Years

I N ORDER TO understand the immense achievements in heart surgery that took place largely in the period 1938 to 1982, we need to take a brief look at the relevant developments in medicine and surgery that took place before this time, i.e., in the 2,500 years or so before 1938. As New York physician Benjamin Franklin Sherman stated in 1896, "The road to the heart is only 2 or 3 cm in a direct line, but it has taken 2,400 years to travel it." In the words of the great British physiologist Ernest Starling, "Every discovery, however important and apparently epoch-making, is but the natural and inevitable outcome of a vast mass of work, including many failures, by a host of different observers."

## THE BEGINNING

This is a complex and compelling story that goes all the way back to the ancient Egyptians, who were aware of the heart's pumping action and the pulse. For more specific observations we must thank Claudius Galen, the second-century A.D. physician to Emperor Marcus Aurelius, who moonlighted by tending to injured gladiators. By virtue of this sideline, he gained the critical insight that death was rapid when the heart was wounded, particularly if the injury was in the left side (the left ventricle) (Figure 1), and was somewhat delayed if the wound did not actually penetrate the chamber. Galen also experimented on animals, which, unfortunately, led to conclusions that were not entirely accurate — some were wildly inaccurate — but that were nonetheless accepted as gospel by physicians and surgeons for the next 1,500 years.

New ideas came with the Renaissance, but the rebirth of interest in anatomy and physiology was actually led by artists, including Leonardo da Vinci, who wished to draw and paint the human body as it really was. Professional anatomists, such as Andreas Versalius, professor of surgery and anatomy at Padua, Italy, began to question Galen, but it was a risky business in a world dominated by reverence for tradition. Miguel Serveto, a Spaniard, was one of the first to note that there was a circulation of blood to the lungs that was quite separate from that to the rest of the body. He made the mistake of publishing his anatomical findings in a theological treatise that was condemned as heresy by John Calvin, and he was burned at the stake in Geneva. Even though he had been rash enough to criticize both the Protestant *and* Catholic churches, the treatment Serveto received must certainly have been a powerful disincentive to research in those days. Today, if one desires an academic career in medicine, the pressure to publish one's research findings is considerable, which has led to the dictum of "publish or perish." In those days, it seems it was "publish *and* perish."

The Englishman William Harvey, having learned from Serveto's example, for a long while let his theory of the circulation of blood become known only little by little through his lectures and dissections. Later, when he published his studies (in 1628), he went out of his way to cite Galen in support of his work. Nonetheless, he demonstrated for the first time that the two pumping chambers of the heart (the right and left ventricles) beat together, that the blood passes from the right ventricle through the lungs and back into the left side of the heart, and then is circulated around the body. He conducted a large number of animal experiments to support his observations in humans. He suspected, but could not confirm, that the blood, supplied to the tissues through the arteries, reaches the veins through capillaries, which he called "pores in the flesh." It was not until the invention of the microscope a few years later, however, that Marcello Malpighi of Bologna was able to document the existence of these small blood vessels.

When surgeons first ventured near the heart, it was quick, cut-and-thrust stuff, carried out in the conscious patient. Before the introduction of anesthesia in the mid-19th century, most surgical operations were performed with the patient tied or held down by the surgeon's assistants, often under the "numbing" influence of alcohol to reduce the exquisite pain that must have been inflicted. Under such horrendous conditions, it must have taken extreme motivation and real courage to be the patient, and special qualities to be the surgeon. Not surprisingly, the quickest surgeons were considered to be the best; the amputation of a limb could be carried out routinely in seconds, rather than minutes. Although this perhaps reduced the period of maximum pain to which the patient was exposed, his or her troubles were by no means over. As neither the principle of antisepsis nor asepsis (sterility) had been introduced, almost every operation was complicated by a foul-smelling wound infection that was not infrequently fatal. Modern-day man — and surgeon — has no idea of the privileged world in which he lives.

At some point during the first two decades of the 19th century, an obscure surgeon from Barcelona, Francisco Romero, attempted to drain excess blood and other fluids that accumulate in certain diseases from the "sac" in which the heart lies. At the prestigious Faculty of Medicine in Paris, the "authorities" felt that Romero lacked sufficient stature to advocate such a hair-raising procedure and refused to publish his report. Accordingly, it is unclear whether the honor of being the first surgeon to operate for this condition was Romero or Dominique Larrey, chief surgeon of Napoleon's elite Imperial Guard. While Romero's report remained in the "silence of the archives," Larrey became famous and was made a baron, demonstrating the multiple hurdles that may need to be overcome if one is to achieve academic recognition.

It took almost a century for the next major milestone. In 1896, a German surgeon named Ludwig Rehn successfully repaired a stab wound of the heart. Such a significant invasion of the body probably could not have succeeded without two crucial advances in the intervening years: the introduction of anesthesia, and the introduction of antiseptic, and subsequently aseptic (sterile), surgical techniques. Surgery to repair diseased or deformed hearts had to wait for further crucial advances to take place — the development of special anesthetic techniques to allow the patient to be oxygenated with the chest open (when the lungs would normally collapse), the introduction of blood transfusion and the evolution of blood banks, and the development of techniques for suturing blood vessels together. Temporarily stopping the heart, or supporting the circulation with a mechanical pump such as the heart-lung machine, required the introduction of heparin, an agent that prevents the clotting of blood.

These developments took place in the late 19th and early 20th centuries, and enabled the surgeons portrayed in this present book to take their giant steps forward. The surgeon's task was also greatly aided by the improved preoperative diagnosis that became possible after the introduction of cardiac catheterization, which in itself is a remarkable story.

## THE HUMAN GUINEA PIG

Cardiac catheterization is a diagnostic technique that allows cardiologists and heart surgeons to know exactly what needs to be done before subjecting a patient to the rigors of more invasive procedures, such as heart surgery. It involves threading a long, thin tube either through a vein or an artery (usually in the arm, leg, or neck) into the heart to allow pressure readings to be taken inside the various chambers. Blood can be withdrawn through the catheter for other measurements, such as oxygen saturation.

A young German physician named Werner Forssmann, aware that primitive cardiac catheterization had been carried out in experimental animals, became convinced that catheterization of humans could be conducted without danger. In 1929, he suggested catheterizing a patient, but his chief at the hospital where he worked in Eberswalde turned him down. Forssmann then volunteered to perform the procedure on himself, but that also was vetoed. Undaunted, Forssmann persuaded a nurse named Gerda Ditzen to assist him. Beyond that point, the details have become clouded by legend. In one version of the story, she appeared to develop cold feet and refused to participate, and Forssmann was forced to tie her to the operating table to prevent her from interfering. A second version suggests that he tied her down in order to catheterize her arm, but then changed his mind and decided to experiment on himself.

What we know for certain is that Forssmann injected a local anesthetic into the crook of his own arm and inserted a catheter into a vein. When he had passed the catheter about 12 inches into his arm, he untied Gerda Ditzen and asked her to call the nurse who was in charge of the X-ray machine. With the catheter protruding from the vein, Forssmann then walked down a flight of stairs to the basement of the building, where the nurse took several X-ray films to confirm the presence of the catheter inserted all the way up to the shoulder. He then pushed it a few inches farther until he was sure it was in his heart, after which they took more X-rays. By this very personal experiment, Forssmann clearly demonstrated the safety of the procedure.

Eventually, Forssmann conceived the idea of injecting a radioopaque dye into the chamber of the heart through the catheter, thus making it possible to create an image of the individual heart's unique anatomy, including any defects, abnormalities, or disease in the major coronary arteries. He wanted to test this idea in dogs, but none of the hospitals with which he was affiliated had canine facilities. This problem was solved by his mother, who offered to look after the dogs in her own apartment, keeping them in the bathtub because they were often incontinent. Forssmann would sedate the dogs in his mother's home, put them in a sack, drive them to the hospital where he could carry out his experiments, then return them to his mother's care.

In time, Forssmann placed a catheter in his own heart once again, injected the contrast material, and had more X-ray films taken. The quality of the pictures was very poor, but at least he had demonstrated that the technique was safe and was accompanied by only brief dizziness and temporary blurring of vision. In 1931, he presented his study at a surgical congress, but the expectations were so low that his speaking time was cut in half. In fact, the audience paid little attention, and his talk engendered snickers of derision.

Afterward, Forssmann lapsed into obscurity. His work was largely forgotten and, after World War II, even his whereabouts were unknown. The distinguished British physician Sir John McMichael, himself a pioneer in this field, tracked Forssmann down at a small country hospital in Germany, where he had been working as a urologist. McMichael invited Forssmann to visit England, following which his reputation was reborn. Forssmann was never appointed to a high position in academic surgery; however, in 1956, he shared the Nobel Prize in Medicine or Physiology with André Cournand and Dickinson Richards of New York, who had by then established cardiac catheterization as a routine procedure.

By using meticulous sterile technique, the preliminaries to true heart surgery were already underway before the introduction of antibiotics, which, from a practical perspective, was a post–World War II advance. However, the more complex open heart surgery, particularly when foreign materials such as mechanical heart valves were inserted, was undoubtedly facilitated by the availability of an increasing number of antibiotics.

These numerous advances in medicine and surgery, developed over centuries but particularly during the first half of the 20th century, set the scene for the revolution that was to take place in the surgery of the heart. As the great Austrian surgeon Theodor Billroth said in 1850, "Only the man who is familiar with the art and science of the past is competent to aid in its progress in the future."

Winston Churchill put it more succinctly when he said, "The future rests on the foundations of the past."

## CHAPTER 2

# The First Steps Forward: Boldness and Delicacy

### ROBERT GROSS AND CLARENCE CRAFOORD

T HE BEGINNING OF heart surgery is considered by most to have started with Robert Gross (Figure 2) in Boston in 1938, with a procedure he developed to correct a condition known as the patent ductus (an abnormal connection between two major blood vessels close to the heart). This was followed in 1944 by the successful excision of a coarctation — a narrowed obstructive segment of the body's major blood vessel, the aorta — by the Swedish surgeon Clarence Crafoord (Figure 3). Neither of these operations was on the heart itself, but they nevertheless corrected structural abnormalities that caused heart failure. Although relatively simple operations by today's standards, they were major milestones that opened up an entirely new field of surgery.

The two surgeons, Gross and Crafoord, were rivals, and Gross privately accused Crafoord of stealing from him both the idea and technique for repairing coarctation of the aorta. Crafoord countered that he had been planning an operation for coarctation for some years, and indeed this seems to be likely. Crafoord was enough of an innovator and such a highly skilled surgeon in his own right that he almost certainly did not need Gross to give him ideas. Nonetheless, it was said that Gross never again allowed visitors into his experimental laboratory for fear they would steal his ideas. Whatever the truth of the matter, these two men deserve our recognition and thanks as being the founders of modern cardiovascular surgery.

Gross was an extraordinary person, highly gifted but someone who did not tolerate competition. Because of his difficult personality, he was finally forced from his position as surgeon-in-chief at Boston's prestigious Children's Hospital. Crafoord, with his Scandinavian reserve, was described to me by one surgeon who remembered his visits to the United States as being "absolutely brilliant" as well as "extremely pleasant and likable." Yet Crafoord also had his quirks; he reputedly had a policy of quietly stimulating competition, rivalry, and dissent between his immediate subordinates, which some thought was a means of maintaining his own predominant position.

## ROBERT GROSS —
## THE ENIGMATIC HARVARD MAN

The glory of being remembered by all subsequent generations of heart surgeons as one of the great founders of their specialty could well have gone to one or two earlier surgeons who attempted unsuccessfully to tie off (ligate or occlude) a ductus (Figure 4), but it was Robert Gross (Figure 2) who was the first to succeed. On August 26, 1938, at the young age of 33, Gross successfully tied a patent ductus in a seven-year-old girl, Lorraine Sweeney.

In his book *The Evolution of Cardiac Surgery,* Harris Shumacker states that before this operation, "so little could be accomplished that cardiac surgery hardly seemed a viable method of therapy. The operative conquest of the patent ductus arteriosus changed everything dramatically. One success led to another, then to a host of others, and suddenly an entirely new age of cardiac surgery was born. It was a period of successes, ideas, accomplishments, and the realization of dreams.... Most of all, this was an era of enthusiasm, hard work and opportunism. Difficulties that seemed insurmountable would be overcome. New achievements were around the corner."

## Young Days

Robert Gross was born in 1905. His father was a piano maker in Baltimore. In the book *The Work of Human Hands,* author G. Wayne Miller describes Gross as "a shy child, a reader, a scholar, one of eight children, an outdoorsman, and tinkerer who loved to take things apart and put them back together. Bob could break down and rebuild an automobile engine. He could mend clothes. He loved hammers, screwdrivers, motors, pumps, and knives. He was good with his hands, very good. His father encouraged him to take clocks apart and then put them together again."

Gross went to Carleton College in Minnesota because he wanted to attend a small liberal arts school. He originally intended to be a chemistry major, but he read Harvey Cushing's biography of Sir William Osler, an outstanding Canadian physician, and this turned him on to the idea of being a doctor. After graduating from Harvard Medical School, Gross spent time as a pathology resident because at first he could not obtain a surgical residency. As a pathology resident, he performed numerous autopsies on children who had died with patent ductuses, and he began to believe they could have been cured by an operation, even though at that time very few operations were carried out in the chest, let alone in or around the heart. In the few previous attempts to ligate the ductus, the children bled to death or died soon after.

In the womb, the developing fetus has no need of a blood supply to the lungs to pick up the essential oxygen and dispose of the toxic carbon dioxide, since its mother provides this gas exchange for it through the placenta (afterbirth). The circulation of blood in the fetus is therefore rather different from that after the baby is born. In the fetus, the blood is directed away from the lungs to the rest of the body. This "shunting" from the pulmonary artery to the aorta takes place through what is formally called the ductus arteriosus.

With the dramatic first deep breath after birth, which is associated with the opening up of the circulation of blood to the lungs, the blood is directed through the lungs, and the ductus arteriosus fairly rapidly constricts down through muscular activity in its wall. Within a short time, it becomes a solid fibrous band through which blood can never pass again.

In some babies, the ductus fails to close down. As a result of the much higher blood pressure in the aorta and the lower resistance to blood flow in the vessels of the lungs, the blood flow through the ductus reverses, flowing from the aorta to the pulmonary artery rather than from the pulmonary artery to the aorta (Figure 4). This has the effect of flooding the lungs with blood, rendering the infant more susceptible to shortness of breath and lung infections. It also places a strain on the heart, since much of its work is being wasted, blood intended for other organs being misdirected into the lungs. The symptoms of heart failure may not develop for weeks, months, or years, although the child is at increased risk from bronchitis and pneumonia throughout his or her young years. There is also the risk of infection affecting the walls of the ductus itself, which can lead to infection in the blood throughout the body (septicemia) and untimely death.

Robert Bartlett, a distinguished surgeon who trained in Boston, recorded, "By the age of six to ten years, the child would begin to cough up blood and become breathless; heart failure led to hospitalization and a miserable death of drowning in bloody secretions."

After successfully obtaining a surgical residency in Boston, Gross worked his way up the junior ladder until he became chief resident at Boston Children's Hospital. He suggested to his chief, William Ladd, that they tie off the ductus, but Ladd expressly forbade him to attempt it. Undeterred, Gross waited until Ladd was out of town (on a ship to Europe), then brought in not one but two patients, figuring that if the first one died, he could operate on the second the next day. Ladd had barely been gone two days when Gross performed the first operation successfully. The second patient also survived. According to

Hardy Hendren, the Robert Gross Distinguished Professor of Surgery at Boston Children's Hospital, a man who had received his surgical training under Gross and whose career had been greatly influenced by Gross's extraordinary personality, "Gross certainly had nerve and confidence; not many chief assistants would attempt to carry out an entirely new operation without their chief's full support. To do so when the chief was out of town took real 'chutzpah.' Gross put his entire career on the line. If his patient had died, Gross's career may have received a hammer blow from which he would never have recovered."

When Ladd got home, he fired Gross.

Robert Bartlett told me, "Everybody in the hospital had spent their lives seeing children die with patent ductuses. It must have been just awful because these kids had progressive pulmonary hypertension [an increase in the blood pressure in the lungs causing increasing shortness of breath] and would live to be about seven or eight. So here were two children who were cured of that terrible problem, and so all of the pediatricians, cardiologists, and surgeons went to Ladd, and said, 'That might have been outrageous, but it's really important. You have to get him back.' So Ladd finally relented, called Gross up, and invited him back. But Gross, who had gone to his farm in Framingham to build a barn, wouldn't come back until he got his barn finished. They [Ladd and Gross] subsequently shared a practice together." Nevertheless, according to Hendren, Ladd never forgave his junior colleague.

Hendren continued the story: "During the war, Gross somehow got deferred from the military. We later learned that the basis of his deferment was probably because he had only one eye through which he could see. He had been born with a cataract. As a little boy, he discovered that he couldn't see when he closed one of his eyes. So his entire surgical career was achieved with one eye, which was remarkable because depth of vision is clearly important to a surgeon."

According to Hendren, "When Ladd retired in 1945, Gross was the obvious heir apparent, but Ladd did everything he could to work against him and to downplay him. Edward Churchill [surgeon-in-chief at the Massachusetts General Hospital at that time] told me that he was the chairman of the search committee that picked Gross, and he said, 'We deliberated about it for two years because we were worried about his emotional stability.' I find that hard to translate, but Churchill was concerned about Gross's emotional self. He said that Sidney Farber, who was the chief of staff and head of pathology, said, 'Don't worry, we'll keep him in check. We'll keep him reined in, and not let him run quite so roughshod over people.' Churchill said, 'We couldn't deny Bob the job because he was head and shoulders above the others being considered.' Gross had done the patent ductus, and had written a book with Dr. Ladd, *Abdominal Surgery of Infancy and Childhood*. That little book is a classic. So Gross was appointed in 1947 as the Ladd Professor."

The William E. Ladd Professor of Children's Surgery at the Harvard Medical School was the first such chair in the nation. Miller describes Gross's appearance at that time: "What a figure Gross cut, with his red bow tie and starched white lab coat and spit-polished shoes and perfectly slicked hair. How he spoke — eloquent, educated, totally in command of his audience. This bunch of Harvardians. A true giant in their midst."

In Allen Weisse's book *Heart to Heart,* John Kirklin (chapter 8) recollects his early days as a medical student when he first had contact with Robert Gross: "He walked in, the very image of a surgeon; probably five feet eight or nine, with his hair in perfect order, immaculately dressed in a beautiful blue suit and red tie...he was the world's opinion of a surgeon in appearance."

Hendren continued: "Gross was a very busy surgeon. In those days, when I was a medical student, he would operate on two or three ductuses every day (as well as doing all other forms of surgery on children). In fact, he employed other surgeons as sort of silent partners, and they would do all of these operations for him with his name attached. They, of course, resented that quite a lot. Gross didn't like anybody else to share the professional spotlight with him. If anybody came along who had any gumption, he saw to it that they didn't stay with him long. He was a curious man, because the attitude of many other leaders in surgery at that time was just the opposite. They trained the best, and they kept the best. Gross had an opportunity to train many of the best, but none of them stayed with him. He made it hard for them. If you were one of his residents, you were just great. As soon as you finished as a resident, you'd better get going.

"When I finished as a chief resident here, it was July 1960. I had been offered a job in Kansas City [Hendren's hometown] as head of pediatric surgery at this fledgling children's hospital, which was at that time a real dump of a place, although they were making plans to improve it. Gross said, 'No, don't do that. You should stay here.' So I turned down the job in Kansas City, and said I would stay with him.

"Soon after, his secretary said, 'You know, you'd better be careful; you did more cases last month than Dr. Gross did.' I laughed, and said, 'Well, for God's sake, don't tell him.' She said, 'Oh, he knows. He knows exactly how many cases everybody does. He looks at all the schedules.' I didn't think much of that at the time, but a few days later I came in to operate one morning and found I was canceled on the schedule. A red line had been drawn through my name for the cases I had booked for eight A.M. and nine A.M. The chief of anesthesia came out, and sort of chided me, 'Why did you cancel your cases without giving us a warning?' The operating room supervisor said, 'Dr. Gross was here a little while ago, and he did that.'

"So I went around to see Gross, who was sitting at his desk. He pretended to ignore me for a minute, but then finally he couldn't because I was standing right in front of his desk, waiting to get his attention. He looked up and said, 'Yes?' I said that I had just come from the operating room and found my name crossed off the schedule. He said, 'Yep, I did that. You're doing too much. Somebody who has just finished as a chief resident should not have two private cases scheduled. I suggest you go on down the street and do some lab work or something else for awhile. Just lie low clinically.' I said, 'What exactly do you mean by that?' He said, 'Just that. Go find yourself an office someplace else. You can work here, but not too much.'

"Other surgeons before me had been banished to other hospitals because Gross was jealous of the fact that they were doing a lot. He would call them in and say, 'I don't want you operating here anymore.' He ruled his department like a kingdom. Apparently, he was not answerable to anybody. So, at any rate, he cancelled me off the schedule. That afternoon I went to see Churchill, who said, 'Hardy, come and start pediatric surgery here, because Bob will never let a young person come up under him. It's just not in his nature.' So I moved to the Massachusetts General Hospital that afternoon. You can imagine how I felt. Of course, the rumors flew that I had been fired, and so forth.

"Although it didn't occur to me at the time, in retrospect, as I look at Bob Gross's career, he was clearly a manic-depressive. He managed to control it pretty well, so that not many, except a few who knew him closely, were aware of it. He would have a bad thing happen in the operating room, a death, for example, and he would disappear for two or three weeks. Just gone. His wife wouldn't know where he was, and his secretary wouldn't know where he was. He would just disappear. Now that's not the behavior of somebody who is in control.

"He was an irascible genius. He was a superb technician, but he would get himself into technical trouble because he wouldn't slow down. I remember many instances. Gross would whiz through, expecting to be able to do every ductus in 55 minutes. Well, you know, there are some you can do in 35 minutes, but there are some that if you have to do them in 55 or 60 minutes, you're going to get into big-time trouble."

I suggested to Dr. Hendren that it must have been impossible to work with Gross.

"Some survived many years because they never opened their mouths, never wrote a paper, never did anything in the lab, just quietly worked behind the scenes. Others, who were not very able technical surgeons, never threatened Gross. But the behavior that Gross exhibited finally brought him down. They got a new president here at Children's Hospital, Leonard Cronkite. Leonard was an older guy who had been a colonel in the Army during World War II, and subsequently the commanding general of the entire National Guard here in New England. So Leonard was a tough military guy. When Gross ran up against Leonard, he met his match.

"I remember one night Leonard Cronkite came to see me at the Mass. General, and said, 'I've come to see you because I want to know why you suddenly left Children's so abruptly.' I told him what had happened. He said, 'Gross just did that? That wasn't legal and he couldn't do that.' I said, 'Was I, the youngest person on the staff, in a position to question what Gross did? There was no way I could have done that. I was nobody and he was everybody.'

"Cronkite sort of mulled it over. When Gross tried to do the same to another fellow, who was a very good surgeon who was coming along about two years after me, Cronkite went to Gross and said, 'Lay off, or the hospital will sue you.' I think the figure he mentioned was $2 million, which was a lot of money in those days. So the surgeon stayed and worked on the staff for ten years, but he never had any medical school appointment because Gross wouldn't let him have one. So you never could tell what Gross was going to do. He was literally a riddle wrapped in an enigma."

## Achievements

Robert Gross was very industrious throughout his career, and went on to make further important contributions to the surgery of the major blood vessels in children. He corrected a coarctation of the aorta soon after Crafoord, and his team worked on replacing segments of the aorta (the main blood vessel of the body) with grafts taken at autopsies from other patients (homografts). He was the first to treat a condition known as aorto-pulmonary window, similar in ways to the ductus but more difficult to correct. The surgical treatment of abnormal blood vessels that surround other structures in the chest, such as the esophagus (gullet) or trachea (windpipe), was another of his contributions.

By 1953, in fact, he had described most of the vascular malformations that a child could be born with, and had outlined surgical techniques for correcting them. In that same year, he brought out his monumental book on pediatric surgery, *Surgery of Infancy and Childhood,* a definitive tome that covered the entire field of surgery in children.

In recognition of his contributions to pediatric cardiovascular surgery, Gross received the prestigious Albert Lasker Award for Clinical Medical Research, not once, but twice, in 1954 and 1959, the only physician at that time to have won the award on more than one occasion. He was also elected to the U.S. National Academy of Sciences, a very rare honor for a surgeon.

With the introduction of the heart-lung machine (a machine that takes over the function of the patient's heart and lungs) in the mid-1950s, Gross, like many of his contemporaries, was less able to master the techniques of "open" heart surgery, and his surgical results were no longer outstanding. The situation of these older surgeons was not dissimilar to that of the stars of silent movies, many of whom could not make the move to the "talkies" successfully. Operations using the heart-lung machine required teamwork, and many of the older surgeons were prima donnas who could not adapt.

I asked Dr. Hendren what eventually happened to Gross.

"He got fired as surgeon-in-chief. It was probably in 1967. When a general in the National Guard, Cronkite, comes up against a 'general' in the surgical field, it had to be a knock-down drag-out. Cronkite could say, 'I've got the trustees with me and you do not.' In retrospect, I think that was the wrong thing to do. It would have been much better to somehow let Gross down more easily."

If he had been in charge, I asked Dr. Hendren, would he have fired Gross much earlier from the staff of the Children's Hospital?

"No, I don't think so. Gross was too brilliant a man to treat in that manner."

After what would appear to be the outrageous manner in which he had been treated by Gross, this statement spoke volumes about both men—the younger, despite his ugly treatment, magnanimously still recognizing the immense qualities of the older.

## Unpredictability

Hendren returned to Gross's unpredictability. After Hendren had been forced to leave the Children's Hospital, "Gross and I had no communication for five or six years. Suddenly, one Sunday night I got a telephone call. 'Hello, Hardy. It's Bob Gross.' I thought I was having a goddamn nightmare. I jumped out of the bed and stood. My wife wanted to know why I was doing that. Gross said, 'I'd like for you to do me a favor.' I said, 'What did you have in mind?' He said, 'You know Wednesday night I'm getting the Bigelow Medal [a prestigious honor awarded by the Boston Surgical Society, which involved giving a lecture]. I need somebody reliable who I can call upon to run my slides. I wonder if you would do that?' I was thinking why didn't he ask one of those he hadn't run out of town, but I said, 'Okay, I'd be happy to.' He said, 'Go and purchase a new projector. Be sure you have a spare bulb. Be sure you have a hemostat [a surgical gripping instrument] to retrieve a slide if it gets stuck. Be sure you have a dime to take the carousel off, if you have to lift it off. I want everything in duplicate. Meet me in my office at three in the afternoon, and we'll go down and practice.' You see, you couldn't fathom Gross.

"I picked up Gross, and we drove down to the place where he was going to give the lecture. He ran through his whole talk with an audience of one, myself, running his slides for him. That evening [at the formal lecture] Kenny Welch [who, like Hendren, had also been "run out of town" some years previously by Gross], realizing that I was going to do the projection, walked up, pulled a $100 bill out of his purse, and said, 'I'll give you this hundred if you'll drop the bastard's slides.'" However, Hendren ensured that Gross's lecture proceeded without a hitch.

Dr. Hendren showed me a framed letter from Gross, congratulating him on an excellent paper he had presented to the American Surgical

Association in 1970, some ten years after the two had acrimoniously parted company. He explained the story behind the letter: "I was due to present a paper, and Dr. Gross was attending the meeting. It was the last meeting he ever attended. I bumped into him, and he said, 'I notice you are going to present a paper. Do you have a copy of it I can read?' I said that I had, and so he came up to our room about five o'clock in the afternoon. My wife was in the shower, getting ready to go down to the reception. He read through the paper, and said, 'Very good.'

"By then, my wife was ready, and we went downstairs to the reception together. I'm sure a lot of people were looking over and, knowing the history of our relationship, were wondering what was this whale-and-water combination standing there together at the reception — the two of us, Gross and me. As we were going in to dinner, he said, 'Do you mind if I sit with you? I don't know anybody here anymore. All my cronies are gone.' So in we go, and we're sitting at dinner, my wife, Gross, and me. During dinner, Gross turned to me and suddenly asked, 'What was the name of that Italian fellow that was such a good artist?' I said, 'Are you speaking about Leonardo da Vinci?' He said, 'That's the one, yes.' That was the end of that. He didn't elaborate at all. Well, you didn't say to Gross, 'Why did you ask me that?' He was such a commanding figure that you didn't do that.

"The next morning, I gave my paper. Gross had told the Chair that he wanted to discuss the paper. So Robert Gross stepped up on to the platform, and said, 'As I get to the end of a career in academic surgery and look at what the young people are doing, it's clear that things that we did in the past were not the best for the patient. It's refreshing to see one of the young people pick up the ball and carry it further than we did in the past. Clearly, the work that has been presented by Dr. Hendren shows originality and technical skill.' He used several words that were very flattering, and then he said, 'I am reminded of the words of Leonardo da Vinci...' — and suddenly it was like a mallet hit me in the head — '...who said that a good teacher will be outshined by a brilliant pupil.' I couldn't believe what I was hearing. The entire audience stood and applauded him. Have you ever seen people stand and applaud a discusser? I was dumbfounded.

"As we were walking out of the auditorium, Frannie Moore [Francis Moore, the distinguished Harvard professor of surgery] put his arm around my shoulder, and said, 'Hardy, you may have thought that what Bob Gross was doing was discussing your paper, but that's *not* what he was doing. What he was doing was apologizing to you in front of the American Surgical Association, and that's why they all stood up and applauded him.' What a curious evolution of events!

"In 1982, I was appointed as chief of surgery here [the Boston Children's Hospital], and the first person who telephoned me was Gross. I was away, but my wife talked to him for a half hour on the phone. He said, 'Tell Hardy to call me as soon as he gets back. I want to talk to him. I don't know why he didn't go back to the Children's Hospital years ago.' Gross clearly just didn't put it all together somehow.

"He was a very unpredictable man. For example, he once walked out on his wife. Six months later, she was having dinner with a guest, and suddenly the front door of the house opened and Gross walked in, went upstairs, changed, came down, and sat at the table as if he had never been gone. The guest told me that in person. Gross had a long-standing affair with a nurse-anesthetist with whom he lived for several years. He never did marry her; Mrs. Gross wouldn't give him a divorce. He was also estranged from his two daughters; they didn't have much to do with him. He retired at age 65, went up to Burlington, Vermont, and never did anything after that. It wasn't a whole lot of years after that that he got put into a nursing home down in Plymouth, Massachusetts. He had rapidly deteriorating Alzheimer's, which was so sad because he was such a brilliant man. So here he was, a man all alone in his last years. He died there in 1988, at the age of 83, unable to use the telephone or do anything."

## Conflicting Opinions

Not everybody paints quite the same picture of Gross as did Hendren. Charles Hufnagel (see chapter 9), who worked in Gross's laboratory and played an important role in many of the surgical advances that came out of it, knew him well. He said, "Bob Gross was one of the most skillful surgeons of his time. He was a man who I found rather easy to get along with. I had very good relations with him until the very time he died. But he was also a very ruthless man. He would protect his own territory with all of the vigor that he could muster. He was not averse to making someone else's idea his own, but I think that that was the fashion of the day. I don't think that there's anything very peculiar about that. The story of his ligating the first ductus while his chief was away points out the aggressiveness of the individual."

According to Robert Bartlett, "You will hear conflicting opinions for a whole variety of reasons. From my point of view, he was an absolutely wonderful man who is a deity in surgery. Gross, to most people, seemed somewhat aloof, somewhat cold, less-than-caring with regard to patients and nursing staff but, from my point of view, it's absolutely not the case. He was a very shy person. The residents generally were totally intimidated by him, but the residents who knew him well came to love him, as just a warm, wonderful person — but there weren't very many of them.

"Dr. Gross used to do a lot of things to subsidize the residents, oftentimes without their knowing. He always seemed to be aware when someone was short of money or someone was ill or someone had a sick child in their family, and he would come up with things that would be helpful. It wouldn't be unusual to have a check for $500 just appear in your locker one day, perhaps from a friendly patient, but it always came through Dr. Gross. In the early days of cardiac surgery in the mid-1960s, the pump-oxygenator [heart-lung machine] was reusable, but had to be cleaned thoroughly after every case, reassembled, and then autoclaved [sterilized] for the next day's operation. He would hire one of the residents' wives to do that job and pay them $4 a pump. Some days there were two or three pumps to clean, so $8 or $12 a day was just phenomenal for residents on a pittance salary."

When relayed to Dr. Bartlett that I had been told that Gross did not treat the junior faculty well because he saw them as competitors, he replied, "That's not true at all. He fostered the career of a whole lot of people who came through the Children's. There was never, to my view, any fear of competition. Now you can imagine that some of the junior faculty might have seen it as competition because he was so very good at what he did, and just head and shoulders technically above anyone else who I've ever seen operate, then or since. That's intimidating to young guys. He was really magnanimous. He fostered everyone's career. If patients got referred to him personally, he took care of them. He operated on them, and was very responsible. He was not a person who would distribute his personal referrals to the more junior faculty. But if someone wanted to develop something that wasn't in his particular area of interest, then they were welcome to it. He maintained superb faculty there, but you had to be good at what you did."

A quite different story from that of Dr. Hendren. Which are we to believe? Perhaps there is truth in both. Gross probably did much to foster the careers of his former residents, if they were planning to move away from the Boston Children's Hospital, where he did not feel directly threatened by them, but perhaps he could not tolerate local competition by junior faculty.

I asked Dr. Bartlett whether Gross had any weaknesses, professionally or privately.

"Professionally, his seemingly aloof, detached attitude often came across to patients and families, but most of his patients and families were absolutely devoted to him....If a child died in the middle of the night—and in the year I was there the mortality for complex congenital heart lesions was about 50%—he would not come in and talk to the family. As a junior resident, that seemed to me to be uncaring. I'd be in there with the family. The kid would die and I'd have to go talk to the parents. 'What does Dr. Gross say?' You'd call him up and tell him. But he lived 45 minutes out of town at his wonderful farm in Framingham. He would just say, 'Well, tell them I'm sorry,' and that would be it. But he would always contact the family later—send a letter or talk with them on the telephone. As I got to know him well, I learned that was just because he didn't tolerate it [death] well. He was just emotionally distraught, and had a hard time dealing with families because he might break down. When the children did really well, he was equally quiet, but clearly very pleased about how things had gone."

Gross was obviously a man with conflicting sides to his personality, and changes in mood. For example, John Kirklin, who was a great admirer of him, admitted that at times he could behave in a way that alienated people: "Some people didn't like him and didn't know how to get along with him. I loved him, and got along with him great. I learned a tremendous amount from him, probably more than I have ever learned from any single individual, especially in the operating room. Dr. Gross was a difficult person. He could not really tolerate any very bright light around him. He was very good to me because I was going back to the Mayo Clinic, and so I wouldn't bother him. But he was a great man in every way."

Dr. Kirklin gave me an example why a lot of people seemed *not* to get along with Gross. "There was a little amphitheater [or gallery] over the operating table. One day we were operating, and the amphitheater was filled with famous surgeons. I don't remember who they all were, but they were people from all over the world traveling after the war. Somebody in the gallery dropped a newspaper on the floor. Gross said, 'Clear the gallery. Get out, and I don't want to see you again today. Go, please, *now*.' The fellow who dropped the newspaper said, 'I'm really sorry.' Gross said, 'The whole outfit of you, get out.'"

Several other eminent surgeons expressed their regard for Gross to me, and added that, when they had visited his department in Boston, he had been very "kind" and "generous" as a colleague.

## Perspective

I asked Dr. Hendren whether he could put the ductus operation into perspective in relation to the development of the surgical treatment of heart disease.

"It was clearly the opening wedge, wasn't it? Two or three people had tried to do a ductus before, and so it wasn't an original idea. Gross alone didn't have the idea, but he was the first to pull it off. It's fine to have talked about it, or tried it and failed, but the guy who pulls it off gets a lot of credit. I know Gross's first patient. As a matter of fact, I gave a talk about pediatric surgery in 1998, and one of the things that I said was that pediatric surgery is different from adult surgery in that we're trying to treat a patient who we hope will be alive sixty to seventy years later. Then I asked this lady who had been Gross's first ductus patient if she would stand up. My nurse had gone out and picked her up that afternoon. I said, 'This is the first ductus that was done by Robert Gross in 1938, and she is with us tonight.' That really poignantly put home the point. The audience thought that was great. I told a lot of people that the only thing anybody will remember about that talk is that Dr. Gross's first ductus patient stood up."

## CLARENCE CRAFOORD — THE INNOVATIVE SWEDE

Along with Americans Robert Gross and Alfred Blalock (see chapter 3), Clarence Crafoord (Figure 3), a Swede, was responsible for the initial surgical attempts to operate on large blood vessels close to the heart, although not on the heart itself. Working in Stockholm, he was one of the first to perform operations for patent ductus arteriosus; indeed, along with Gross, he advocated clamping, dividing, and oversewing the two ends of the ductus when ligation (tying) might be hazardous. Of more significance, Crafoord was the first surgeon in the world to carry out resection of a coarctation of the aorta in a human subject.

Coarctation of the aorta is another condition with which babies can be born, in which the aorta, the main artery that carries blood from the heart around the body, is greatly narrowed at the site where the ductus originally entered it (Figure 5). Blood can no longer pass easily from the heart to the lower part of the body, although the supply to the upper part of the body is intact. The obstruction, of course, leads to a strain on the heart and to a high blood pressure in the upper part of the body with a low blood pressure in the lower part. This difference can be detected by taking the blood pressure in the arm and comparing it with that in the leg. Children born with this problem often show relatively poor development of the legs unless the obstruction is corrected early in life. Furthermore, if the child successfully reaches adulthood, there is a high risk of rupture of blood vessels in the brain due to the persistently high blood pressure in the upper part of the body.

## The First Operation

Clarence Crafoord took the bold step of resecting (cutting out) the obstructed portion of the aorta and then suturing the two divided ends together. Although this sounds like a simple operation, it took a bold man to carry it out initially. Any technical error could have led to massive bleeding and loss of the patient's life; any infection of the suture line would have almost certainly resulted in rupture and death. However, Crafoord had technical ability on his side. According to Viking Bjork, one of his trainees, "Crafoord was a meticulous surgeon. What he did was always perfect.... The way he did coarctations was very good. He was excellent for the patient. He put all his energy into the patient's care."

Crafoord was already a highly respected chest surgeon when, on October 19, 1944, he operated on his first patient with coarctation of the aorta at the Sabbatsberg Hospital in Stockholm. The patient was an 11-year-old boy with high blood pressure, the only child of elderly parents. The parents were informed that the outlook without an operation was poor and that such an operation had never been performed before. After a long consideration, they permitted an exploratory operation, and gave Crafoord freedom to decide during it whether or not a resection and repair of the aorta would be feasible. This was indeed carried out, an exceedingly bold operation in those days.

It involved clamping the aorta above and below the coarctation, cutting out the narrowed segment, and stitching the two cut ends of the vessel together. As all the blood passing to the lower trunk and legs passes down the aorta, and as the blood pressure within the vessel is high, there was clearly a risk that, after joining (anastomosing) the two ends of the aorta together, the two cut ends could tear apart and the patient bleed to death. Fortunately, the operation was carried out successfully and the postoperative course of the patient was uneventful. The boy was discharged home two weeks later. Records indicate that, 32 years later, the patient remained well, without high blood pressure.

The surgical treatment for coarctation of the aorta, a relatively uncommon birth defect, was important for one other reason. It demonstrated to surgeons that, if the largest and most important blood vessel in the body could safely be clamped, a segment excised, and the two ends repaired successfully, then surely other abnormalities of the aorta and other major arteries could be dealt with similarly.

## Controversy

This first operation was swathed in controversy since Robert Gross claimed that Crafoord had obtained the idea when visiting his laboratory in Boston, and had seen him perform such a procedure in a dog. Crafoord and his supporters countered by saying they had been thinking of this procedure for some time, and it did not result from Crafoord's visit to Gross's laboratory.

Crafoord claimed he gained the idea for this daring operation a few years earlier, during a ductus operation when he had severe bleeding that could not be arrested until he put clamps on the aorta above and below the site of hemorrhage. The clamps were applied for 28 minutes and, in spite of this long interruption of the circulation to the lower part of the body, there were no problems afterward. For example, the lack of blood supply to the lower part of the body did not lead to damage of the spinal cord with resulting paralysis of the legs. He reached the conclusion that a patient with a coarctation would stand an even longer period of aortic cross-clamping. He reasoned that, in a patient with a coarctation, at least a small blood supply to the lower part of the body must have developed by abnormal routes through what are called "collateral" vessels. As blood flow down the aorta was already greatly restricted or even occluded, clamping the aorta would have little extra effect. The experience stimulated him to practice dividing and repairing the aorta in dogs, which, if massive bleeding was to be avoided, was anything but easy in those days of very primitive needles and suture materials.

Credit has been given in some American medical literature to Gross for performing the first operation for coarctation. However, he did not perform his operation until June of the following year, having heard of three of Crafoord's successful cases from an American cardiologist who had attended one of Crafoord's earliest operations. According to Charles Hufnagel, who was working with Gross at the time, Gross had been asked to act as a reviewer (for an American journal) of Crafoord's report on his first cases. Gross and Hufnagel already had a paper due for publication that outlined their experimental work on resection of coarctation in dogs. Gross immediately admitted two patients with coarctation and successfully operated on one of them, adding these two cases as an appendix to the experimental paper when he received the proofs. In this way, his two patients were actually reported before Crafoord's, whose own paper was not published until some weeks later. However, Crafoord's cases predated those of Gross. I have no reason to doubt this story, because Hufnagel was certainly in a position to know the facts. According to Hardy Hendren, "Gross wouldn't have done that if he weren't trying to get primacy of publication. Gross was a very competitive man who didn't like to be one-upped in any sense of the word."

Erik Berglund, a Swedish physician who worked with Crafoord, informed me, "Crafoord carried out some dog experiments on coarctation but, when he visited Gross in Boston, who was doing experiments on coarctation, he didn't mention this. When he returned to Stockholm and published his first case of coarctation in a patient, Gross was very upset and angry because he thought that Crafoord had stolen his idea."

Robert Frater, another distinguished cardiac surgeon, commented that Gross "was somewhat irascible and jealous of his reputation. He never quite forgave Crafoord for doing the first coarctation. It was silly of Gross to be so jealous of Crafoord. He should have been happy that Crafoord validated his ideas."

## Sabbatsberg and the Karolinska

After this historic first operation, Crafoord continued to be the central figure in the development of heart surgery in Sweden and, indeed, in Europe. Crafoord took Stockholm to the forefront of thoracic surgery, first at the Sabbatsberg Hospital and subsequently (after 1957) at the Karolinska Institute. He and his colleagues kept up with all of the innovations emanating from elsewhere, and made major contributions to the diagnosis of heart disease and the care of very sick patients. For example, artificial ventilation (by a machine that inflates the patient's lungs) developed greatly through the work of Crafoord's colleague Carl-Gunnar Engström; Crafoord placed great emphasis on its use during heart operations and the postoperative period. The electrical cardiac pacemaker was also pioneered in his department by his junior colleague Ake Senning, in collaboration with Rune Elmqvist at the Elema-Schönander Company (see chapter 6).

Crafoord was later to become the second surgeon to successfully use a heart-lung machine (chapter 6). Early on in the development of heart surgery, he had sufficient vision to realize that open heart surgery was the future. As early as 1946 he directed his juniors, initially Viking Bjork and subsequently Ake Senning, to design and build a heart-lung machine in the laboratory. As we shall see later in our story (chapter 6), Crafoord and Senning performed the second successful operation in the world using the heart-lung machine in 1954.

Despite his advancing age by the mid-1950s, Crafoord, unlike Gross, adapted to open heart surgery relatively well, which was unusual for the older generation of surgeons, although Ake Senning mentioned that "we operated together," suggesting that Crafoord benefited from having a younger man with him. Crafoord had a highly active and innovative mind that kept him in the forefront of surgical advances over many years.

## Crafoord, the Man

Crafoord was born in 1899. By the age of four or five he had already decided he wanted to be a doctor. Although his mother supported his ambition, his father wanted him to join the Swedish Navy; he compromised by saying that he would become a ship's doctor (which he never did). He studied medicine at the Karolinska Institute in Stockholm, and began his surgical training in 1922.

In those days, "surgery" covered almost the entire body, and Crafoord gained experience in abdominal surgery; ear, nose, and throat surgery; orthopedics; and almost every other aspect of surgery. However, his chief had a special interest in the developing field of thoracic (chest) surgery, and this is what probably stimulated Crafoord's interest in what would become his chosen field.

From photographs taken in his later life, Crafoord can be seen as a slim, ascetic man with thinning gray hair and glasses. Surgeon Bill Bigelow (chapter 5) described him as "tall, alert, and energetic, with the rugged features of an outdoorsman." Although he added that Crafoord "displayed the degree of arrogance that was expected of a European man of his station in those days," it has been difficult for me to gain a clear picture of his personality. It would appear that he was a modest man, particularly about public attention, and was always nervous about speaking in public, particularly when it was in English. Those who knew him best, his former pupils Bjork and Senning, did not provide me with many details of Crafoord as a person, but only as a surgeon. Bjork was very forthcoming, but was inclined to talk about his own work and achievements rather than those of others. Senning was the ultimate "man of few words," and I found it rather difficult to persuade him to talk about anything at all!

Bjork did recount one story to me relating to his time as one of Crafoord's juniors: "I had sometimes to care for Crafoord's private [fee-paying] patients. Once he was late [for an operation]. I didn't like the patient to be asleep so long. I had opened [the abdomen], as I was allowed to do. When he didn't come, I took out the gallbladder. I had seen it done many times. I closed up. He was so angry. He spent a long time shouting at me. I never did anything again if I was alone."

Bob Frater met Crafoord and remembered, "He seemed a very genial fellow, but he was very senior by then. One never quite knows what sort of efforts they had to make in their early years to get prominence, and then they became benign as they got more senior. He was very well respected. Crafoord was a very energetic, very far-looking fellow. It was under him that Bjork and Senning started to develop a heart-lung machine. So he must have been a man who knew what it took to make advances in this difficult field. There were these stories about the hierarchy in Sweden — Crafoord, Senning, and Bjork, all battling for attention. Absolutely. The Swedish story was that Crafoord went hunting for deer, and Senning was following behind hunting for Crafoord, and Bjork was behind hunting for Senning." Evidently, Crafoord used to admit that he ruled by "splitting up people." If two of his juniors were similarly gifted, as were Senning and Bjork, Crafoord would try to heighten their competitiveness, often to the detriment of their relationship.

## Later Life

"I think it was in 1956 or 1957 that Crafoord had an injury," recounted Viking Bjork. "He got out of a car, a door hit his head, and he got a severe head injury. He had to be operated on by my wife's uncle, who drilled some holes and let out the blood. It was an epidural hematoma [a collection of blood outside the brain]. Then he was away from surgery for more than half a year, nearly sick all through the year. Crafoord didn't do much work after he had his brain operation."

Berglund confirmed that "Crafoord never had quite the drive and energy after [his head injury]. In 1963, he developed atrial fibrillation [an abnormal heart rhythm], which also slowed him up. In his later career, he continued operating when he was really no longer quite so good at it, and his reputation suffered."

Eventually, Crafoord retired, dying in 1983, at age 84. His contributions, along with those of Gross, had laid the essential foundations to the newly evolving field of cardiovascular surgery on which others could build. Very soon, two more surgical giants would appear on the scene, again one on either side of the Atlantic.

## CHAPTER 3

# Blue Babies:
# The Battle to Save Their Lives

———

## ALFRED BLALOCK AND RUSSELL BROCK

I N THE MID-1940S, the torch lit by Gross and Crafoord was carried further by Alfred Blalock (Figure 6), an American Southerner who was chairman of the department of surgery of the Johns Hopkins Hospital in Baltimore, and Russell Brock (Figure 7), a leading chest surgeon at both Guy's Hospital and the Royal Brompton Hospital in London. Blalock was an outwardly relaxed man, socially charming and very much at ease, who surrounded himself with gifted young surgical residents. Brock was a much more socially reserved and introspective man, and yet with a streak of showmanship, who strove for professional perfection throughout his life.

Both men were involved in the development of operations for the treatment of what were, and still are, known as "blue babies," the name given to babies and young children whose skin is a dusky blue color. The blue color (cyanosis) results from an abnormally low level of oxygen in the blood, which is caused by both an obstruction of blood flow to the lungs and abnormal mixing of blue (deoxygenated) blood with pink (oxygenated) blood. Because the amount of oxygen in the blood is far lower than it should be, the baby or child may be breathless even on slight exertion, when he or she takes on an even darker blue appearance. Before Blalock and Brock, these children led a miserable existence, usually dying in childhood with progressive and distressing shortness of breath.

In an interview with William Roberts for the *American Journal of Cardiology* in 1998, David Sabiston, a surgical resident with Alfred Blalock in the 1950s, described the impact Blalock's new operation had on these young patients: "These children would pass in a wheelchair or be carried in the hallway panting for breath, nail tips and lips blue, very cyanotic [dusky blue], and often with oxygen tanks." Two weeks later, he reported, "They would walk out of the front door of the hospital pink and running around. It was almost like a miracle." Brock's quite different operation had a similar miraculous effect. These two men therefore initiated surgical approaches for treating an abnormality of the heart itself, rather than that of the major blood vessels outside of the heart, as Gross and Crafoord had done.

However, Blalock's operation was again a manipulation of the major blood vessels arising from the heart, and not an operation on the heart itself. He constructed a new blood supply to the lungs to *increase* blood flow — in effect, he did the opposite of Robert Gross in that he *created* a ductus. Although Blalock's operation was not a heart operation as such, it was the first time that an abnormality *within* the heart had been "bypassed." The operation made the surgical world even more aware that surgery on the heart itself might be possible.

Brock actually took this great step. He believed the obstruction to blood flow to the lungs should be attacked directly, just as a plumber would open a blocked pipe. He designed knives and other instruments that could be introduced into the heart to cut through or "dilate" the narrowed valve that was the source of the obstruction. Although Brock could not actually see what he was accomplishing inside the heart (hence the term "closed" heart surgery), but was guided largely by feel, this bold approach took surgeons actually *inside* the heart for the first time. It was therefore an extremely important conceptual advance. One more milestone was passed.

## ALFRED BLALOCK—
## THE SOUTHERN GENTLEMAN

I never had the good fortune of meeting Alfred Blalock, unlike Russell Brock, who for a time I worked under at Guy's Hospital. However, several of Blalock's trainees have written extensively about him and his life, in particular the distinguished surgeon William Longmire Jr., who assisted Blalock at the very first "blue baby" operation and subsequently performed many of the operations himself. Longmire's biography *Alfred Blalock, His Life and Times* is an invaluable overview of Blalock's career, his contributions to surgery, and his personality and character. Similarly, the autobiography of the remarkable African American Vivien Thomas, a laboratory technician who played a major role in the experimental development of the operation in Blalock's department, contributes much insight into Blalock's life and persona.

Blalock was born in 1899 in Culloden, Georgia. He was bright and did well in school. He enjoyed sports, and was good enough to make the high school tennis team and to be the pitcher on the baseball team. Upon completing high school with a grade of 99.5 on his report card, he attended Georgia Military Academy for one year, took some additional summer courses, and entered the University of Georgia as a sophomore, graduating when he was 19 years of age. "Al," as he was known throughout his life, was a popular young man and had many friends. He progressed to the prestigious Johns Hopkins Hospital Medical School in Baltimore in 1918, which had already gained a reputation second to none as a place of medical learning.

Longmire describes Blalock as "a good looking—some said handsome—man; certain features, such as a somewhat prominent nose and protuberant ears, were a bit incongruous, but his overall appearance and manner suggested elegance. He was slender, of above-average height, and well muscled, with full brown eyes and dark hair that had a slight, gentle wave. With his mild, unpretentious manner, he quickly and easily made friends. Even after he became a world-renowned figure, he was equally at ease with people in all stations of life. With his great sense of humor he enjoyed either hearing or telling a good story. As one might imagine, these pleasant ingredients made him both a charming host and a gracious guest."

In his youth, Blalock was popular with girls, to the extent that a friend, Tinsley Harrison, who was an excellent tennis player and played doubles with Blalock (winning the doubles championship of Nashville in 1925), wrote, "Alfred Blalock was a Casanova. He was Don Juan. Really a lady's man." Throughout his life, Blalock always had a ready smile and a pleasant word for an attractive lady. He also maintained a great interest in sports. When on vacation, it was golf in the morning, then a swim, then lunch, and fishing or tennis in the afternoon. As a medical student, he was known as "playboy Al," and it was not thought he would pursue an academic career. But what Al had, according to one contemporary, "was character and drive. He was not among the first-class minds I have known, but he was willing to work longer than anybody. Al would stay in the lab until midnight and then go out on a date." So he was something of a chameleon — "playboy Al" and yet hardworking at one and the same time.

## Tuberculosis — Enforced Rest

The development of a problem with Blalock's left kidney (which was surgically removed in 1923), from a structural abnormality with which he had been born, certainly did not prevent a full life. But this immense zest for life caught up with him at a fairly early age. After graduating in medicine and an aborted surgical residency at Hopkins, he transferred to Vanderbilt University School of Medicine in Nashville, Tennessee, in 1922. There, while running the experimental surgical laboratory as well as serving as chief resident, he worked and played too hard, and developed pulmonary tuberculosis. He was working in his laboratory every night until midnight, and then carousing and "raising hell" until 3:00 or 4:00 in the morning. He became so run down, he lost his resistance to the infection and developed a tuberculous lung lesion. The young Blalock was sent to the Trudeau Sanatorium at Saranac Lake, New York. He was given total bed rest, the standard treatment of the day, and spent the better part of the next year, summer and winter, in bed on an outside porch.

After approximately a year at Trudeau, Blalock became so disenchanted with his forced inactivity and discouraged by his lack of apparent progress, as well as by the unwillingness of his physician to opt for more aggressive treatment (artificial pneumothorax, in which the infected lung is purposefully collapsed by the injection of air into the chest cavity), that he discharged himself from the sanatorium. Cashing in his life insurance policy, he used the money to travel to Europe to visit various physiological laboratories. While in Germany, he suffered a severe hemorrhage from the lung and coughed up a great deal of blood. The people in Berlin apparently ignored his request for medical assistance, leaving him alone in a foreign country, weak and frightened. Longmire reports that Blalock remained bitter that he had not received help at this critical time. Fortunately, the hemorrhage spontaneously abated, and he slowly regained sufficient strength to make his way back to the United States. With considerable difficulty, he managed to get to Saranac, where his physicians finally agreed to initiate pneumothorax treatment.

In Longmire's opinion, this period away from his career may have been beneficial to Blalock, as it provided him the opportunity for reflection and introspection. Another famous American surgeon, Evarts Graham, is quoted as saying, "Withdrawal gives opportunity for a man to develop powers within himself which otherwise may remain dormant in a life crowded with the pursuit of limited objectives.... To such a person, withdrawal provides an opportunity for the mind to be receptive because it is released from the pressing demands of the toils and distractions of ordinary life." Henry Bahnson, who trained under

Blalock and got to know him well, is quoted by Longmire as saying, "His work in life was more focused than that of many of us and he had considerable tenacity to pursue the goals he selected. I had thought this stemmed from his session with tuberculosis and a conscious decision on his part to concentrate his efforts in selected endeavors." As we shall see in subsequent pages, one or two other surgeons profiled in this book were able to "benefit" from an enforced period of withdrawal necessitated by their developing tuberculosis.

Blalock had many pneumothorax treatments, both at Saranac and after his return to Nashville. The procedure was repeated every two weeks or so for approximately 13 months. Even with one lung collapsed, his energy was such that he was able to reactivate his laboratory and continue his studies of the circulatory system. In exploring reasons for Blalock's tremendous drive and experimental activity during his early Nashville days, those who knew him have suggested that he had a strong conviction that he wasn't going to live very long. The fact that his insurance company paid off his life insurance seems to suggest that it felt the same way.

When Blalock was training to become a surgeon, there was no general acceptance of just what constituted proper preparation. The surgical experience he gained at Vanderbilt, even by the standards of most academic institutions of that day, was minimal. After completing the residency in 1925, Blalock progressed steadily through the academic ranks at Vanderbilt to become a full professor by 1938. During his time at Vanderbilt, he married and had three children.

A significant player in the development of the "Blalock" operation for blue babies was Vivien Thomas, a laboratory technician hired by Blalock in 1930, who remained with him until Blalock's death in 1964. Thomas, born in 1910 in Lake Providence, Louisiana, was one of five children. His parents moved to Nashville in 1912, where his father worked as a carpenter and contractor. Thomas went to a good local school and also learned his father's trade of carpentry, being required to report after school and on Saturdays to help him with whatever job he had in progress. Thomas planned to attend Tennessee State College but, after working one summer as a carpenter at Fisk University, he was asked to stay on in the job. Shortly thereafter, he lost his job because of a seasonal slowdown in construction and the collapse of the stock market. Through a friend he had heard there was an opening in Blalock's laboratory at Vanderbilt, but his friend said that Blalock was "hell" to get along with and he didn't think he would be able to work with him. Thomas told him that things were so tight he would have to take his chances, since he had to have some source of income.

Blalock told Thomas that he was getting busy with patients and so needed somebody to continue his laboratory work, someone who could get to the point where he could do things on his own even if he, Blalock, were not around. Thomas took the job, intending to work until he had saved enough to go to college, and then try to go to medical school, but in fact, he never left Blalock's employment.

Thomas's autobiography, published in 1985, is a good social history of the problems faced by a black man in Nashville at that time. For example, he reports that in the 1930s, white men doing the same work were classified as technicians and were paid significantly more than he was, because all of the African Americans were classified as janitors. He mentioned this to Blalock, and a few days later his pay was increased.

Rollin Daniel, a young Nashville friend of Blalock, wrote that Blalock "often worked at night, much of the time doing paperwork and dropping into the laboratory at occasional times to check on an animal involved in a chronic experiment. [Although] most of the preparations were carried out by Vivien [Thomas], Dr. Blalock would think the thing through. He and Vivien would operate together on the dog, or a few dogs, and then Vivien would take over, Dr. Blalock dropping by, making suggestions and corrections and Vivien performing the operative procedures and setting up the experiments with tremendous care and attention to details."

With the help of Thomas and a series of young research fellows,

Blalock's laboratory was highly productive. Perhaps of most importance were their seminal studies on cardiovascular "shock" — the collapse of the blood pressure and cardiac output that can occur after blood loss following injury or in certain other conditions. Blalock recommended massive transfusions and fluid replacement for those in shock, a radical concept at that time. He wrote more than 50 scientific papers on the topic of shock, mostly while at Vanderbilt. This work, which proved invaluable particularly in the care of those with war wounds, was, in Blalock's opinion, by far the best work he ever did.

Sanford Leeds, who worked closely with Blalock as a research associate during this period, wrote, "He was a master at working with people and making them productive. He stimulated productivity to a large degree by his personal example of hard work, and by his careful planning and directing. Although his forceful personality enabled him to dominate, he was never domineering. He always seemed to sense the right thing to say at the right time with magnetic charm." However, "no attempt to portray Dr. Blalock would be complete without mentioning that he had human failings. Although a quick temper was usually well-controlled, it would flare up occasionally to subside quickly. Annoyance or impatience would occasionally show and would lend contrast to his usual good humor and pleasant manner. He could be strongly partisan when anything which concerned the South or a close friend was involved."

In 1938, in a decision that was to have immense relevance to his future work on blue babies, Blalock determined to study a condition known as pulmonary hypertension. In this condition, which is still relatively poorly understood today, the blood pressure in the vessels supplying the lungs is greatly increased; in the usual form of hypertension (high blood pressure), it is the blood vessels in the rest of the body that are involved. In order to have an experimental animal model that mimicked the disease in humans, Blalock wanted to increase the blood pressure in the lungs of a dog. He thought that by bringing an extra blood supply to the lungs, and thus greatly increasing the blood flow through the lungs, this would cause the blood pressure in the lungs to be increased.

Blalock therefore asked Thomas to perform a series of operations in which the artery that carries blood to the dog's foreleg was diverted to take extra blood to the lungs. This could be accomplished by joining (anastomosing) the artery that supplies blood to the left foreleg to that supplying the left lung. Although Thomas accomplished this operation successfully, subsequent studies revealed little or no change in the blood pressure in the pulmonary artery. The increased blood *flow,* therefore, was not associated with an increase in blood *pressure,* a very important observation when some years later Blalock was asked to develop an operation to treat blue babies.

## Johns Hopkins Hospital

In 1941, Blalock accepted the chairmanship of the department of surgery at Johns Hopkins Hospital in Baltimore. Thomas moved with Blalock to Baltimore, where he did not find life very different from Nashville since Baltimore remained a deeply segregated city at that time. (Despite Thomas's advanced technical and research skills, it was not considered in any way "politically incorrect" for Blalock to ask Thomas to act as bartender when he gave parties at his home.) Thomas found much of the equipment in the Hopkins experimental surgery laboratory to be primitive and outdated.

When he began at Hopkins, Blalock said to Longmire, "This [surgical] residency [program] needs some new blood. I'm going to bring in some good Southern boys to turn it around." To do so, his first step was to shorten the training of the existing senior residents so that he could bring in new people. The outraged surgical residents held a meeting and wrote a strong letter of complaint to him, signed by each member of the surgical house staff. Blalock interviewed each house officer in turn, curtly repeating on a take-it-or-leave-it basis the offers he had made the day before with no changes. He could be very tough when he needed to be.

According to Sabiston, Blalock made very few mistakes in selecting his residents: "He had the ability to pick people who were really scholars and gentleman." He selected young men who were hard workers, and he put a lot of emphasis on character.

Al Starr (chapter 9), who also was a resident under Blalock, told me, "He was a very caring individual for the residents, and he developed strong personal relationships with them. The residents would name their children after Alfred Blalock. He was a real father figure. He felt a sense of responsibility for anyone who worked for him, and he would go out of his way for them. It was extraordinary to see this, because he was world famous and yet the people that worked around him were very important to him."

One surgical resident subsequently under Blalock was Tom Starzl, later to become one of the great pioneers of organ transplantation. In his autobiography, *The Puzzle People,* Starzl writes about the highly competitive, even ruthless, surgical residency training program at Hopkins at that time, where the intern was on duty 24 hours a day every day of the year except for a one-week vacation: "The training program was 'pyramidal' in that only two of the 18 starting interns could be retained for a full six—or seven—year residency....The extras were culled....It was a ruthless educational philosophy. The average level of technical surgery and the opportunity for clinical experience during that era at Hopkins were unparalleled....For some it was heaven, and for others hell. I found it to be purgatory."

Although Blalock's department trained many of the future leaders of surgery in the United States, New Zealand surgeon Sir Brian Barratt-Boyes (chapter 10) was critical of the residency program at the Johns Hopkins, saying, "I knew Blalock well. I was visiting professor at Johns Hopkins on several occasions. He was a charming man...[but] I have to be very critical of his teaching methods. The chief residency system that they had developed at Hopkins wasn't in the patients' interest. It was in the *surgeons'* interest, because the residents learned by their mistakes on their patients. I used to be absolutely appalled at what went on, and at the decisions that were made by these guys [the residents] who really didn't know much about it at all. They ran the department. But, of course, a number of them turned out very well."

## Helen Taussig and the Problem of Fallot's Tetralogy

One morning in 1943, Blalock called Vivien Thomas to a meeting he was to have with the children's cardiologist Dr. Helen Taussig. This was to prove a fateful meeting of immense importance in the development of heart surgery. Taussig described the blue babies and children she saw in her clinic, the little patients for whom she could do so little. She explained that in a condition known as Fallot's tetralogy, there was not sufficient blood getting through the lungs to be oxygenated. She had made an astute observation, noticing that those patients who also had a persistent ductus (which enabled more blood to reach the lungs) did fairly well until the ductus closed. Taussig expressed her belief that, by surgical means, it should be possible to direct more blood to the lungs. However, she gave no hint as to how this could be accomplished, leaving Blalock to think about the problem. It is noteworthy that Taussig had previously met with the great Robert Gross in Boston and had asked him whether anything could be done for her blue babies. Gross had either been too busy to consider the problem seriously or had dismissed it as impossible; reportedly, he regretted this lost opportunity for the rest of his life.

Fallot's tetralogy is a collection of four heart abnormalities originally described in 1671 by the Danish physician Niels Stensen, who was also a bishop and later became a saint, one of the few physicians to be beatified. Numerous other cases were reported before the French physician Etienne-Louis Fallot reported two more cases in 1888, and, yet mysteriously, it is by his name that the condition is known. There are two primary abnormalities in the heart and two that are secondary (Figure 8). The first of the primary abnormalities is an obstructive narrowing (or stenosis) of the valve between the right side of the heart and the artery that takes blood to the lungs. The condition affecting the pulmonary valve is therefore said to be pulmonary stenosis. The second is a hole in the wall (or septum) between the two pumping chambers (ventricles). The other two abnormalities are secondary to these primary ones, and need not be elaborated here.

One of the major problems with Fallot's tetralogy is that the blood supply to the lungs is greatly reduced. Because of the pulmonary stenosis, the blood intended to go to the lungs is instead shunted through the ventricular septal defect, to be pumped once more into the aorta and around the rest of the body. There is, therefore, mixing of the little blood that has passed through the lungs (pink or oxygenated blood) with the much greater volume of blood that has *not* picked up oxygen in the lungs (blue or deoxygenated blood). This means that blue blood reaches the organs and tissues of the body, and is manifest by the skin appearing blue, hence the term "blue baby."

A blue baby was destined for a short and distressing life since the lack of oxygen getting to his or her muscles and organs caused the baby to grow inadequately, remain physically weak, tire easily, and become breathless from only minor activity. Eventually, the heart failed, partly because it was receiving poorly oxygenated blood itself and partly because it was being forced to put out a much greater effort than usual — and the child died a very unpleasant death.

Today, with the availability of the heart-lung machine, the stenosed pulmonary valve is opened or enlarged and the hole in the septum is repaired with a patch of synthetic material. This complete correction of the condition is carried out by the surgeon under direct vision. Before the advent of the heart-lung machine, however, and indeed before any operation inside the heart was deemed possible, Fallot's tetralogy could not be corrected.

Blalock's proposed answer was to direct extra blood to the lungs by creating an artificial ductus (chapter 2). This would result in the organs of the body receiving much more oxygenated blood, just as occurred in Helen Taussig's patients who also had a natural ductus.

After some preliminary studies, Blalock and Thomas solved the problem by redirecting the artery to the left arm to the artery to the lungs (Figure 8), the very operation they had developed in dogs in Nashville some years previously in their efforts to produce pulmonary hypertension. As Dr. Taussig had hoped, they, like plumbers, "changed the pipes" around to get more blood to the lungs. Thomas quotes Robert Pond Sr., who, in a discussion of scientific creativity, stated, "It is completely possible to invent something and never know what the need is, never know what problem you had solved." It seemed to Thomas that the creation in 1938 of their operation might well fall into this category—a use for it did not become apparent until 1943.

## The First Patient

Blalock and, particularly, Thomas worked hard in the laboratory on the Fallot project for over a year, but there were still some unanswered questions. Although the artery to the foreleg in the dog could be tied off with impunity, without jeopardizing the blood supply to the leg, would a patient tolerate tying of the artery to the arm? Would the arm be damaged by this reduced blood supply? Would the arm continue to grow adequately? At worst, the arm could become gangrenous, and this could be accompanied by great pain. Would the patient, with an already diminished flow of blood through the lungs, tolerate anesthesia and the occlusion of the right or left pulmonary artery while the anastomosis was being performed? It would, of course, be impossible to answer these questions until the operation was performed in a blue baby or child.

Since Thomas and the surgical research fellows had done all the laboratory work in dogs, on November 29, 1944, Blalock planned to join them to practice the operation so that he could perform it on a patient. He wanted to assist Thomas on one dog, and then do one or two himself with Thomas's assistance. However, on the day he was scheduled to practice the procedure in the laboratory, the condition of the little girl on whom he planned to do the operation, Eileen Saxon, was deteriorating so rapidly that he felt that if he were to save her, he would have to operate that day.

Thomas was asked to go to the operating room to make sure all the necessary surgical instruments were available. One point we tend to forget today is that the sophisticated instruments, specialized needles, and fine suture materials used for vascular surgery today were not available in 1944. Even the facilities in the operating room were primitive by today's standards. For example, the lighting was poor for such fine work, and an auxiliary portable spotlight needed to be brought in. The temperature in the operating room in the summer months was almost unbearable, even to those who were there only to observe.

As the child was in such poor condition, the chief of anesthesiology initially refused to give her an anesthetic, believing the risk of operation was too high. However, Blalock insisted. He had discussed the situation with the family, telling them the operation had never been attempted before and that the chance that the child might die on the operating table was high. Blalock's assistants were the resident, Longmire, and a young intern who was one day to become famous in his own right, Denton Cooley (chapter 13). Helen Taussig stood near the head of the table with the anesthesiologist. Vivien Thomas stood on a stool where he could look over Blalock's right shoulder and, during the course of the operation, he gave his chief a number of helpful suggestions in regard to the technique of the procedure (Figure 9).

One might think that joining two blood vessels together would be a simple procedure, but the vessels were small and surrounded by abnormal dilated blood vessels, called collaterals, that had developed in the body's effort to resolve the problem itself. This region of the body, in the depths of the chest, is also home to many important structures — blood vessels, nerves, et cetera — making the operation extremely hazardous.

In Longmire's opinion, "The operation was one of the most difficult in which I have ever participated.... There were a number of times during the procedure when I must say it looked as if it would be impossible to complete the proposed operation. If I had been the operator I probably would have withdrawn, but with the tenacity that was so characteristic of Alfred Blalock, he persisted and the anastomosis [the joining of the two blood vessels] was completed. As soon as the anastomosis was opened and the occluding bulldog clamps removed from the vessels, Dr. Harmel [the anesthesiologist] reported a marked change in the patient's color."

In the postoperative period, when she was cared for by the surgical resident, Henry Bahnson, the child's condition was extremely critical, but she slowly improved and was able to go home after about two weeks.

Sadly, however, that first historic patient was eventually to die. After some months, the anastomosis probably constricted down and the child became blue again. A repeat operation was attempted, but the child died, less than one year after the original operation. In the meantime, however, a large number of other children had been operated upon successfully, and the benefit of the procedure had become well established.

Longmire notes that, before the first operation, "Dr. Blalock was still a bit on trial as far as his surgical technical ability was concerned because he had come there [Johns Hopkins] as a relatively young man and was noted for his experimental work rather than his clinical accomplishments. In the preceding couple of weeks, he had attempted several rather complicated, major operative procedures that had not gone well.... He was discouraged.... I have always suspected that these unsatisfactory operative results led him to push ahead with a dramatic move into an exciting new and unexplored field. The 'blue baby' operations certainly consolidated Blalock's position at the hospital."

On the topic of Blalock's surgical skills, Thomas records that Blalock could be impatient, tense, and irritable when under stress in the operating room: "The atmosphere became tense the moment he entered, and he seemed to have a different personality." Even when things were progressing smoothly, he would find something to complain about, and would whine in his Southern drawl, "Won't somebody 'hep' me?" Thomas attributes Blalock's behavior to the fact that he knew he was not technically an outstanding surgeon. However, when he did get into operative difficulty, he was reputedly a master at getting out of it.

In the words of one doctor, the report of the first three patients at a clinical conference at the hospital "was one of those experiences one cannot forget. To everyone it was apparent that a great historic event had taken place."

News of this successful operation spread rapidly, and "blue babies" began to be referred to Blalock in greater and greater numbers. Before long, he was operating upon one heart case daily, then two, and sometimes three. The babies were profoundly ill, and the mortality at first was considerable. The surgical and pediatric house staff were literally working night and day taking care of these critically ill patients before, during, and after operation. Blalock evidently did not fully appreciate the tremendous workload the house staff carried, which led to some dissension among his juniors. Surgeons from all over the world visited Baltimore to learn the surgical technique. Newspaper reporters, especially local ones, were always around.

Blalock's operation had a profound effect on the medical profession as well as on the public, because it brought *instant* improvement in the state of health of the baby or child. Before the operation the babies were dusky blue and breathless, whereas *immediately* after they were pink and their recovery had begun. This dramatic change in appearance had much more impact on both physicians and the public than did the operations for closure of a ductus or correction of a coarctation that had been carried out in the preceding few years. It was primarily Blalock's operation, therefore, that alerted surgeons to the fact that it might be possible to operate on the heart itself. As a result, Blalock received immense professional and public acclaim, certainly more than almost any surgeon who had preceded him.

It was not just that Blalock's operation benefited these young children. The *concept* of performing an operation to correct abnormal physiology (function) was revolutionary. Blalock's operation to a large extent corrected the performance of a structurally abnormal heart. It was a *constructive* operation, rather than *destructive*. Before it, surgery had been largely limited to removing diseased tissue — excising tumors, draining pus, and so on. Even tying the ductus, though it corrected a defect, was not truly constructive in the way that Blalock's operation was. It was this new concept of doing something constructive that made it such an important surgical advance.

## Visit to Europe

In 1947, three years after his first successful operation, Blalock was invited to lecture and demonstrate his operation in Europe, initially as an exchange professor at Guy's Hospital in London. (Longmire notes that Blalock, whose fingers were deeply stained with nicotine, had great difficulty in getting enough cigarettes to take with him to England; it was almost impossible to obtain American cigarettes in Europe at that time.)

Europe proved a triumphal tour. Blalock was a good lecturer, reputedly having "a magnificent resonant speaking voice which, combined with a pronounced Southern drawl, made his public presentations memorable to all who heard them." The great American pioneer of lung surgery Evarts Graham, who was in London when Blalock made his visit, reported, "There has never been anything quite like Al Blalock's triumphant tour of Europe....The prestige of Johns Hopkins was enormously increased by Al's visit. All of us Americans were proud to claim him as a fellow American. His unassuming personality captivated everyone as much as his epoch-making surgical accomplishments."

Helen Taussig clearly felt some bitterness at first that Blalock was receiving so much adulation for performing an operation that she had suggested to him. Late in her career she did receive numerous honors, including the U.S. Presidential Medal of Freedom. Some of this recognition, however, was for the leading role she had played in ensuring that the sleeping pill thalidomide, which was suspected to be associated with the development of limb defects in the developing fetus, was not used in pregnant women in the United States. She was killed in a car accident in 1986, just before her 88th birthday.

## Later Life

The great advance in the treatment of congenital heart disease made by the Blalock operation was recognized in 1954, when Blalock shared the prestigious Albert Lasker Award for Clinical Medical Research with Helen Taussig and Robert Gross for their "distinguished contributions to cardiovascular surgery and knowledge." Blalock was also one of relatively few surgeons elected to the U.S. National Academy of Sciences.

Soon Blalock became aware that the lead in surgery was moving to other centers that were developing heart-lung machines (chapter 6). He assigned the responsibility of developing open heart surgery to two of his juniors. After years of conscientious effort, in March 1956 they performed their first open heart procedure with the use of a heart-lung machine. Blalock did not actively participate in the open heart operations, believing that younger men could do a better job.

Thomas continued to run the surgical laboratory. Blalock maintained an interest in the laboratory, but perhaps found it difficult to keep up with advances in the basic sciences. Thomas seems to have gone through a period of dependency on alcohol, although he ultimately shook off this need. Blalock retired from his position at Johns Hopkins in 1964; Thomas did not retire until 15 years later.

Sadly, Blalock lived only a few months after taking retirement. As early as April 1948, he had developed chills, a fever, difficulty and frequency in urinating, and general aching. For the rest of his life he continued to be plagued by urinary tract infections, the cause of which was never clearly established. (It must be remembered that he had only one kidney, the other having been removed in 1923.) During this period of 16 years, his various medical advisors, who included several of the brilliant young men he had personally trained, misguidedly treated him for conditions as varied as slipped disc, hepatitis, and disease of the large bowel, but none of them ever made the correct diagnosis. After his death in 1964, it was found that he had an undiagnosed cancer in the remnant of the left ureter (which had drained urine into the bladder from the kidney before it was removed), which was almost certainly associated with the chronic infections from which he had suffered. The cancer had spread to his liver. It is ironic that someone who did so much to train surgeons, and who, at Johns Hopkins, was surrounded by some of the best medical minds in the world, died from an undiagnosed condition that had troubled him for years.

The story of Vivien Thomas, the boy who left school at 13 yet who played a significant role in the development of the blue baby operation, has a happier ending. First, in 1971, the former fellows and residents at Hopkins decided to present him with a portrait, which publicly recognized his role in surgical research and in the development of the skills of many young surgeons. Second, Hopkins awarded Thomas an honorary degree. Third, he was made an instructor in surgery, an appointment normally reserved for fully trained surgeons. He served in this capacity until 1979, when he retired. He died at age 75 in 1985, the year in which his remarkable autobiography was published.

## RUSSELL BROCK—
## THE ENGLISH LORD

Russell Brock (Figure 7) was an immense early influence on me as a medical student and junior hospital doctor. It was his pioneering work that initially captured my imagination and influenced my choice of heart surgery as a career. Brock was honored by the Queen of Great Britain, first with a knighthood (so that he was addressed as Sir Russell), and subsequently by being elevated to the peerage (becoming Lord Brock), one of the few British surgeons to receive this recognition. Despite his distinguished career, Brock's appearance was not at all distinguished. He was relatively short, had slightly bandy legs, and wore heavy spectacles. During my time at Guy's, a junior nurse, who did not know him, once thought he had come to the ward to repair a radiator; to his credit, he took the mistake with good humor.

Brock was one of the most stimulating characters I have had the privilege of knowing. Others, however, might remember the experience of working with him slightly differently, since his juniors frequently took a verbal beating. One former trainee recollected, "My time with Brock was perhaps the most stimulating period of my training—and I still have the marks on my back to prove it." He demanded very high standards, was a hard taskmaster, and did not always treat his juniors fairly. As one eminent British surgeon rather bluntly put it, "Brock could be a real shit." Nevertheless, the majority of his trainees feel as I do, and retain great admiration and regard for him, possibly mixed with a tinge of trepidation.

Brock was a thinker and innovator. In his prime, he drove his team relentlessly. Like several other eminent surgeons, including Blalock, when he was under stress in the operating room he could sometimes treat his assistants particularly harshly. John Wright, a Brock trainee who later became a leading London heart surgeon, related an interesting story of an occasion when one of Brock's colleagues, Norman Barrett, who had known Brock since they were "boys" together, came into the operating room when Brock was "getting all stewed up and everybody was terrified. Barrett looked over at the operative field, and said, facetiously, 'You know, Russell, your problem is you are not temperamentally suited to cardiac surgery.'" As Brock was by this time in his 60s, the opinion came too late for him to take it into consideration in his choice of career.

Like Blalock, Brock's difficult behavior was partly a result of his technical limitations in the operating room. In the opinion of Sir Terence English, a Brock trainee who did much to establish heart transplantation in the United Kingdom and a great admirer of Brock's work, "He was irrational, very difficult. Whatever you did, it wasn't quite right. That was an expression of his frustration that he couldn't do things better. If he had control in an operation, he wouldn't be cussing his assistants all the time. He was a rough surgeon. He knew what needed to be done, but he couldn't do it. But, inevitably, everyone who worked with him ended up with a huge respect for him."

As John Wright succinctly put it, "Everybody had this mixture of respect and fear for him. You never spoke if you weren't spoken to, and you never engaged in 'small talk.' He had no time for small talk at all. If you engaged in anything like, 'It's pretty warm today,' the response would be, 'No small talk.' The impression simply was that he didn't value it. It was of *no* value. He only had time for clinical conversations, assessment, accuracy. Personal comments and everything else were a waste of time, so you did not engage in any small talk. You would walk together in silence unless there was something meaningful to discuss. Whether it disguised an inability on his part to engage in small talk, I can't answer."

During the nine months in which I worked closely with Brock, although he could be irascible and difficult when under stress during surgery, I felt his complaints were unreasonable on only one occasion. I was assisting him at an operation and he repeatedly — and unfairly and unpleasantly, I thought — complained about the assistance I was giving him. However, once the patient was safely in his room, Brock came to me and warmly and genuinely thanked me for the help I had provided. I realized then that his bad humor and unnecessary comments during the operation had been the result of his personal stress rather than solely due to my inadequacy, and that his complaints need not be taken too seriously.

During operations like this, he was the epitome of the surgeon who could be pleased by nothing. The apocryphal story among trainee surgeons is that whenever the "chief" ties a surgical knot and the assistant dutifully cuts the free ends of the knot, the chief's complaint is either that the ends have been left too long or, alternatively, too short. At such frustrating times, all junior assistants are tempted to ask their chief, "How would you like this one cut, sir — too long or too short?" Few of us ever had the nerve to do so, particularly when operating with someone like Brock, although I have heard this retort once from a junior colleague — an Australian, of course — when we were both assisting another of Brock's former trainees, Ben Milstein, who had something of Brock in him in this respect.

## The Young Man

Russell Brock was born in 1903. Little is known about his childhood and youth. He attended a historic and well-known "public" (i.e., private) school in England called Christ's Hospital school, and won a scholarship to Guy's Hospital Medical School of the University of London at the age of 17. It was already clear that he was a brilliant pupil. As a medical student, he won many prizes and medals, and graduated with distinctions in 1927. He passed the examinations for the Fellowship of the Royal College of Surgeons of England within a year of graduating (which was not that unusual in those days) and focused his attention on a career in surgery, particularly in chest (thoracic) surgery. Heart surgery had not evolved at that time, but this ultimately became his major interest.

In 1929, Brock was awarded a Rockefeller traveling fellowship, which he spent with the renowned surgeon Evarts Graham, in St. Louis, Missouri. Graham was recognized as the first surgeon to successfully remove an entire lung (pneumonectomy) for cancer, which he did in 1933. In one of those twists of fate, Graham's famous patient, himself a physician, lived a long life after this operation and, indeed, outlived Graham, who was a heavy smoker and, ironically, died of cancer of the lung in 1957.

On his return from the United States, Brock quickly rose up the surgical ladder, and he was appointed surgeon to Guy's Hospital and also to the Royal Brompton Hospital in 1936. He was one of the few surgeons in the United Kingdom of that era to develop an experimental surgical laboratory. In his early career, Brock made significant contributions to the surgery of the lung, particularly in elucidating the precise anatomy of the airways in the lungs that facilitated surgical approaches to removal of part of one lung, which was particularly important in the days when tuberculosis was common. In the mid-1940s, despite the pressure that was on him as a practicing surgeon in London during World War II, Brock's interests turned to the surgery of the heart. This may have been stimulated to some extent by seeing Dwight Harken remove a shrapnel fragment from the heart of a U.S. serviceman (chapter 4).

## Direct Attack on the Pulmonary Valve

After the war, there is no doubt that Brock was greatly stimulated by the visit of Alfred Blalock to London in 1947, where Blalock demonstrated his new operation for blue babies with Fallot's tetralogy. Although Brock began performing the Blalock operation on his patients, he had other ideas about treating the condition. Rather than bypass the narrowed pulmonary valve with an artery "shunt," Brock — along with another London surgeon, Thomas Holmes Sellors — believed that a direct attack on the pulmonary valve itself would be preferable (Figure 8). By opening the narrowed valve (an operation known as pulmonary valvotomy), blood flow to the pulmonary artery would increase, and the patient's condition would improve. Brock (and Holmes Sellors) advocated pulmonary valvotomy rather than the Blalock shunt since, although they were both intended to relieve the same condition, he felt his approach led to better development of the blood vessels in the lungs, which was important for the patient. He also used this approach in children born with pulmonary stenosis alone, i.e., not associated with the other features of Fallot's tetralogy (Figure 10).

In 1948, Brock reported three successful operations for pulmonary stenosis performed through an opening (incision) in the right ventricle, the first having been carried out on February 16, 1948. As with Harken's work during World War II (as we shall see later), the fact that patients would tolerate an incision being made in the muscle of the right ventricle was a significant stimulus to further heart surgery since it demonstrated the heart' s tolerance to direct surgical intervention.

Holmes Sellors had actually performed a similar operation a few weeks before Brock, but Brock's drive and dedication in pursuing heart surgery have, in the opinion of many British cardiac surgeons, given him a greater stature than his erstwhile competitor. For example, in Ben Milstein's opinion, Holmes Sellors "wasn't a man with the same sort of drive [as Brock], but he did some quite clever things." John Wright told me that Holmes Sellors "behaved entirely differently to Brock. He did not have Brock's dedication. He was in there at the beginning [of heart surgery] but, in my limited experience, I would not rate him on the same level as Brock." Nevertheless, both men contributed significantly to the development of heart surgery in the United Kingdom.

There is an interesting anecdote about them that illustrates their different outlooks on surgery. The story goes that they were both being considered for a consultant surgical post—a senior faculty position—at a London hospital. As heart surgery was still in its infancy, the selection committee consisted entirely of physicians (predominantly cardiologists) rather than surgeons.

Brock was interviewed by the committee first, and was asked by one cardiologist when he would operate on a patient with mitral stenosis (a life-threatening sequel to rheumatic fever in which one of the valves in the heart becomes narrowed and obstructs the blood flow—see chapter 4). Brock, the great scientific surgeon, whose career was based on detailed clinical diagnostic skills and precise physiological measurements, gave a comprehensive and lucid dissertation on the various clinical symptoms, physical signs, and chest X-ray appearances that would determine whether or not he would operate on a patient with mitral stenosis. He would operate only, of course, if the disease were advanced enough to be causing clinical and hemodynamic disability, et cetera. The committee thanked him, and he left the room.

Holmes Sellors was then invited in for interview. The same cardiologist asked him the identical question, "When would you operate on a patient with mitral stenosis?" Holmes Sellors's immediate and brief reply was, "I would operate on the patient when the cardiologist told me to." Holmes Sellors got the job. Although I strongly suspect this story is apocryphal, it does aptly illustrate the difference in philosophical approach to surgery between these two gifted men.

Shortly after his initial operations on the pulmonary valve, Brock played a major role in the development of surgical treatment for mitral valve stenosis, a much more common condition, performing an operation to open this obstructed valve within six weeks of Bailey and Harken in the United States in 1948 (chapter 4). His contribution was fully independent of theirs since he was completely unaware of their efforts.

## Clinical Skills

Brock's clinical acumen, i.e., his skills at diagnosis and treatment, based on years of experience, was legendary. Sir Roy Calne, a major pioneer in organ transplantation, wrote, "I was privileged to be taught by the most outstanding clinician that I have encountered." As a clinician, Brock was his own man; he did not accept what he was told by a physician or cardiologist, but needed to prove it for himself. I heard Brock say many times that "a cardiac surgeon must know enough cardiology so that the cardiologist doesn't make a fool of him." By this he meant that the surgeon must be as sure as he can be that the diagnosis the cardiologist has made is correct. Otherwise, he will open the patient's chest and find himself faced with a defect or problem that he didn't anticipate, placing him in a very difficult position.

Although he placed immense emphasis on always examining the patient carefully, Brock had no patience with physicians who went on at length describing the various heart murmurs and other noises that could be heard through the stethoscope. "The heart is a pump, not a musical box," he would say. These observations, like many that

Brock made in his lifetime and which his former trainees know as "Brockisms," seem so simple and obvious today that their importance to the development of heart surgery can easily be overlooked. In the 1940s and 1950s, however, few of Brock's contemporaries on either side of the Atlantic were so clear-thinking or enlightened. Like most of the pioneers of heart surgery, he experienced considerable resistance from some of his medical colleagues.

Neither did Brock like the attitude of some very cautious cardiologists after a successful operation had been performed. At the time of the patient's discharge from hospital, he claimed that even when the operation had cured the condition completely, they would sometimes advise the patient, "Go home and lead a completely normal life. Do whatever you want to do. But for God's sake, don't run for a bus or you'll drop down dead." In contrast, however, whenever a patient was not progressing as well as expected, Brock would advise his colleagues and juniors to think of the worst complication it could possibly be, and work back from there.

## Patients' Deaths

Brock's early heart operations, like those of his American counterparts, carried a high mortality rate. Ben Milstein, an early trainee of Brock, recollects a disastrous period when "eight or nine out of ten consecutive mitral valvotomy patients died." Brock was a man who felt deeply for the well-being of his patients, and those early failures and deaths caused him great anguish and must have given him many sleepless nights. In 1948, Brock wrote of the day after his fourth death in succession: "Despair stalked before us and everyone's morale was low. I said to my team that we could only do one of two things — give up or go on — and that it was impossible to give up as we were certainly in the right. The only thing, therefore, was to go on."

On the occasion of his being presented with the prestigious Gairdner Award, he gave a lecture entitled *The Philosophy of Surgery* in which he describes the difficult times that a surgeon can experience when pioneering a new field of surgery as unforgiving as heart surgery. He quotes the great American surgeon Rudolph Matas, and these words are worth repeating here as they well illustrate the anguish that surgeons can suffer:

"If in the course of an operation the surgeon is assailed by violent emotions the rapidity with which they follow each other and the physical exertion in which he is engaged, sometimes the very gravity of the circumstances in which he is placed, absorb all his energy and suffice to divert his mind from all other preoccupations. These violent and often terrible experiences do not possess, however, the poignancy and intensity of the more deliberate reflections which come on after the tragedy is over. Then the merciless self-imposed, direct cross-examination begins, in which the surgeon, standing before the bar of his own conscience, asks himself what part of the disaster may be attributable to his own sins of commission or omission; or if the outcome of the fatality is merely the result of an accident, that which no man can possibly alter or divert." Brock added, "It is the repetition of such experiences that leave their mark on the surgeon and inevitably influence his life permanently."

Those of us who worked with Brock know how heavy was the *permanent* mark he had to bear. Terence English was one of many who emphasized to me that the deaths weighed heavily on Brock's shoulders: "He was conscious of death all the time. I can remember an apocryphal story of Brock looking at himself in the mirror each morning, and saying, 'Well, Brock, who are you going to kill today?' I think those early surgeons were very conscious of that. Brock certainly was. He felt it very strongly, particularly with regard to children. Many of them died."

Perhaps it was because of the high mortality rate of heart operations in those days that Brock thought of them as battles—the surgeon against the enemy. When considering whether a diagnosis was accurate or not before he embarked upon an operation, he would point out that he needed to know whether he was going to be confronted in the operating room by "a boy on a bicycle or a full armored division." During the operation, when he perceived he was not getting the assistance from his juniors that he needed, he would question "whether Wellington would have won the battle of Waterloo if he had been assisted by the troops that I have." If, during the course of an operation, he found that preparation for the procedure had been in some way inadequate, he would explode into a tirade about the necessity of "keeping your powder dry, and checking your musket before firing it." His juniors would never forget to prepare fully on future occasions. A senior trainee remembered the occasion when he was performing an operation, without Brock's guidance, that went horribly wrong and, although he got control of the situation, Brock was called in to give advice. Brock asked, "Do you know what the politicians do when a general has been defeated in battle?" The young surgeon replied that he did not, to which the response was, "They send for another general. Go and have a cup of coffee." Brock took over the operation.

## Later Career

Brock and his trainee and, subsequently, colleague, Donald Ross, were among those who introduced open heart surgery relatively early in the United Kingdom at Guy's Hospital, particularly by the use of hypothermia (chapter 5), but Brock was never as comfortable with open heart surgery as he was during the closed cardiac surgical era. He found it difficult to adapt to the use of the heart-lung machine, as did many of his generation of surgeons; they were individualists rather than team players, and open heart surgery required a team. Ross told me that Brock "was number one, two, and three, with no interference or advice. He couldn't work as a team. He never could and he never would."

Although Brock continued to give a wonderful service to his patients, by 1960 his era of innovation was largely over, and it was left to younger men, such as Ross, to expand open heart surgery fully in the United Kingdom. However, Brock continued to operate for several more years and to follow his early patients. Brock was a big enough man not to feel threatened by his junior colleague's undoubtedly superior technical skills. Terence English remembers one such incident when Brock had been asked by one of his cardiology colleagues to advise on surgical treatment of a very sick woman: "Brock came to the ward, and went into the whole case very thoroughly, as he always did, and decided that he wouldn't operate on this woman. He wrote in the patient's notes that, in his opinion, the risks would be too high, but he did suggest that Mr. Ross might be asked to see the patient and offer a different opinion. I was hugely impressed by this. That took a lot for a man who was naturally shy and reserved to ask for his former senior registrar to see the patient. I think this showed his greatness."

## The Man

Throughout Brock's life, his natural reserve made it difficult for others to get to know him well. He was very shy and reserved, yet inwardly passionate.

When I asked John Wright what Brock's strengths and weaknesses were, he replied, "He was a very clear thinker and that was his great strength. Tremendous attention to detail. As you know, as a surgeon he wasn't particularly gifted. But he was very, very good at working out exactly how to do it — drawing up the detailed protocol — probably because he wasn't like Denton Cooley, to whom everything was so easy he couldn't remember how he did it anyway. It wasn't easy for Lord Brock, and so he worked it all out in detail, and then followed it through.

"He was quite sure of himself — he was quite certain that if he felt something was right, then it would be. He had these hard-and-fast rules, and he carried them through. In my experience, he was usually correct.

"I don't know whether you would call it a weakness or not, but everybody who worked with him or for him seemed to fear him. They respected him enormously, but there was also this tremendous element of fear. When he arrived at the Royal Brompton Hospital in the morning, the doorman at the gate would immediately telephone the operating suite to say that his car had entered. When he went past the receptionist, another phone call would come through to say he's arrived, and the whole operating theater would come to attention. There was a good deal of fear.

"But his other side was equally amazing. For example, he often liked to do a ward round on a Saturday morning. One Friday, he said, 'I'll be here at nine o'clock tomorrow.' I said, 'Actually, tomorrow is my boy's birthday, sir. I was going to take the day off, and take him out somewhere.' He immediately said, 'Family matters are extremely important. They come first. You will *not* come in tomorrow. You will do your family duty.' So, although he generated fear, he could be equally gentle. His personality and his character were Jekyll and Hyde."

It was Brock's persistence toward the attainment of perfection that perhaps gave him and his juniors the most personal anguish. Eminent British surgeon Lord (Rodney) Smith wrote of Brock, "Throughout his life he allowed neither himself nor those with whom he worked any margin for uncertainty or inaccuracy, and he gave the impression of perpetual disappointment at the unattainability of universal perfection. Anything remotely smacking of the slipshod or the neglectful was anathema to him and he would never offer a patient less than his best — and did not see why anyone else should either."

Brock tried equally to be a perfectionist in his use of the English language, and indeed tried to instill its correct usage in his juniors. John Wright remembers an occasion when he wrote a manuscript he was hoping to submit for publication in a surgical journal, which he asked Brock to read. After reading it carefully, Brock commented, "You said here that you had '*lost* one of your patients.' Do you mean he's dead? If so, say so. 'He's dead.'"

Although Brock demanded perfection from his staff, he would, in the words of Sir Thomas Holmes Sellors, "do anything to help a young surgeon's career if he felt that he lived up to his own standards." One of his trainees commented that one epitaph for Brock might be "A man who had no time of his own, but would always find it for others." Like Blalock, Brock had a genuine concern for the welfare of his junior staff.

There is one very nice anecdote that possibly illustrates Brock's inherent reserve and formality. His personal secretary for his entire career, Miss Jones, would follow him on all of his ward rounds and outpatient clinics, with her own personal handwritten charts and records, which she would serve up to him as he saw each patient. One of his trainees has described "the faithful Miss Jones as the erstwhile equivalent of the modern day computer." Late in life, after the death of his wife, Brock married Miss Jones, and so she ended her days as Lady Brock. However, even after their marriage, for some time she continued in her role as secretary. When they were together in the hospital, Brock would sometimes have difficulty in adjusting to her new role in his life. For example, when she was helping him on with his white coat, he once turned to her and said, "Thank you, Miss Jones."

## Sense of Humor

In Ben Milstein's opinion, Brock "did not have much of a sense of humor." My recollection, and that of many of Brock's trainees, is otherwise. For someone who was inherently shy and reserved, examples of his humor — albeit often subtle — abound.

Denton Cooley, who spent a year training with Brock in London, recalled that when he told Brock that a surgical procedure could be done in a certain way and, indeed, was frequently done that way, Brock answered, "Cooley, people commit adultery frequently, but that doesn't make it right."

During one operation in which Brock felt his assistant was rather getting in his way, he said, "If you do that again, a great spike will come up through the floor and strike you." When the assistant asked whether the spike would strike him in the foot, Brock responded, "With luck, somewhat higher up."

Even under stressful conditions, he could occasionally — *very* occasionally — find his sense of humor. One junior trainee remembers that during an operation, he was instructed to keep an eye on the heart in the open chest while Brock and his other assistants cannulated the femoral artery in the leg in order to connect the heart-lung machine. To the trainee's distress, as he watched the heart, it suddenly stopped beating. He immediately relayed this dramatic information to Brock, whose tongue-in-cheek response was, "Now then, no small talk."

Brock once told me a story that has intrigued me for more than 35 years. A British chest surgeon, an early colleague of Brock, pricked his finger during an operation for an infectious condition (an empyema). In this pre-antibiotic era, the infection spread through his hand and arm. The unfortunate surgeon's medical advisors were faced with the question of whether they should recommend amputation of the arm in an effort to try to save their patient's life. Brock pointed out to me that the surgeon was right-handed and that the infection was in his right arm. The implication was that to amputate his right arm would mean that he would no longer be able to work as a surgeon, which to Brock would clearly have been a personal disaster. I have never been quite sure that I heard him correctly, but I am almost certain that Brock commented, "*Fortunately,* the surgeon died." I took this to mean that he felt it was better to be dead than to no longer be able to perform surgical operations. Such was Brock's dedication to his work that I believe I heard him correctly.

Russell Brock died at the age of 76 in 1980, having, with Blalock, introduced two constructive operations to correct heart defects. In particular, in Brock's case, he had taken the attack into the heart itself. Coupled with the work of Bailey and Harken on the surgical treatment of mitral stenosis, as we shall see, this was a landmark step in the development of heart surgery.

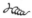

# CHAPTER 4

# The Seeing Finger:
# Opening Obstructed Valves

———

## CHARLES BAILEY AND DWIGHT HARKEN

THE SURGICAL RELIEF of a commonly obstructed heart valve, the mitral valve, is primarily the story of two of the most flamboyant and controversial characters to stride across the surgical floor. One, Charles Bailey (Figure 11), was from a poor background and a lowly regarded medical school, a true maverick who bucked the system. The other, Dwight Harken (Figure 12), the son of a respected country doctor, had trained at Harvard Medical School and, although his ego alienated some, remained a Boston establishment figure. Whether a result of the differences in their backgrounds or the flamboyance of their respective personalities, or both, they were the major players in one of the great feuds of 20th-century medicine.

Both were born in 1910, and, intriguingly, died within days of each other in 1993. Their willingness to push ahead in the face of immense criticism, and sometimes censure, from many of their medical colleagues advanced closed heart surgery from a treatment for the relatively few children born with heart defects to an option for the far greater number of adult patients with heart disease acquired later in life.

## Rheumatic Fever and the Mitral Valve

Rheumatic fever is a condition that largely affects children as a sequel to certain infections. Today, in Western countries (though not in some other parts of the world), rheumatic fever occurs far less frequently than it did in the early part of the 20th century. This is a result of the better environmental conditions in which we live and the availability of antibiotics, which have greatly reduced its incidence. Rheumatic fever often causes the valves of the heart, particularly the mitral valve, to become red and swollen, rather like the edges of a wound when the skin has been lacerated. Subsequently, scarring takes place and the valve becomes shriveled, its orifice becoming narrowed, or stenosed (Figure 13).

Stenosis results in reduced blood flow through the mitral valve, with accumulation of blood in the chamber of the heart (the left atrium) that drains through the valve. The distension and increasing pressure in the left atrium in turn leads to the accumulation of blood in the lungs. Lung congestion leads to shortness of breath, initially on exercise and subsequently even at rest, and causes the patient to cough up blood-stained sputum. The patient slowly deteriorates, usually over a number of years. Eventually, the lungs become "waterlogged," the patient suffocating through an inability to take air into the lungs. Mitral stenosis leads to a slow and miserable death.

In the 1940s, mitral stenosis was a common and debilitating affliction, seen widely in Europe and North America. Today, we have forgotten how it could ravage the patient. Francis Moore, the legendary Harvard professor of surgery, commented to me, "I don't think the world today has any glimpse of the effect of advanced mitral stenosis on a patient—cyanosis [blueness], wasting—they lost lots of weight—absolutely bedridden." Bill Bigelow (chapter 5) went so far as to say, "After a long period of lying propped in bed, gasping for breath, or after severe angina pain, death to many of them was a blessed relief.... [Such patients] are not encountered in present-day heart surgery because surgical treatment is available at an early stage of their disease." It was no wonder then that, according to Russell Brock, "The great pressure to aid the development of mitral valve surgery came not from the doctors, but from the patients."

Heart surgeon Bob Frater attested to the dramatic improvement that could occur in the patient's condition after a successful mitral valvotomy, the operation to relieve the obstruction: "Of all the operations that I have ever done in my life, the one in which the quickest acknowledgment of an improvement in symptoms comes is mitral stenosis. If you asked a mitral stenosis patient two days after surgery, 'How are you feeling?' 'I'm feeling good, doc.' 'What's the difference?' 'Well, I can breathe easily now. I can take a breath.' They would notice the improvement so quickly."

In 1902, a London physician with the rather fine name of Sir Lauder Brunton urged that the mitral orifice should be enlarged surgically. Many physicians strongly condemned this suggestion, largely because they believed that rheumatic fever weakened the heart muscle and that this, rather than the narrowed valve, was the major cause of the heart failure that developed. In the 1920s, Elliott Cutler, surgeon-in-chief at one of the Harvard hospitals in Boston, carried out a number of operations intended to relieve mitral stenosis, the first in 1923, but the technique he used resulted in a state of "regurgitation," or leaking, of the valve. This exacerbated rather than improved the patient's heart failure, and all eight of his patients died at surgery or soon after. However, in 1925 Sir Henry Souttar, a surgeon at the London Hospital (famous for the story of the "Elephant Man"), performed the surgical procedure successfully, and the patient, a teenage girl named Lily Hine, survived for many years. He never performed another similar operation and, when asked why, he responded that it was because the physicians never referred another patient to him. However, this single successful operation did allow Souttar later to honestly claim, "I am the only surgeon in the world who has operated on the heart with *no* mortality."

The controversy as to the cause of the heart failure following rheumatic fever still raged, and many physicians were adamantly opposed to any form of surgery for the condition. It was more than another 20 years before Bailey and Harken, along with Russell Brock, took up the challenge once again. As Souttar later wrote, "...it is no use to be ahead of one's time!"

## CHARLES BAILEY— THE PHILADELPHIA MAVERICK

Charlie Bailey (Figure 11), as he was universally known by his colleagues, was high on my list of pioneer heart surgeons to interview when, by sheer chance, the opportunity came to me "out of the blue" when I was living in Oklahoma. I was attending a banquet that formed one of the social events associated with a medicolegal conference in Oklahoma City in early October 1989. Charlie Bailey, who, unbeknownst to me, was attending the meeting and was present at the banquet, was brought to my table by Nazih Zuhdi, who had stimulated my interest in the history of heart surgery, and I had the privilege of being introduced to him. The 80-year-old Bailey was rather taller and slimmer than I had imagined, and wore hearing aids and spectacles. He greeted me affably with the words, "I hear you think I'm dead." This had indeed been true until some weeks previously, when I had been assured by Zuhdi that Charlie Bailey was still very much alive.

Bailey was born on September 8, 1910, in Wanamassa, New Jersey. "At that time, it was a fairly primitive, undeveloped area," he told me. "I grew up as a barefoot boy with cheeks of tan. My father started out as a bank clerk, but he didn't want to be tied down to that, and so he left the bank and worked for or with a number of different companies. He had a habit, which his son manifested later, of telling his bosses how to run their businesses. When the confrontation became acute, he would say, 'Well, here's my resignation, and I hope you have good luck doing it your antiquated way.' I'm probably the only doctor you know who has told the deans of two medical schools where they could stick their professorships.

"My mother wasn't Jewish, but she was a 'Jewish mother' in the sense that, before I was born, her son was to be a doctor. I grew up knowing I was going to be a doctor, and therefore I played with sick animals — frogs with broken legs and birds that couldn't fly. Although I knew I was going to be a doctor, I really wasn't sure what sort of doctor I would be. Finally, as a child, I had come to the decision that I would become a cancer researcher and solve the problem of malignant disease. At twelve, I had a violent change in this aspiration when my father [who was age 42 at the time] died of rheumatic heart disease in my mother's arms in front of me. Since the heart is obviously a mechanical pump, it seemed to me it ought to be possible to do something for a sick heart, and so I decided I was going to devote my energy to doing that. From then on, that was my effort." Bailey's father died coughing up blood, a result of mitral stenosis. This tragic event must have been a frightening — and ineradicable — experience for the 12-year-old boy.

After college at Rutgers University in New Jersey, Bailey proceeded to Hahnemann Medical College in Philadelphia, graduating with an MD degree in 1932. Hahnemann at that time was a mix of medical school and college of homeopathy (an alternative form of medical therapy) and not highly regarded as a center of medical education.

Bailey recalled, "I was the second youngest and one of the top students in medical school. In my sophomore or junior year of medical school I realized that, if I wanted to do anything for the heart other than drug treatment, I would have to become a surgeon. But during my internship year, because of an inadvertently mistreated patient, I got into very bad grace with the medical director of the hospital. It could well have ended in my leaving before completing my internship. As a result of that, I became somewhat embittered with organized medicine and decided I was going to be a general practitioner.

"I ran a general practice in Lakewood, New Jersey, for almost five years. By the end of that time, I decided that I was definitely going into surgery and, indeed, into heart surgery. Although there was no heart surgery going on at that time, I felt that, if I became a chest surgeon, I would be able to gradually spread into the field of heart surgery. So I applied to the graduate school of the department of surgery at the University of Pennsylvania, and was accepted and entered it in 1937. I had made quite a few contacts among my medical colleagues and, within a couple of months, I was offered a residency in chest surgery at the Seaview Hospital. Upon completion of my training program, I was invited to become a member of the faculty of my alma mater, Hahnemann Medical College. I would be active in general surgery, but I was to handle the special discipline of chest surgery, which meant everything under the skin of the chest except breast surgery, which was part of gynecology. I did all that, and I also worked in the animal laboratory and in the pathology laboratory, particularly studying heart valves. I took a special interest in the mitral valve, which was the one that had affected my father."

## The Lady's Girdle

Bailey continued, "I must here go back to the time when I was fifteen and working my way through college selling newspapers and working Saturdays and afternoons at a grocery store. In the summer vacations, I took various jobs, one of which was with the Realsilk Hosiery Company of Indianapolis, Indiana. This job consisted of going from door to door selling ladies' silk stockings, which weren't so available at that time as they are now. I also sold ladies' underwear.

"At that tender age, I became intimately aware of the anatomical structure of the old-fashioned lady's girdle. This girdle is a cylindrical garment with four sets of garters, one set for the front of each stocking and one set for the back of each [Figure 14]. It is semi-elastic, usually of woven material, sometimes of nylon. When I was studying the mitral valve, it struck me that this valve is built almost exactly the same as a lady's girdle. It doesn't have garters, but it does have groups of little strings [the chordae] that attach to the papillary muscles. The deformity of the mitral valve caused by rheumatic fever reminded me of what would have happened to a nylon fabric girdle if someone had ironed it with an iron that was too hot. It would have frizzled up the material, and thickened and hardened it all around. The opening where the legs come out would have become much diminished in size, to the extent that the lady wouldn't have been able to get her legs through it.

"So with this combination of fantasy and the obvious disease of the mitral valve, which I had seen at autopsy in patients who had died from the disease, it was obvious to me that the way to open up such a narrowed valve would be to cut between the front and back strings [or garters] on either side. The obstruction would be overcome. This operation worked very well in dogs, and it seemed to work well on the valves of dead people who had had this disease. It was certainly far superior to the methods used by Dr. Cutler in Boston twenty years previously, where some of the valve tissue had actually been excised.

"There was one other incident that impressed me. One night, on my way home from a house call, I was following a truck when it struck a deer. It knocked the heart and lungs of the deer completely out of the body, so that the heart lay on the roadway beating away. I took the heart and lungs home, and found that the deer heart beat for almost two hours. Before that, I had thought that only the reptilian heart would beat for such a long time after being taken out of the body. The deer heart is almost identical to the human heart in its structure. I now became impressed that the mammalian heart is a very strong organ, and quite capable of taking all kinds of insults. The human heart must be strong or it wouldn't last for seventy-odd years, as it does in most of us in America.

"This led me to speculate about how we could cut the mitral valve. It seemed to me that, since doctors use their fingers for examining patients — and the gynecologists perhaps take that to the ultimate degree — we might well examine the heart that way. We didn't have any heart-lung machines and so we couldn't stop the heart to open it and look inside, but we could put a finger into the heart." (Because the heart could not be opened and the operation performed under direct vision, this type of operation became known as "closed" heart surgery. Brock's "blind" operation on the pulmonary valve is also an example of a closed heart operation.)

"There happily exist two appendages, one on the right and one on the left side of the heart, which open into the respective atria ["receiving" or "collecting" chambers of the heart] [Figure 13]. By making an opening in the tip of the left atrial appendage, one could insert one's finger and immediately feel the mitral valve from its top side. One should be able to recognize whether it were obstructed or not, where the extremities of that arcuate line of closure were, whether or not there was any calcification of the valve [i.e., whether the valve was so diseased that patches of bonelike thickening had developed], or any blood clot in the atrium. As long as there was a snug purse-string stitch around the opening in the atrial appendage through which one put one's finger, there should be no bleeding. The heart should readily tolerate such an examination of the valve and, if one didn't obstruct the blood flow for more than two to three beats, there shouldn't even be a drop in blood pressure. After performing this procedure in dogs in the laboratory, it wasn't too much for me to consider extending this to human beings."

This seems a simple and logical procedure and, indeed, today it is just that, but, in the mid-1940s, it was considered unconscionably reckless by many of Bailey's contemporaries. The mind-set of surgeons, even chest surgeons, was quite different then from now. I can well remember one of my surgical mentors in London in the 1970s mentioning that, during his own surgical training in the 1930s, he had been strongly advised *never* to touch the heart because of the risk of ventricular fibrillation, a life-threatening irregular rhythm. Dwight Harken also wrote of how he was "confounded" by the reluctance of the great surgeons he trained under to touch the heart.

Bailey has written in the surgical literature that, having conceived this approach to the surgical correction of mitral valve stenosis, it remained only for a suitable patient to present himself or herself. This involved much discussion with his medical associates, some of whom were outraged, others skeptical, and a few intrigued or even impressed. In the transcript of a taped 1981 interview with some of Dr. Bailey's colleagues at Hahnemann, Dr. Victor Satinsky said, "Charlie literally grabbed physicians by the lapel and pleaded with them for patients with severe mitral stenosis, but nobody would trust him with this radical idea of operating on the heart. However, his perseverance finally paid off."

## The First Patients

"In 1945," Bailey continued, "a very sick man was brought to my care. He had severe mitral stenosis with heavy calcification of the valve [i.e., the valve was so scarred that calcium had become deposited in it, rendering it bonelike and noncompliant — the calcification would have been seen on a chest X-ray], and he obviously wasn't going to survive with medical treatment alone. He was treated medically until he improved as much as we could expect, and then he was turned over to me for an operation. I opened his chest, and put my finger into the atrial appendage through an opening surrounded by a purse-string suture. I examined the valve, which was heavily calcified, almost like shark's teeth, and wondered whether the calcium would split satisfactorily. Before I could try to do this, my assistant — a very able, indeed outstanding, young surgeon, but who had unfortunately not worked with me in the experimental laboratory and had no real knowledge or understanding of what I was going to do — became so upset, so disturbed at the sight of seeing his chief with his finger in a heart that was still beating, that he pulled so vigorously on the purse-string suture that he actually tore off the appendage, which in these cases is often somewhat fragile. Of course, massive bleeding occurred. There was no way we could stop it, and the patient expired on the table."

Two more attempts over the next three years were also unsuccessful and proved fatal for the patients. Bailey subsequently wrote, "By this time the foregoing deaths with this unheard-of surgical procedure had caused considerable animated discussion among our medical colleagues." The chief of cardiology at Hahnemann, Dr. George Goeckeler, was instructed to advise Bailey that he would no longer be permitted to operate on any such patients at their hospital. Dr. Goeckeler has been described by Victor Satinsky as "a very proper, stiff Quaker.... Everything that was righteous in life he was for, and everything that was 'waspy' in life he was for. All other things were rather strange to him." Dr. Goeckeler said to Bailey, "It is my Christian duty not to permit you to perform any more such homicidal operations." Replied Bailey, "It is my Christian duty to perfect this operation. Nothing could be worse than what mitral stenosis does to people."

Bailey's operating privileges at several Philadelphia hospitals were withdrawn, severely limiting the number of hospitals where he could attempt this surgery. He came up with a bold idea for improving the odds in the future. If two such patients could be operated upon on the same day, the chances were that at least one of them would "make it." If the operations were done at different hospitals, the probability was that news of the patient's death during the first operation would not reach the second hospital in time to interrupt the performance of the second procedure. So he arranged to operate on two patients on June 10, 1948, the first at the Philadelphia General Hospital at 8 A.M., and the second at the Philadelphia Episcopal Hospital at 2 P.M. Word of this plan was not likely to reach the ears of Bailey's critics because neither of these hospitals was at that time affiliated with the Hahnemann Medical College, and there was very little communication between members of their respective staffs.

The morning patient was desperately sick. Even Charlie Bailey hesitated to go ahead with the operation, but the patient's cardiologist, Dr. Tom Durant, said, "Charlie, if you can help him, you can help any of them." The operation proved to be a surgeon's nightmare. Every time Bailey touched the heart, its rhythm became extremely irregular. Bailey suggested that they abandon the operation, but the cardiologist had with him (from his work in the research laboratory) a preparation of quinidine for intravenous administration, which would reduce the "irritability" of the heart. He urged its use, and this advice was reluctantly accepted. As the quinidine was being given, the heart contractions became slower and weaker and finally ceased altogether. Despite manual massage of the heart, its contractions could not be recovered. The cardiologist urged that something be done to the mitral valve to relieve the intense congestion of the lungs. Bailey insisted that the patient first be "pronounced dead," presumably hoping that this would absolve him from the accusation that he killed the patient. This was done. Bailey then inserted his finger into the heart and tried to open the valve. Although he did this successfully and the heart began to beat for a period of some minutes, the patient did not survive.

With this fourth death, Bailey, his operating team, and the attending cardiologist hurried across town to the Episcopal Hospital. There, the patient was a 24-year-old housewife and mother who had been known to have a heart murmur for many years and had progressively become incapacitated from mitral stenosis during the past two years. Fortunately, the operation went well, and Bailey was able to open the valve orifice not with his finger, but with a special hooked knife that he had designed (and which he passed along the index finger between two gloves on his right hand). The patient was out of bed and walking on the third day after the operation. On the seventh, she was transported by rail approximately 700 miles to a medical convention in Chicago at which Bailey was speaking. To subject the patient to this stress so soon after the operation illustrates Bailey's boldness — or, some might say, recklessness.

Bailey took up the story: "Her name was Claire Ward, and she came from New Jersey. She lived for 38 years after the operation, during which time she had two more children. She worked during nearly all of that period. My paper on this operation wasn't published promptly, because the American College of Chest Physicians was reluctant to publish it. They thought it was fantasy, and didn't want to publish something in their journal that they considered unscientific. However,

Dr. Dwight Harken in Boston had a successful survivor from a quite similar technique six days after my operation, and he had stronger support from the Harvard group. Eventually, it was decided by the authorities that both of us would be allowed to publish. So the paper was finally published. The reaction at first was that I had spent time in a mental institution and obviously hadn't recovered, because everyone knew you couldn't touch the heart without it stopping. So there were scurrilous things said for awhile.

"Russell Brock, of London, had the same idea that Dr. Harken and I had. It was entirely independent of our work, and he did his first successful operation about two months after Dr. Harken and I had done ours. It became established that the three of us — Harken, Brock, and I — had all done just about the same operation. If any two of us hadn't been born, the other one would have done the same thing at the same time, and 'closed' heart surgery would have been developed because its time had come."

## The Sad Story of Horace Smithy

Apart from Bailey, Harken, and Brock, there was one other surgeon who has to a large extent been forgotten, but who was very early into this field. This was Horace Smithy of Charleston, South Carolina. In 1948, he performed operations for mitral stenosis in eight patients, of whom five survived and were able to leave the hospital. Smithy deserves immense credit for his vision and boldness. Why is his name not as well remembered as those of Bailey, Harken, and Brock? Smithy was one of the most tragic figures among this group of pioneering heart surgeons. Within a few months, he was dead himself (at the age of 34) from stenosis of the aortic valve, having failed to persuade any of his surgical colleagues, including the intrepid Charlie Bailey, to operate on him.

## The "Golden Age"

Following this initial success, there was a steady flow of more suitable candidates to Bailey for this form of surgery. After several further successes, the restrictions on performing this surgery at Hahnemann were rescinded. The reports of similar surgery by Harken and Brock also did much to overcome the initial hesitancy felt by many in the Philadelphia medical community. Even the cautious Dr. Goeckeler became supportive of Bailey's work and, indeed, had nothing but praise for him.

"My successive reports to various medical groups," continued Bailey, "in which I communicated to them our increasing experience with this operation, were at first largely ignored. However, about a year or two later, other chest surgeons began to visit me in Philadelphia. It became a very exciting period for me, which lasted for quite a number of years until open heart surgery became feasible. Then, of course, the heart could simply be opened and the valve looked at."

Victor Satinsky reminisced, "Charlie began to have people come to him from all over the world. We really didn't realize we were in a golden age then; it was just like doing our everyday work, although with great excitement. We were like a bunch of little kids having a good time with something new, and I don't think we realized until much later that this was really a breakthrough. Charlie was not only very, very innovative, but he gave everybody else a chance. As soon as someone had an idea he would say, 'Go do it.' He always encouraged people to be creative."

Bailey spent his own money on buying equipment and building up the facilities at the hospital. He also equipped an experimental laboratory. Then a great personal tragedy occurred. His eight-year-old daughter died of acute hepatitis. Satinsky suggested that, instead of sending flowers, people should donate money to establish a Mary Bailey Institute for Cardiovascular Research in honor of Bailey's daughter. This was done, and the institute was established.

## The Feud

Bailey gave me his thoughts on his erstwhile surgical competitor, the Boston-based Dr. Dwight Harken. "Dwight Harken was a very brilliant man. Initially, he was a bit on the arrogant side. Since I was a graduate of Hahnemann, which was a homeopathic medical college at that time and even gave a degree in homeopathy as well as an MD degree, he was inclined to look down on me. He was a Harvard graduate, and one of those 'great Bostonians.' And he was much annoyed that I had done my first successful operation five or six days before he did his. This was purely accidental, as I happened to get a patient earlier than he did. Both of us had had some unsuccessful efforts before that, I believe. It was hard for him to believe that this unscientific, improperly trained man could be doing the same thing as he did, and even with a few days' advantage.

"We had some differences of opinion. Besides that, Boston doctors fight in their medical meetings. Philadelphia doctors are very respectable and considerate of each other. I was shocked when we first met in San Francisco at a medical meeting and each of us presented our operation for the mitral valve. He spoke after me, and harshly criticized what I had done. I was shocked and, in my discussion period, I didn't defend myself. Not too long after that, we met at a medical meeting in Chicago, where again he lacerated me publicly. Again, I didn't defend myself. Then I got to thinking that the 'Good Book' says you should turn the other cheek, but it doesn't say what you should do when that cheek gets slapped also. So the next time we met, I was prepared. From then on we both gave as good as we got, and people invited us to medical meetings not only for our scientific presentations, but for the enlivenment we would bring to the audience. This went on for several years."

On one occasion, Bailey forced Harken to admit that his reported statistics were incorrect. "I said to him, 'You didn't give us the truth about your statistics.' He finally got around to saying, 'I have just found — I didn't know when I came here yesterday — that there has been an additional death in that group.' With stumbling and bumbling, he had a very poor defense.... It was important to me that I should knock off his arrogance. Well, when I got back, I thought that was a hell of a thing for me to do, a guy who used to teach Sunday school and who I thought was a decent human being. Yes, Harken had said awful things about me, but that's the way they are in Boston, and he has always been a Bostonian. Well, I'm a Philadelphian, and I should be more of a gentleman. I never said anything against him again.

"Many years later, after I had told my medical school dean where to stick his professorship — by the way, you always have to do it quick before they can say 'You're fired' — I had been sued for malpractice. A patient of mine had died, and the plaintiff's lawyer kept hammering away at me. In particular, he kept quoting Dr. Harken, who had written an article that included the results of about nine hundred cases. 'Dr. Harken says you have to do it so and so, and you *didn't* do it so and so.' The lawyer really gave me fits. We two, me and Harken, were the only true authorities on the operation. Finally, my lawyer said to me, 'He keeps quoting that fellow Harken. Could you get Harken to come down here and testify on your behalf, because if he says that what Dr. Bailey did in this case was perfectly all right, then you're out free. But at present the jury thinks you did terrible things that this great authority, Dr. Harken, says you shouldn't have done. You didn't write a paper on as many operations as he did, did you?' I said, 'No. I've done that many, but I haven't written a paper yet.' My lawyer said, 'Do you think Harken would come?' I said, 'I know he's very upset about medical malpractice and he may be tempted to try to help a fellow doctor, but he and I haven't been very good friends.' My lawyer said, 'I think we're going to lose this case if you don't try.'

"So I made the call. I mean, what could I lose? I got Dr. Harken on the phone and told him exactly what the plaintiff's lawyer was saying about him. Dr. Harken said, 'That isn't what I said. That isn't what I meant.' I said, 'Well, Dwight, nobody but you could turn this case around for me, and my lawyer has asked if you would be willing to come down and testify.' He said, 'Charlie, when do you need me?' I said, 'It would be tomorrow morning or early afternoon.' He said, 'Charlie, there is a shuttle at such and such a time and I can get into

New York at eleven A.M. I'll be there. But Charlie, you've got to understand this, you can't pay me one cent. I'm doing this because I feel this
medical malpractice has got to be squelched.' What could I say?

"He came into the courtroom and told the jury that everything
Bailey did was right, and that we were the two guys who had the most
experience in the world and so forth. 'Unfortunately, we do have a
certain number of patients who die, and the patient in this case just
happened to be one of those who did die.' Dwight Harken saved the
case for me. We won it. Well, naturally, you can imagine how I felt
after he saved my bacon. I wrote him a nice letter.

"Later, after my altercation with my second medical school dean, I
was sort of 'retired' for nine months. That's when I learned that retirement is 'death on the installment plan.' Never, never retire. I'm going
to get back on the horse and, when I fall off, it doesn't matter whether
they bury me or leave me at the side of the road — that's my motto.
Anyway, here I was 'retired' for nine months, and I finally get a chance
at a hospital in the Bronx. But they were troubled because I had trouble at two medical schools. I needed a strong recommendation, and I
called up Dwight, and he said, 'Charlie, have them write to me.' They
did. He told them that he had known me for many years and I was one
of the great men of our time. By this time we weren't fighting anymore.
In fact, I had said a few good things about him that had gotten back
to him. What could I do after he saved the lawsuit? So we became, if
not bosom friends, at least very good friends in our autumn years."

Interestingly, Harken told me the same stories about him and
Bailey but, despite his support for Bailey at crucial times, he never
felt they became friends. He retained a poor opinion about Bailey's
character until the day he died. Indeed, opinions on Bailey among the
other surgeons I interviewed for this book were very mixed.

## Further "Experimental" Operations on Patients

For several years, Hahnemann became a leading center in cardiac
surgery. For example, Bailey probably performed the first open heart

operation under hypothermia (chapter 5), but it was not successful. However, he did perform the world's second successful procedure. For several years, Bailey was willing to operate on patients with almost any heart condition, and he became involved in surgical developments in the correction of congenital heart defects, hypothermia, and the heart-lung machine. Heart surgeon Bill Bigelow commented that Bailey "was a wild man, with an insatiable desire for notoriety. He lost so many patients, but he made a tremendous contribution." He "did a lot of operations, many of them strange things." After the introduction of the heart-lung machine, Bailey's group investigated coronary artery surgery and even heart transplantation in dogs.

It was his foray into surgery for coronary artery disease, well before most other surgeons had taken an interest in this field, that led to one of Bailey's most disastrous "public" appearances. He had developed the operation of coronary endarterectomy, in which he reamed out the atherosclerotic plaques (obstructions) from the inside of a coronary artery while the patient was supported by the heart-lung machine. He passed an instrument down the coronary artery and blindly tried to scrape out the diseased tissue. This was clearly an extremely hazardous operation. He accepted an invitation to demonstrate the operation on closed-circuit television to a professional audience at a major surgical congress; few other surgeons would have been so bold as to accept such an invitation. The operation went horribly wrong and there was immense bleeding from the heart, which Bailey could not control. Finally, the organizers felt it best to discontinue the television coverage, and faded Bailey out. Obviously, this type of experience, though well-meaning in that Bailey was attempting an experimental procedure to help a patient, did nothing for his reputation among his peers, many of whom thought it the height of recklessness.

Bob Frater remembers watching Bailey operate after he had moved to St. Barnabas Hospital in the Bronx: "He had moved to New York because it more or less became impossible for him to work in Philadelphia. He was going to fix an aortic valve, but he was going to do it with the patient's own tissues.... The operation was a disaster, and the surgery failed. After the patient's death, Charlie went straight into a room across from the operating room, and didn't invite me in with him. Hanging around at the entrance to the operating room was a whole bunch of the patient's relatives. I didn't quite know what to do. Then a nurse came out to the family, and said, 'I'm terribly sorry to tell you, but your family member didn't survive the operation. We worked all day. We tried our best, but we couldn't save him.' They were obviously pretty upset. The nurse said, 'And Dr. Bailey is so upset that he can't see you for the moment. He's reflecting about the case in private. In awhile, I'm sure he will see you.' By the time they saw him, the family was apologizing to *him* for the terrible trauma he had been through during the day. It was the most remarkable performance I'd ever seen. Charlie actually managed to make them feel sorry for *him,* for the struggle he had gone through to try and save their relative. It was astonishing. I could see that Charlie actually believed it himself. It wasn't an act or contrived. I think he was genuinely upset when this patient died. But he got their sympathy. They were actually patting him on the shoulder. It was so bizarre you couldn't put it in a movie.

"Charlie was doing these extraordinary operations — all sorts of cockeyed experiments with horrendous mortality. And yet he was messianic. He really believed he had a job to do, which was to help these poor people. In one way, he experimented unreasonably, but I think you needed people who were willing to do that sort of thing to get heart surgery going."

In 1955, at the height of his intense surgical activity, Bailey found time to write a book, *Surgery of the Heart,* which must have been one of the very earliest — if not the first — books in this field. Although surgery of the heart was still greatly limited at that early stage, the book runs to over 1,000 pages, and was undoubtedly a major contribution toward this rapidly developing field. The entire book, with the exception of a handful of chapters, was written by Bailey himself.

In March 1957, Bailey's leading position in the field of heart surgery, and possibly his flair for publicity, gained him greater public recognition by being featured on the cover of *Time* magazine (Figure 15).

## Later Life

Bailey received honorary degrees from the colleges he had attended, Rutgers and Hahnemann, but not as much professional recognition as he might have expected.

He observed, "I've received pretty good recognition. I didn't get some of the positions of presidencies of medical societies that perhaps I might have. You see, I was sort of a maverick. I was bringing in new ideas, whereas the fellows who get to the top are the ones who get a consensus of folks supporting them. Walt Lillehei [chapter 7] didn't have anything like the positions that you would have thought he should have had because he was also a sort of maverick. That's often the case, but if I had my choice, I would much rather be a maverick and do something that would eventually be accepted than be president of a society."

I asked Dr. Bailey whether, if he was able to relive his life, he would do anything differently.

"Oh, yes. I would have tried to go to Harvard Medical School and get the recognition that that would have given me. I would have tried to go to the Mayo Clinic to get the recognition that that would have given me. But perhaps it's an advantage for a white Anglo-Saxon Protestant — I think that's the way they put it — to go to a homeopathic medical school and become a member of a 'minority,' and have the discrimination and disadvantages that it brings. It makes you work like heck to show what you know. Why do you think I went back and got my doctor of science degree from the University of Pennsylvania? I didn't need it, but there were rumors that I was a low type and not well educated and all that. So I went on and got it. At the time I got it, only five people had done it. So you see, there is some advantage in achieving 'minority' status."

Eventually, in his late 50s, Charlie Bailey turned his attention to medicolegal matters.

"When I got sued three times, even though I won the lawsuits, I was so disturbed by spending two weeks in court each time and hearing the plaintiff's lawyer saying such awful things about me, and telling the whole world that everything I had done was a fraud and that I was incompetent, that I thought someday, when the kids get out on their own, I'm going to go to law school and find out what this is all about. Neither my medical colleagues nor my lawyer friends seemed to be able to tell me. Well, I got to be 56 and I looked in the mirror, and I thought, my God, I'm getting old, and law school will never take me. But eventually, I did pass my LSAT with the help of my daughter, who knows how these things work, and then I did get accepted into law school at Fordham University in New York. I was lucky, for one of my patients was a member of the board of Fordham University." Dr. Bailey took a course in the evenings while still practicing surgery during the day.

"So in 1973, at the tender age of 62, I became a lawyer. I worked for two different law firms thinking I would become a courtroom lawyer, a defense attorney, but the firms had different ideas. They knew it didn't matter how much law you knew. The facts don't count in a courtroom very much. The important thing is whether you're a good actor and can persuade the jury to think the way you want them to think. I was past sixty, and how was I going to learn to be a courtroom lawyer? It takes you fifteen to twenty years. I became persuaded that they were right."

Bailey subsequently formed a group that persuaded an insurance company to make major changes in the way that doctors are insured against medical malpractice suits. He was still working in this field when I met him.

In 1991, two years after I had met with him, ironically Bailey developed heart valve disease himself and needed replacement of his aortic valve. He asked Denton Cooley (chapter 13) to perform the operation, which was successful.

What drove him to make the contributions he did? His father's death when Bailey was at a young age must have been a great stimulus, but there were other factors. Satinsky reported that "as a child, Bailey had had an Uncle Charlie. In Bailey's early years, his mother used to say, 'You're just like your Uncle Charlie,' who was a kind of ne'er-do-well. I believe that Charlie had to show to his mother that he wasn't. He constantly had to prove over and over again that he was an achiever, and that he wasn't like his Uncle Charlie.... Charlie was always doing new things, many of which annoyed others, and yet his contributions were appreciated. You can't split a person. The very thing people don't like about him, his aggressiveness, is the very thing that makes him what he is, a pioneer."

Charlie Bailey died in 1993, at the age of 82, having led a very full life as both surgeon and lawyer, the only surgeon included in our story to have two distinct professional careers.

## DWIGHT HARKEN— THE FLAMBOYANT BOSTONIAN

Dwight Harken (Figure 12) made three significant contributions to the development of heart surgery. First, he successfully removed numerous bullets and fragments of shrapnel from U.S. servicemen's hearts during World War II, demonstrating that the heart would tolerate significant surgical manipulation. Second, he performed a successful mitral valvotomy within a few days of Charlie Bailey's first success. Third, he carried out one of the first replacements of any valve in the heart using a mechanical prosthesis (artificial valve).

Robert Bartlett, who was a surgical resident under Harken in the 1950s, described him as a "fantastic character...very loud, very bombastic, extremely egotistical." He was certainly one of the most flamboyant personalities among pioneer heart surgeons, and it was possibly for this reason that he clashed so frequently with Charlie Bailey, who was equally extroverted and flamboyant. Sir Brian Barratt-Boyes (chapter 10), perhaps less charitably, described Harken as "a very brash guy, very opinionated, very much in charge of his department. But he made major contributions in the valve area, no question."

I met Dr. Harken in November 1988, in his office in Mount Auburn Hospital in Cambridge, Massachusetts. It was a small room, containing an old desk and chairs, the walls completely covered by framed certificates, diplomas, and honors. On the windowsill were examples of artificial prosthetic heart valves in whose design he had been involved, and a book edited by Denton Cooley with an inscription to Dr. Harken on the front page.

I had met him originally when I was a young research fellow at the Peter Bent Brigham Hospital in Boston in the mid-1960s. Then, he had been at the height of his powers — well built, auburn-haired, vigorous, energetic, and almost hyperactive, with "personality" written all over him. I remember how impressed, almost awed, he had been when I told him that the British heart surgeon Sir Russell Brock had been elevated to the peerage, and was now Lord Brock. I had the feeling that Dr. Harken would have enjoyed such an honor and title himself.

Now, in 1988, he was retired from surgery — moderately tall, slim, and white-haired, with sunken cheeks mottled with red veins. He wore heavy-rimmed glasses, as opposed to the rimless glasses I remembered he had worn as a younger man. His sight was clearly deteriorating, and he was also slightly hard of hearing. He remained, however, vigorous and energetic, and he welcomed me warmly. He was friendly, articulate, extremely courteous and considerate, and clearly enjoyed recounting his story. At his suggestion, I had timed my visit to coincide with a small celebration that was taking place in the hospital to mark his contributions to cardiac surgery.

Afterward, we walked through the early darkness of evening to his home, which was not far away. His large, old-fashioned house — much dark wood, rather like an old English manse — was full of period furniture, books, and ornaments. It was comfortable rather than elegant. His study contained many memorabilia of his life, including medals, trophies, and photographs, all on display. He had traveled extensively, and had been awarded almost every honor you could expect. He enthusiastically showed me bits and pieces from his past, and related a story associated with each autobiographical item.

## Father and Son

When, in 2002, I spoke with Dr. Harken's son, Alden, himself a well-known heart surgeon, his childhood recollection of his father was of "a very dynamic, very dedicated guy who spent a huge amount of time at the hospital with patients, and who loved what he did. He thought what he did was important, and that the luckiest people in the world are people who are doing something that not only they think is important but that the rest of the world thinks is important. When my sister and I would make rounds with him on weekends, we would walk into a hospital and see patients who were exceedingly grateful to him. They would tell my mom and us what a contribution he had made to their lives. I think that I saw somebody whose compensation for what he did was not material."

However, the young Alden did not see as much of his busy father as he would have wished. "When I was a small boy, he didn't spend a lot of time with us. I can remember looking out the back window of our apartment to see if his car would pull into his parking space before I had to go to bed. Usually, I had to go to bed before he came home. I saw him some on the weekends, but usually that was at work. We would go in and make rounds with him. I learned to ride my bicycle in the Boston City Hospital parking lot. We spent most of our time as kids involved in hospital patients, medicine, or medical-related things. I do remember going to a baseball game with him. I do remember fishing with him once. And, when I was probably a late teenager, I do remember going up to a place in New Hampshire that he loved. That would have made him in his late fifties. As he was beginning to decrease his activities, we spent more time together, but by then I had more extramural interests of my own. But as a small boy, it was not a lot of time.... But we were proud of what he was able to accomplish, and I certainly don't think it marred my relationship with him. I think the message he was sending was very important to me."

Dwight Harken and I left the study and went through to the drawing room, which was comfortably furnished in period furniture and could have been an English academic's home. Indeed, the Harkens' neighbors were largely academic lawyers from Harvard Law School. Over supper, we began our discussion of his career. Dr. Harken also gave me a copy of a book, *To Mend the Heart,* by Lael Wertenbaker, that is to some extent a biography of him as well as being the story of the early days of heart surgery. It is written in a rather adulatory style, but is well documented and includes many stories that he repeated to me.

## Boyhood

Dwight Harken was born in 1910, and grew up in Osceola, Iowa, where his father was the town doctor. According to Alden Harken, his grandfather "graduated from high school in Iowa, sold encyclopedias for about a year and a half, and decided that wasn't what he wanted to do. At night, there was no television, nothing on the radio, and nobody to talk to, so he read the encyclopedia. About that time, he decided he wanted to go into medicine. He had spent a lot of time with the encyclopedia so he took the Iowa State Medical Board Examination, and passed it. He never went to college and never went to medical school. Then he settled into southwestern Iowa, where he developed a huge practice, not because he was very effective — although I think he was — but because he was the only physician of any variety there. He then became the railroad doctor."

Dwight Harken remembered his father as being handsome, dignified, and always well dressed. The father, Dr. Harken Sr., began taking his son Dwight with him as "anesthesiologist" when he was seven. "We would set out in the early days by horse and carriage," recollected Dwight, "and later by automobile, to an outlying farm to deliver a baby. The woman would be given a cloth soaked in chloroform to hold over her nose and mouth. When she fell asleep, it was my responsibility to take the cloth away to prevent excessive anesthesia. If she began to feel pain, I would replace the cloth over her face." This was quite a responsibility for a seven-year-old boy, as chloroform was a dangerous agent; in those days, anesthesia probably caused as many deaths as the surgery.

It was Dwight Harken's father's dream to emulate the already-famous Mayo Clinic in Rochester, Minnesota, which had been established by Dr. Mayo, the father, and was by then run by his two sons. He wanted to establish the Harken Clinic in Iowa. His plan was that his two sons would assist him, Dwight as the surgeon and his younger brother as the physician. As Lael Wertenbaker writes, Dr. Harken Sr. was "more autocratic than fatherly," and he "assumed he would remain the undisputed head man at his clinic." He ran his extensive practice as he did his family, accepting neither criticism nor opposition. Alden Harken described his grandfather as "a very real taskmaster."

For a small-town general medical practitioner, Dr. Harken Sr. was clearly very different from many of his counterparts, since he made every effort to keep up with, and even contribute to, medical and surgical advances. By the age of 12, Dwight was driving his father in his car every Sunday evening to take the train to Chicago, where he would watch new surgical techniques on the following day. Dwight would meet the returning train early on Tuesday morning. As the railroad doctor, Dwight's father was able to travel free to Chicago. That was his "continuing medical education." He also read voraciously.

Even more remarkably, Dr. Harken Sr. set up a small research laboratory in the local hospital, actually in the attic over a garage. It must surely have been most unusual for a rural general practitioner in the 1920s and 1930s to be sufficiently interested in research to set up an experimental animal laboratory. Dwight Harken explained to me that, since animal experiments were carried out there, the laboratory was kept a secret from the community. It was accessible only through a trap-door. He recalled, "The local sheriff was paid by the county to dispose of stray cats and dogs, but my father paid him extra so that he brought the animals to us. I gave the anesthetic while he operated on them."

## Harvard

Dwight's son, Alden, explained that "my dad graduated from Osceola High School, as did my mother. Both of them were very eager to get away from the very rural lifestyle of southwestern Iowa. In that era, if you graduated in the top 10% of your class in high school, you automatically got accepted to Harvard. So he went to Boston as an undergraduate and medical student. The first couple of years were pretty rough and stressful because, when you had come from Osceola High School, your preparation for an undergraduate career at Harvard was inadequate. At Harvard College, he wasn't a very effective student. He was certainly not a brilliant student. He was always a very hard worker, always a very innovative guy, but those are not the attributes that are rewarded when you're taking Greek and Latin and the other studies in the very rigid curriculum of the late 1920s and 1930s. I think he probably did just well enough to get into Harvard Medical School. He graduated from Harvard College in 1931, and from medical school in 1936."

After a couple of years at the medical school, Harken took a year off and went to art school. He was not doing too well academically at the time and, as he feared he might fail the exams, decided to opt out for a year. He claimed he had difficulty with reading.

"I think he was horribly dyslexic," Alden told me. "My mother was a very avid reader, very capable with words, and very fluent. I'm dyslexic, and all three of my children are dyslexic. My father read very, very slowly, as do I, but at that time the concept of dyslexia didn't exist. So he just had to plod through his educational programs. I can understand that, because I did the same thing."

After a year at the Massachusetts School of Art, Harken returned to repeat his second-year medical training. Once he had contact with patients, rather than books, he did extremely well.

On his son's graduation in 1936, Dr. Harken Sr. was deeply disappointed that Dwight did not immediately return to join the family practice. Despite his son's subsequent success as a surgeon, it seems that Harken Sr. never really forgave him. For the rest of his life, he remained somewhat bitter that Dwight had chosen another route. His disappointment was made ever greater when his other son contracted multiple sclerosis and died. According to Wertenbaker, Dr. Harken Sr. never accorded Dwight any parental accolade for his later work in heart surgery. When, many years later, Dr. Harken Sr. visited the Brigham Hospital in Boston to watch his now famous son in the operating room, he left before the end of the operation. Somebody who was there at the time concluded, "That monumental effort he [Dwight] was putting out, hypertensive, aggressive, wild, erratic, was designed to succeed in his father's eyes. He was looking for that word of approval which he was *never* going to get."

Alden Harken, however, was less certain that his father's immense drive had been stimulated by his grandfather's expectations of him. He felt that Dwight's energy came "more likely from some kind of inner drive." Dwight's expectations of his own son, Alden, were always very high, "but he was vastly more supportive of me than his father was of him."

## Early Career

Instead of returning to Iowa, Dwight Harken, by now married, took up an internship at Bellevue Hospital in New York in 1936, where he earned $15 per month; his father refused to give him any financial support. The highlight of his experience was the month he spent on the ambulance, which he found very exciting. In those days, it was important for the young physician or surgeon to learn about the causes of their patients' deaths by obtaining autopsies on those who died. Harken threw his full energy into obtaining this permission from relatives. Wertenbaker reports that "he would promise them anything in the world — and deliver what he promised. Arrange the funeral, get the embalming done, send his wife out to beg clothes for the corpse."

After two years, Harken returned to Boston, and ended up on the Harvard service in the Boston City Hospital. Edward Churchill (one of the Harvard professors of surgery) recommended that Harken gain some experience at the Royal Brompton Hospital in London, which was the first institution in the world devoted exclusively to chest diseases, and was also one of the first to recognize the need for surgeons who concentrated on thoracic surgery. Dr. Harken and his wife greatly enjoyed their time in London; he described it to me as "one of the greatest experiences of our lives."

## The War Years — Bullets in the Heart

In 1939, when it became apparent that war was inevitable, the Royal Brompton Hospital began preparing to take in the wounded; all existing patients were discharged from the hospital. Although Dr. Harken was offered a position in the British Medical Corps, as a U.S. citizen he decided to return to Boston, where he set up in surgical practice. By 1944, however, at the age of 34, he had joined the U.S. Army. In view of his experience in thoracic surgery, he was sent back to the United Kingdom as the surgeon to a team who were to specialize in treating American soldiers with chest injuries; the team set up the 160th General Hospital near Cirencester in Gloucestershire.

It was there that Harken made his first major contribution to the development of heart surgery. Among the patients he admitted to the hospital were a number who had bullets or fragments of shrapnel embedded in their chest, in and around the heart. Most of these fragments were located either within the right ventricle or adjacent to the walls of the great vessels arising from the heart. Few fragments were found in the left ventricle since, if that were penetrated, it was generally fatal and the man died on the battlefield from exsanguinating hemorrhage. In total, Harken removed 78 fragments within or in relation to the great vessels (e.g., the aorta and great veins) and 56 in or in relation to the heart, a total of 134 operations, without a single death. Given the relatively primitive suture materials and postoperative care facilities available then, these outcomes say much for Harken's surgical skills. On reviewing a film that I had seen originally with Dr. Harken in 1988, in which he demonstrated one of these operations, I was reminded how difficult many of them must have been.

Harken used to locate the exact site of the fragment in the heart by touch, gently feeling it through the heart wall. When he had located it, he would put "stay" sutures in the heart muscle on either side of the place where he was going to make his incision. He would then cut through the wall of the heart, quickly push in a grasping instrument to grab the foreign body, and pull it out. His assistant would immediately pull the stay sutures together, thus effectively closing the hole in the heart wall, to minimize bleeding. Harken would then place sutures to permanently close the incision he had made.

This sounds simple enough but, when I reviewed Harken's film of his operation, it was clearly very tricky. Fishing about with a long clamp for the bullet or piece of shrapnel through the wall of the heart while the heart was beating vigorously and pumping out blood must have been a frustrating and nerve-racking experience. Under such circumstances, it seemed amazing that the surgeon would ever locate and grasp the object.

A young American military physician, Paul Zoll, who was later to play an important role in the development of the artificial cardiac pacemaker, monitored the electrocardiogram during many of Harken's wartime operations. One interesting story recounted by Wertenbaker relates to an innovation that Zoll and Harken introduced in an effort to make the surgery easier: "At one time Harken and Zoll thought that perhaps a giant electric magnet could be used to transfix the metal fragments instead of clamps. A special model was ordered and sent over from the States. When it was turned on in the operating room, the results were disastrous. The regular electric equipment in the operating room went immediately awry and, worse still, every metal instrument in the magnetic vicinity migrated at top speed towards the magnet." The idea was abandoned.

It is clear that only healthy young men would have stood up to this procedure as well as they did. Obviously, the patients the hospital received from the battlefield were those fortunate enough to have survived the initial injury without bleeding to death or suffering other fatal complications; the unfortunate others never made it back from the continent of Europe to Harken's hospital. The patients were therefore in a stable state when he saw them. Nevertheless, to remove so many pieces of metal from the heart or its close proximity without losing a single patient says much for the expertise of his entire team.

Harken later wrote that when he first observed the strong beating of the heart, "I wondered about the reluctance of these master surgeons to touch it. It seemed incomprehensible that we surgeons, who are considerably mechanically oriented, should not attack this significantly mechanical organ."

Harken's operations, which predated Brock's pulmonary valvotomies, contributed the first major series that demonstrated that the heart would withstand considerable manipulation. This experience certainly provided optimism, if not complete confidence, that the heart could be operated on without the procedure necessarily proving fatal to the patient. This was an immensely important learning experience for the surgeons, including Harken himself, who would, soon after the war, begin their tentative efforts to conquer heart disease.

It was perhaps the first definitive and conclusive step in demonstrating the falsity of the apocryphal statement of the renowned Viennese surgeon Theodor Billroth, in the 1880s, that "any surgeon who wishes to preserve the respect of his colleagues would never attempt to suture the heart."

## Return to Boston

After the war, Dwight Harken returned to Boston. Based first at Boston City Hospital and later at the Peter Bent Brigham Hospital, he began a hectic schedule of operating in several local hospitals, and rapidly gained extensive experience in chest surgery. He was welcomed at some hospitals, but disliked at others.

There is no doubt that Harken was a larger-than-life character. Among some of the residents, he was known as "Dwightee the Almighty." He was enthusiastic and hyperactive. One of Harken's junior colleagues is quoted as saying that Harken acted "like he was walking down Main Street playing a trombone and a drum at the same time!"

According to Robert Bartlett, "To do what he did, develop cardiac surgery in the early days, you had to be supremely self-confident. Harken certainly had chutzpah.... He had mega-doses of self-confidence."

## The Attack on Mitral Stenosis — The Pain of the Pioneer

Harken soon began to consider the surgical relief of mitral stenosis, just as Bailey was doing in Philadelphia and Brock in London. He, like Bailey, examined postmortem heart valves and practiced his new operation in dogs. His first attempt in a patient was unsuccessful, the patient dying on the following day, but on June 16, 1948, only six days after Charlie Bailey's first success, Harken followed Bailey in performing a successful operation.

Harken, Bailey, and Brock began to attract very sick patients with mitral stenosis from all over the world. The mortality was inevitably high, and Harken, in particular, suffered great anguish from his patients' deaths. He called this personal agony "the pain of the pioneer." Wertenbaker quoted Harken as describing the surgeon's pain on losing a patient as the "most heinous creation of Satan in his most diabolic mood. I would ask all to understand it and wish no one to suffer it."

It was a catch-22 situation. It would not be justified to attempt an unproven operation of this magnitude and nature except on a very sick, dying patient, yet the debilitated condition of the patient greatly increased the risk of the operation. The surgical technique could be practiced in healthy dogs, but they did not have mitral stenosis or all of its debilitating sequelae. And it was not only the surgical technique that needed to be developed and proven; the anesthesiologists were on an equally steep learning curve, as were those who cared for the patient after the operation.

After the sixth death in his first ten patients, Harken determined to abandon the operation. He recalled, "I was so distraught and depressed that I went home and went immediately to bed. I decided to give up. I told my wife that I could not take any more pain and distress. My friend Laurence Ellis, a cardiologist who had referred patients to me, came to the house. My wife told him I was in bed. He came upstairs, and sat in my room. 'I hear you're thinking of quitting heart surgery,' he said. I replied that I was, that I couldn't go on with it. He said that it would be criminal for me to do so, as it would waste the lives of the people I had already operated on. I asked him what he meant by 'waste their lives.' He said that I surely must have learned something from these deaths, and that this would help me do the operations better in the future. I replied that, after all of these deaths, I didn't think any respectable physician would send me a patient again. He pointed out that he was considered a respectable physician, and he would refer more patients to me. He said that the patients I had lost from the operation were dying anyway, and that I had given a few of them a new chance at life. He convinced me that I should not waste this experience, and that I would do better in the future. That really was the turning point for me personally."

Not all physicians were as understanding and supportive as Laurence Ellis. Like Bailey and Brock, Harken suffered his share of intense criticism, which led to him being temporarily banned from carrying out heart surgery in some of the Boston hospitals. But once he had bounced back from his initial despair, he was able to withstand these taunts and comments.

Alden Harken confirmed how badly a patient's death affected his father: "He got to know his patients very well prior to the operation and, if somebody didn't do well, it really hurt him. I always look at that as a wonderful example of the relationship a surgeon should have with his patients and their families. If things don't do well, it's gotta hurt, and it hurt him a lot. When a patient died, he was overwrought. It really startled me that he would take these problems so personally and so seriously. I think that was one of the reasons that his relationship with his patients and their families was as close as it was." Francis Moore conceded that most of Harken's patients "just worshipped him."

Robert Bartlett also commented on this aspect of Harken's personality: "He had great compassion for his patients. He felt deeply about every single person. He got emotionally involved with his patients, whether the patient was doing well or doing poorly. He hated bad news. As the resident on the service, you had to call him at ten o'clock every night and tell him how his patients were doing. You quickly learned that the system was to call him and first tell him something really good, even if everything was falling apart. Then, well into the conversation, you would say, 'By the way, Mrs. Jones has had two cardiac arrests and I'm trying to resuscitate her, and Mrs. Green is still bleeding.'"

With increasing experience, the results of the operation steadily improved, and Harken began to accept patients in whom the disease was less advanced. These patients could better tolerate the operation, and so the results improved further. After Harken presented a series of successes at a meeting at the Brigham, the audience broke into applause, and Harken felt that "the dark days were over."

In most Western countries, the operation of closed mitral valvotomy, where the valve is opened without the advantage of direct visualization, has largely been superseded by what is known as open mitral valvotomy. In this procedure, the patient is supported by the heart-lung machine, the heart is opened, and the valve is dilated (or excised and replaced with a mechanical prosthesis) under direct vision. Closed mitral valvotomy is now rarely performed. In some other countries, however, such as India, where they do not have the financial resources to carry out open heart surgery on a large scale, closed mitral valvotomy remains a common and important operation in the treatment of patients who have suffered from rheumatic fever.

## The Feud from the Other "Corner"

From my discussions with Dwight Harken and Charlie Bailey, the reasons for their antipathy toward each other—apart from priority for the first operation—were not absolutely clear to me. Differences in their background may have played a part, but it appeared to go deeper than that. Harken had a deep lack of respect for Bailey, mainly because he viewed Bailey as "unethical and irresponsible." He made mention of Bailey's "lack of respect for human life," referring to the significant number of his early patients who died. But *all* of the true surgical pioneers, Harken included, experienced a high mortality rate in their initial series of patients. And so just why Harken, and several others, were so critical of Bailey remains something of an enigma to me.

Bob Frater's opinion was that "Harken was not as reckless as Charlie Bailey, but some of his early operations were as crazy as Charlie's. The point is that *all* of these early surgeons did crazy things in the days before open heart surgery was developed. Harken was part of that, but he was a more serious character than Charlie. All of these operations were an assault, but they were essential steps on the way. You had to dare to go where someone hadn't gone before. Once somebody had dared to do it, then others jumped in."

But there was no doubting Harken's antipathy towards his surgical competitor. Harken recounted to me the very same story that Bailey subsequently told me with regard to his flying to New York to defend Bailey in a lawsuit. Having heard this account from both parties, I was impressed that Harken, seemingly without hesitation, had been prepared to change his busy schedule and travel to New York on the very next morning. I felt that this indicated a hidden respect, or even affection, on his part for Charlie Bailey. Whereas Bailey told me that, for all their rivalry, which plumbed to the depths of personal attack at times, he knew that Harken was "an okay man at heart," Harken, on the day I met with him, had absolutely *nothing* good to say about Bailey. It appeared to me that Bailey's impression that he and Harken eventually developed mutual respect and became almost friends was fallacious.

Charles Hufnagel knew both Bailey and Harken very well and agreed that "they had a running feud over who got the first surviving mitral [valvotomy] patient, and they argued over the way the operation should be done. Each thought that the other was an unmitigated thief in that they both wanted to claim the first mitral valvotomy. I would see Bailey often, and I found him too forceful and too aggressive for my taste, but that was a part of his personality. He was a very difficult man to get along with, loquacious and forceful, dynamic in pushing his point of view, and Harken was similar, very much the same. They didn't appreciate their similarities."

Alden Harken recollected an interesting point about his father's relationship with Charlie Bailey: "As a little kid, I grew up hearing lots of things about Dr. Bailey. Some years later, but early in my career, I was privileged to participate in a seminar at the American College of Cardiology. To my absolute astonishment, one of the other panelists was Charlie Bailey. After we had given our presentations, I went up to him, and said, 'Dr. Bailey, it's so nice to meet you. I've heard so much about you.' He looked me straight in the eye, and said, 'I bet you have.' He was absolutely correct. I never heard a good word, but I think my father subsequently recognized what a phenomenally capable guy Bailey was."

## Surgery on the Aortic Valve

For several years in the 1950s and 1960s, Harken's surgical practice was immensely successful. He was very busy, combining his increasing cardiac surgical workload with general chest surgery. Possibly because of his obvious professional, and financial, success, Harken soon found himself being criticized by his colleagues — not for his surgical failures anymore, but for the media attention he was receiving for his successes.

With mitral valvotomy established, Harken turned his attention to the aortic valve. Aortic valve stenosis (narrowing and obstruction) and regurgitation (leaking) were other common conditions that resulted in great debility and untimely death. Charles Hufnagel (chapter 9), who had trained at the Brigham, had designed a mechanical (prosthetic) ball-and-cage valve in the laboratory there (Figure 16), with the ultimate aim of replacing the aortic valve. Harken worked on improving Hufnagel's prosthesis and tested his improvements in a machine built for him by an engineer. According to Francis Moore, Harken set up a "wear and tear" operation in his home cellar; steam from his central heating drove a little engine that made these valves open and close hundreds of thousands of times in a week to see if they would wear out. (In life, each heart valve opens and closes something like 35 to 40 million times a year.) He then implanted the mechanical valve into dogs, with generally poor outcome.

By now — the late 1950s — the heart-lung machine had been introduced, and so Harken's plan was to excise the diseased valve and replace it with his valve prosthesis. He realized his prosthesis was imperfect but, in view of the high mortality associated with severe aortic valve disease, he believed he would be justified in implanting it in selected patients; his patients couldn't wait for a perfect valve. One of Harken's maxims was "Perfection may be the enemy of good." He realized he did not have a perfect valve, but he reasoned that implanting it in very sick patients would carry less risk than allowing them to go untreated.

Harken's first attempt at aortic valve replacement with a mechanical valve in a patient was unsuccessful, but on March 10, 1960, he performed a successful operation. The procedure was performed using a heart-lung machine, with cooling of body temperature. His patient, Mary Richardson, proved one of the success stories of early open heart surgery, and the account of her disease and treatment is described in detail by Jürgen Thorwald in his book *The Patients*. Although Harken had to replace her mechanical valve three years later, this second operation provided her with a further 22 years of life. This operation by Harken constituted a major advance in the development of cardiac surgery since it represented one of the very earliest, if not the first, successful anatomical replacements of any heart valve by any surgeon.

There followed two more failures before another success. Harken was faced with another period of anguish over the deaths of several of his patients. For the patients, however, crippled as they were by their valve disease, Harken was offering a glimmer of hope — hope of survival and of a better life. Wertenbaker records one poignant story: "One patient who died on the operating table had left him [Harken] a note which was delivered to his house after he had gone to bed totally depressed. The note said, 'Thanks for the chance.'"

According to Robert Bartlett, Harken, like many of the early pioneers of heart surgery, was never really at ease with open heart operations. And yet he was one of the few early surgeons who was relatively successful in straddling the divide between "closed" heart operations and those that required the use of the heart-lung machine.

## Professional Conflicts

Harken's overpowering personality eventually created problems that could no longer be suppressed. Francis Moore, in whose department Harken worked, told me, "I enjoyed him, and suffered with him, because he was a difficult personality. He was red-haired. I'm not sure just what we mean by 'flamboyant' but, whatever we mean by it, he was it. He got into awful trouble because he was so flamboyant. I would almost say he was 'intolerant' of others who hadn't given as much thought to a problem as he had. Most people felt he had an uncontrollably huge, gigantic, titanic, and hopeless ego. But I think that most ego arises from insecurity, and he certainly had that. When I met his father, who became a patient of mine, I could see where it came from. His father was a very authoritarian Iowan. You could see how Dwight, being brought up in a small town with this very authoritative and very outspoken father, was pretty well beaten down. So he then took that out on his colleagues."

Alden Harken commented that "the relationship between Dr. Moore and my dad was one of mutual respect, but always strained. They were never good friends.... It was not a painless experience for Dr. Moore to have somebody like my dad around who continued to challenge the status quo. I think it took someone who had a lot of self-confidence to tolerate someone like my dad on a service. It's a huge tribute to Dr. Moore."

Robert Bartlett emphasized how Francis ("Frannie") Moore handled Harken's ego well: "Frannie made it possible for him to do what he did. If Harken had bad results, he would talk with Dr. Moore. Frannie would say, 'Well, Dwight, you're doing a great job. Hang in there. This is the way progress is made.' He would encourage him, and send him patients, and so on. Moore was just a marvelous facilitator."

Harken's overwhelming personality and unpredictable behavior ultimately resulted in his leaving the famous Brigham Hospital and confining his practice largely to Mount Auburn Hospital, a less prestigious institution. Dr. Bartlett provided details: "He treated his residents and fellows terribly. If something was going wrong, it was usually their fault. He would blame his complications on the patient, if he could, or on the instruments, or on the nurses, or on the most senior residents around. He was fairly kind to the most junior residents because they would be in the hospital all night looking after his really sick patients and, in those days, they were *really* sick. But when you got to be the senior resident, you fell into that 'if something's going wrong, it's your fault' category. Most of the residents wound up hating him. He would regularly fire residents, and yet expect them to show up the next morning. He was a very hard person to work with and to work for, which, in fact, ultimately led to his, shall we say, 'early retirement.' He treated the cardiologists the same way. He was not aware of this, I'm sure. He was just going through life at his particular pace, and probably never had much of a feeling that he was offending people along the way.

"Every couple of months, when things weren't going his way,

Harken would threaten to quit. He would go down to Frannie Moore's office and say, 'I can't do this. I'm doing these wonderful things. If you don't get a new cardiologist, I'm going to quit.' Finally, in about 1971 or 1972, he had one of these rampages, and Frannie said, 'Okay, Dwight, I accept your retirement.' His ego was so big that he would not say he was sorry. Frannie said, 'You said you wanted to quit, so quit.'"

## Legacy

In 1975, at the age of 65, Harken retired from operating. For the next 18 years until he died in 1993, he devoted much of his time to the development of the American College of Cardiology, of which he had been president in 1964.

I asked Alden Harken how he thought his father would like to be remembered. He responded, "I think that operating electively on a series of patients in whom you could accomplish an intracardiac procedure with success [e.g., removing a bullet] was a conceptual jump, and he would like to have been remembered for that. The next conceptual jump was to operate on a diseased heart, as he did with mitral valvuloplasty. I think he would have looked upon the aortic valve replacement as a technical advance, but not a conceptual jump."

This last statement surprised me somewhat, but perhaps Alden Harken was considering the fact that Charles Hufnagel and others had carried out most of the conceptual and innovative work on mechanical valves. Francis Moore also emphasized this point: "Hufnagel, who should never be overlooked because he was such a central figure, was in the lab with Dwight. Dwight was a developer of ideas, a doer, but not really an inventor, whereas Hufnagel really was an inventor." But Moore added, "Dwight deserves a very secure place in surgical history."

Having been born in the same year, Dwight Harken died just a few days after Charlie Bailey. Their stories, although in many ways so different, were inextricably entwined even until death. It is perhaps ironic that, having performed successful operations for the relief of mitral stenosis within a week of each other in 1948, and having feuded for much of the ensuing 55 years, they should leave this world almost together. But, as Charlie Bailey's widow is quoted as saying, "Charlie beat him in life, and beat him in death."

## CHAPTER 5

# Six Minutes!
# Hypothermia and the
# Race Against Time

————

## WILFRED BIGELOW, F. JOHN LEWIS,
## AND HENRY SWAN

THREE MEN PLAYED major roles in getting open heart surgery — that is, surgery where the surgeon could open the heart
and actually see what he was doing — off the ground: Wilfred Bigelow
(Figure 17), F. John Lewis (Figure 18), and Henry Swan (Figure 19).
Bigelow came up with the concept of cooling the patient's body
sufficiently to allow the heart to be stopped for approximately six
minutes without damaging the brain, and proved its validity in the
experimental laboratory. Lewis was the first to actually use this
approach successfully in the treatment of a patient, and Swan was
the first to report its use in a series of patients. This was the first
time that surgeons had been able to work *inside* the heart under
direct vision, and so their work was a major step forward in opening
the door to open heart surgery.

# WILFRED BIGELOW —
# THE CONCEPT OF HYPOTHERMIA

Wilfred (Bill) Bigelow's major claim to fame in the development of heart surgery is based on the experimental studies he carried out in introducing the concept of hypothermia (cooling). This technique made possible the first open heart surgery in humans. Cooling of an organ — or, indeed, of the whole body — reduces its metabolic rate (the rate at which the various physiological and biochemical processes of the cells turn over), thus reducing oxygen and energy demands. It is the same principle as when we store meat in a refrigerator — cell metabolism is reduced, and the meat stays fresh. Bigelow reasoned that cooling of the entire body would protect the brain and other organs from a temporary lack of blood and oxygen. This would allow the heart to be stopped for a longer period of time than at normal body temperature. This extra period of time, though not very long, would enable operations to be performed *under direct vision* inside the heart.

At normal body temperature (37 degrees Celsius [37°C] or 98.6 degrees Fahrenheit [98.6°F]), if the heart stops beating, the brain will begin to undergo irreversible damage after about four minutes. Cardiac massage or resuscitation of the heart therefore has to begin within four minutes if the brain is to be preserved intact. Bigelow and his colleagues carried out work in dogs showing that, if the body were cooled to a temperature of approximately 30°C (86°F), the heart could be stopped for perhaps six to eight minutes, during which time the circulation could be discontinued without harm to the brain and other vital organs. This six-minute period allowed the heart to be opened and a very simple abnormality in the heart surgically corrected.

The exploration of hypothermia was only one of Bigelow's contributions. Perhaps as important was the development by his group of the first electrical artificial pacemaker for the heart, which he used in experimental animals. As with hypothermia, however, others expanded his pioneering studies and were the first to use the pace-maker in the treatment of patients.

## The Toronto Scottish Enclave

When I met Bill Bigelow (Figure 17) in Toronto in the fall of 1991, he had long been retired. He collected me from my hotel at 7:50 A.M. He had with him in his car a black Labrador, one of his hunting dogs, who sniffed me in a friendly manner. Dr. Bigelow was wearing his "walking-hunting" clothes, namely a flat tweed cap, flannel trousers, English-style sports jacket, sweater, and a sports shirt open at the neck with a scarf inside the shirt collar. We drove the five minutes to his home, which was an elegant brown brick building in an equally elegant inner suburb of Toronto known as South Rosedale.

Dr. Bigelow was rather shorter and smaller than I had anticipated from his photographs. I expected a strongly built, athletic man, not someone small and wiry. I got the sense of a rather reserved person, a very pleasant, decent, honest man with good fundamental Scottish-Presbyterian morals and principles, but not the most exciting personality.

Dr. Bigelow had previously mailed me copies of two books he had written in his retirement, which gave me much of the background to his experimental and clinical work. For *Cold Hearts,* published in 1984, the story of his research into hypothermia, he had been awarded the Jason A. Hannah Medal of the Royal Society of Canada in 1986 for the best history by a Canadian author. *Mysterious Heparin,* published in 1990, recounted the discovery and development of the anticoagulant heparin, much of which took place in Toronto and without which the development of the heart-lung machine would have proved immensely difficult, if not impossible. Indeed, Dr. Bigelow had written considerably more in his retirement than most of the other surgeons who appear in this book.

Throughout his books and his conversation, there was an all-pervading sense of Canada. His books were full of information about Canadian contributions to the various fields about which he was writing. He was clearly a great Canadian patriot, very proud of his country.

Bill Bigelow was born in Brandon, Manitoba, which at that time (1913) must have been barely settled and a very small town indeed. His father was a "horse-and-buggy" doctor there. The young Bigelow was educated at Brandon College and the University of Toronto, receiving a BA degree in 1935 and an MD in 1938. His surgical residency at the Toronto General Hospital was interrupted by service in the military in Europe from 1941 to 1945. He was one of two surgeons in the sixth Canadian clearing station that landed on the Normandy beaches in 1944. Between 1946 and 1947, he was a research fellow at the Johns Hopkins Hospital in Baltimore, where he came under the influence of Alfred Blalock. The remainder of his career, until he retired in 1977, was spent in the department of surgery at the Toronto General Hospital, the major teaching hospital of the University of Toronto.

## "Cold Hearts" — Early Work on Hypothermia

It was at the Johns Hopkins Hospital that Dr. Bigelow first had the idea of using hypothermia.

"During the war [World War II]," he told me, "I was stuck in England for almost two years before the Allies opened the second front. During this period, we were not particularly busy, and I took the opportunity of visiting various British hospitals. I saw many patients who had been sent from the fighting in North Africa and Italy, and the thing that bothered me was to see a patient whose artery had been damaged and who had therefore lost a leg. This stimulated my interest in the effects of local hypothermia [cooling of the limb]. So my interest in peripheral vascular surgery led me to the heart, and my interest in hypothermia stimulated my thinking."

When Bigelow had given the Gibbon Lecture in 1984, he expanded on how he became interested in hypothermia. He found the environment at the Johns Hopkins in 1946 "intensely interesting and involving. After watching the blue baby operation, I thought that surgeons would never be able to correct or cure heart conditions unless they stopped the circulation of blood and operated under direct vision.... One night I woke suddenly with a simple solution: cool the whole body, reduce the oxygen requirements, interrupt the circulation, and open the heart. I could hardly wait to return to Toronto to investigate this simple and enchanting theory." He therefore appears to have had what one could call a "Eureka!" moment, like Archimedes, when the answer to a scientific problem suddenly became apparent.

"To begin research with the aim of cooling the patient went against the usual thinking," Dr. Bigelow told me. "Nobody had explored the use of hypothermia in this way before. However, I was encouraged by the work of a Philadelphia physician, Temple Fay, who had been cooling patients to try to cure their cancer. He took only terminal cases, and so had a high mortality rate. Some of his patients were cooled to low temperatures, but then brought back to life. I thought, gee, that's a neat idea."

By careful experimentation, Bigelow's group found that if shivering (which is due to increased muscle activity) was prevented, oxygen requirements fell with the lowering of body temperature. This was a simple but important fundamental discovery. Furthermore, after rewarming, there was no evidence that an oxygen deficit had been created, i.e., on rewarming, the body did not have an *increased* oxygen requirement. During the next three years of intensive study, Bigelow's group discovered that there was a limit to safe cooling. Their experimental animals generally did not survive if cooled below a body temperature of 20 to 24°C (68–75°F). When cooled to 20°C, the circulation of dogs could be interrupted for 15 minutes, with half of the dogs recovering fully. Bigelow reported this finding to the American Surgical Association in 1950; he described the audience's reaction as "one of intense interest combined with strong doubts." He also found that newborn animals could be cooled to much lower body temperatures with safety—as low as 5°C (41°F) in a newborn dog.

After two more years of research, Bigelow and his colleagues were able to cool monkeys to 18°C (64.4°F) and open their hearts for 20 minutes, with 100% survival. Thus, in 1952, five years after starting research in Toronto, Bigelow was now ready to try his technique in patients with simple heart defects that would take less than six to eight minutes to repair. But before he could do so, John Lewis in Minneapolis reported the first successful heart operation using hypothermia. This was closely followed by successful operations by Henry Swan and Charlie Bailey.

I asked Dr. Bigelow whether, having done the background work on hypothermia, he was disappointed when another surgeon did the first clinical case.

"I had never heard from John Lewis but, when the news of his case came through to us, we were naturally disappointed. However, we had other things going at the time, such as the pacemaker work, and studies on hibernation. Furthermore, we had started doing mitral valvotomies in patients in 1950. Perhaps there were just too many things going on at that time. Our team would have achieved more prestige if we had carried out an operation under hypothermia, but we just followed our nose."

For several years in the mid-1950s, hypothermia flooded the literature and dominated surgical meetings. Although the heart-lung machine was used successfully in a patient by John Gibbon only one year after the first operation using hypothermia, it would be at least a further four or five years before heart-lung machines were in relatively common use. During this period, at many centers hypothermia was virtually the only means of carrying out operations inside the open heart.

## The Enigma of Hibernation

In his book *Cold Hearts,* Bigelow described his later research. His group's inability to consistently cool an adult laboratory animal with safety below a temperature of 20 to 24°C (68–75°F) continued to be frustrating to them. Bigelow felt that this limited the value of hypothermia as a means of performing open heart surgery, because most operations would take much longer than six minutes. In 1951, in order to achieve safe *deep* hypothermia (cooling below 25°C [77°F]), he decided to study hibernation.

His group initially discovered that a groundhog could be cooled to a body temperature of 3°C (37°F), the circulation stopped, and the heart opened for two hours with no ill effect. How was this possible? The groundhog has a hibernating gland, known as "brown fat," and Bigelow's group felt this was worthy of investigation. If they could transfer this remarkable cold tolerance to humans, it would make their six-to-eight-minute open heart procedures obsolete.

They established a groundhog farm where they could study 400 groundhogs sleeping peacefully through the winter months. After four fruitless years of investigation, they made an attempt to isolate an active principle from the blood of the hibernating gland that might give the groundhog the ability to survive at these very low body temperatures. Bigelow's group acquired the cooperation of several basic scientists, and extracts of blood and brown fat were tested at regular intervals throughout the year. One December, at the onset of hibernation, they were able to detect the appearance of a new substance in one of their extracts. A small amount of this substance was injected into test animals, greatly increasing their tolerance to low body temperature. They did not have enough of the extract to identify its structure but, after the period of natural hibernation, the substance intriguingly disappeared from the extracts taken from the groundhog's brown fat.

Their excitement was even greater during the following winter when, as hibernation approached, the same substance appeared in the extract. Had they finally identified an elusive hormone that protected the groundhog from the detrimental effect of cold? Eventually, they were able to identify the chemical structure of the extract, and their chemist synthesized it in the laboratory. The extract was to be called "hibernin." They now had access to an adequate supply to test its action fully. Excitement was so great that Bigelow temporarily stopped his surgical practice. The university applied to patent the substance, and some National Aeronautics and Space Administration scientists made inquiries about it, presumably believing that it might allow astronauts to be maintained in a "hibernating" state on long space flights.

A photograph was taken of the first three guinea pigs to be cooled to a body temperature of 5°C (41°F) under the influence of hibernin and subsequently rewarmed successfully. In view of their impending important announcement to the scientific world, a university photographer took a picture of the research team. In his Gibbon Lecture, Bigelow expressed the optimism they all felt: "Undoubtedly this picture would hang in museums alongside that of Banting and Best and their famous first insulin dog." The Nobel Prize must surely have been in the back of their minds.

Following satisfactory toxicity studies, two patients were successfully operated on using hypothermia with injections of hibernin. They were carefully cooled 4°C (39.2°F) lower than the usual range and, although they recovered satisfactorily, the nurses reported that oddly, in the recovery room the patients acted "as if they were drunk," which subsequently proved a very perceptive observation.

Four articles were carefully and precisely written covering every aspect of this work. But just before these papers were submitted for publication, a letter was received from the patent office in Washington, D.C., stating that hibernin had been patented 20 years before as a plasticizer, a chemical that maintains the pliability of plastic tubes. Bigelow wrote, "We were amazed but not concerned since there was only one inch of plastic tubing used as a connector in the extraction process, and hibernin only appeared during hibernation." However, as a final check, they tried to extract "hibernin" from the blood in the absence of plastic tubing and, conversely, tried to extract it from the plastic tubing itself. The results were shattering. In the absence of plastic tubing, no hibernin was obtained, but it could be extracted directly from the plastic tubing. The hibernin was, in fact, simply a contaminant from the plastic tubing.

"What a disappointment it was, and what a giant effort it had been," stated Bigelow in his Gibbon Lecture. "Then we all laughed.

The absurdity of it all....With further chemical wizardry, the active principle proved to be butyl alcohol," thus explaining the astute observations made by the recovery room nurses. "We finally admitted defeat." (I must admit that I doubt if I would have laughed at such an immense last-minute disappointment.)

Hibernation is still a mystery. What allows the groundhog to survive such low body temperatures? "I think there's something there waiting to be discovered," said Bigelow.

Surprisingly, nobody seems to have followed up on Bigelow's work into the mystery of hibernation and its application to surgery. The ability to cool patients successfully and reduce their metabolic rate would be invaluable in a number of medical and surgical conditions.

## The Concept of the Cardiac Pacemaker

As the body was cooled and its metabolism was reduced, the heart, of course, would beat more and more slowly. Eventually, if the body was cold enough, the heart would almost stop beating completely. The idea for a pacemaker for the heart came during one of these experiments on hypothermia. One day, in 1949, during a routine cooling procedure in the laboratory, the animal's heart suddenly stopped at 22°C (71.6°F). Dr. Bigelow's group found that by poking the heart with a probe, they could elicit a beat, and poking it 60 times per minute produced a blood pressure. An electrical stimulus had the same effect. They hypothesized that this might be the answer to safe deep hypothermia; perhaps the cold heart needed a pacemaker to maintain its function.

Reviewing the literature, they found that back in 1932 one person had purposefully made a pacemaker, albeit of a primitive nature. Bigelow and his colleagues set about designing a new one. By 1950, they were able to report on the successful development of an electrical pacemaker. When the heart was stimulated externally or by electrodes placed inside the heart, it would beat. By modifying the rate of the paced electrical impulses, the heart rate could be increased or decreased at will. Although they found that the pacemaker was not the answer to achieving successful deep hypothermia, they had certainly stumbled on something equally or perhaps more important.

Having heard of Bigelow's work, and in fact having been in direct contact with him, Paul Zoll, the Boston cardiologist who had been a colleague of Dwight Harken in the United Kindom during World War II, was the first to treat a human patient using a pacemaker, in 1952. Bigelow was disappointed that Zoll did not recognize the help he and his colleagues had provided, which included details of the electrical circuit they had used. (Zoll received the Lasker Prize in 1973 for his work in establishing the pacemaker and the closed chest defibrillator.) It was not until 1958, however, with the introduction of transistors, that the pacemaker could be made small enough to be implanted in the body, a procedure first carried out by Ake Senning in Stockholm (chapter 6). It would seem that some surgeons and physicians who subsequently developed their own pacemakers did not acknowledge Bigelow's pioneering efforts, and even claimed the idea for themselves.

Dr. Bigelow told me, "When we first published on our pacemaker, eight universities in Europe and America wrote asking if I would tell them how to make one. One of the most aggressive was a man who I shall not name — let's just call him Mr. X. We sent Mr. X an electrical stimulator. He then wanted to know how to put it together. We sent him a circuit. One of my colleagues went to the National Research Council and said, 'Look, for God's sake, get this damn thing patented. I've been after you for two years to get a patent.' So they said 'okay' and went to the patent office, where they found that it had been patented by the company for which Mr. X was working."

## Opinions

I asked Dr. Bigelow whether his contributions to surgery had been sufficiently recognized. For example, had he received any honorary degrees? He mentioned a couple of honorary doctorates he had been awarded, but added, "I guess the greatest honor, other than degrees, was the affirmation of my peers, which is really all you want."

Dr. Bigelow was too modest to mention the many other awards and honors bestowed on him. For example, he had received the Honorary Fellowship of the Royal College of Surgeons of England and the Order of Canada, the highest honor that can be bestowed by the Canadian government on a Canadian citizen.

Dr. Bigelow's opinion was that "a surgeon involved in innovative work requires a lot of courage to persist when things are going wrong." I asked him to elaborate on what qualities a surgeon on the cutting edge of surgery needs. "You've got to have a toughness and aggressiveness to do pioneering surgery. It doesn't mean that you're unfeeling, but you have to have a moral toughness. You need to keep thinking, but you must tread gently and carefully and not get carried away. Make your own observations very carefully because they may be more important than what you're reading. Intellectual humility is to realize how little we know.

"Actually, the quality you needed, besides courage, in the development of open heart surgery was to be technically reasonably skilled. Particularly in the era of hypothermia, where the speed of the surgery was forced upon us, it was important to do things technically right. You also had to have self-confidence and a good solid feeling of self because, when you're doing new work, there are no guidelines. You're doing an operation that may only have been done a few times previously. You have to have enough self-confidence.

"One of the problems in doing something new is having to make decisions. Shall I tie off this artery? I wonder if it will cause gangrene. Shall I do this? And so on. With regard to heart surgery, we made these decisions in an era when the answers weren't known. One of the problems was doing something and then wondering whether you did the right thing. I'm sure that drained you for the rest of the operation. You had to make a decision and get on with it. There are people who can't do that. The decisiveness, along with the courage, and the feeling that you're doing the right thing, comes from carefully examining the patient and knowing the patient's situation. I always interviewed the relatives before the operation. If a patient dies, you don't talk to the patient anymore, you talk to the relatives. If they're behind you, then that's important."

I was interested to learn how easy or difficult it had been for him to continue when he had made a decision that proved to be wrong. Could he cope with that?

"I guess none of us can do that easily, but you just made the best decision you could. It was tough. We lost a lot of patients from the early heart-lung machines. Afterwards you would get depressed, and if you didn't get depressed, then there was something wrong with you. The key is the length of the depression. There is nothing wrong with a surgeon getting depressed about a bungled surgery and screwing things up. But you've got to get cracking the next day. You may think that a person like that is callous. You might think this dog is crazy because it always wants to start up again. It's what you're born with, and you have to have that. That comes from your genes. You don't get that at training school. There can be no criticism at being terribly depressed or upset. My wife used to say, 'You die with your patients.' I didn't think I was demonstrating that, but I evidently got cranky the next day.

"I'm intellectually agnostic, but I used to pray, you know, just a little prayer. I didn't pray routinely. It was just once in awhile. I would sometimes ask for the patient to do well, and sometimes give thanks that the patient had indeed done well. I think you should pray on both occasions. If you're always asking, and not thanking, I think that's not right. For me, this was just communication, which I thought might help — nothing more in it than that."

After a long and productive retirement, Bill Bigelow died in 2005 at age 91.

## F. JOHN LEWIS —
## THE FIRST OPEN HEART OPERATION

"John Lewis? He was different," said Swedish heart surgery pioneer Ake Senning (chapter 6), when asked to comment on Lewis. And

Lewis *was* different from most of the others involved in the development of heart surgery. He was a man of diverse interests, in some ways an outsider, a bohemian. When he died in 1993 in Santa Barbara, despite his enormous achievement in heart surgey, his life was perhaps largely unfulfilled. After taking one giant leap forward in heart surgery, he soon dropped out of the field entirely. Disenchanted with his career in medicine, he retired early and followed his interests in writing and painting.

Floyd John Lewis was the first surgeon in the world to operate inside the living human heart with an unimpeded view. His operation in 1952, when he was a mere 36 years old, was the true beginning of open heart surgery and initiated the rapid development that took place over the next 25 to 30 years. Rarely has a surgeon taken such a giant step forward in the history of medicine — and rarely has such a surgeon so shortly after simply walked away.

This historic operation was carried out in the University Hospital, Minneapolis, on September 2, 1952, with the aid of hypothermia. The patient was a sickly five-year-old girl named Jacqueline Johnson, who weighed less than 30 pounds (approximately 14 kilograms). She had a hole in the wall (septum) between the two collecting chambers of the heart (the atria), an atrial septal defect (Figure 20). After being anesthetized, she was wrapped in a refrigerated blanket until, after a period of more than two hours, her body temperature had fallen to 28°C (82°F). At this point, the cooling blanket was removed, and the surgeon began the operation. The chest was opened, the blood vessels entering the heart were clamped so that no blood passed through the heart (and therefore no blood was pumped to the brain or other vital organs), and the partially empty heart was opened. With the brain relatively protected by the cold temperature, Lewis knew that he had approximately six minutes to do what he needed inside the heart. If he went beyond six minutes, the child's brain might be irreparably damaged (even if he could get the heart beating normally again). He quickly repaired the hole in the septum and rapidly closed the heart, releasing the clamps so that blood entered the heart chambers once more. The heart soon regained its contractions.

By the time the chest was closed, the patient's body temperature had fallen to 26°C (79°F). To rewarm her, she was placed in a bath of hot water kept at 45°C (113°F). After 35 minutes, her body temperature had risen to 36°C (96.8°F), at which time she was removed from the bath. Her recovery from anesthesia and her subsequent convalescence were uneventful, and she was able to go home 11 days later. This operation proved a major step forward in surgeons' attempts to repair abnormalities within the heart, and assured Lewis of immortality in the history of medicine.

By the time I corresponded with Dr. Lewis in early 1990, he was 73 years old and had been retired and living in Santa Barbara, California, for the past 14 years. In our correspondence, he wrote, "If you do decide to come, let me know and, unless you already have a place in mind, I will give you the name of some nearby hotels and motels. I live in a one-bedroom guest house and therefore could not offer overnight accommodations even to a fellow author."

I was immediately struck by the fact that this former surgeon, who had been the lead participant in an operation of such enormity in the advance of surgery, was ending his days in a one-bedroom guest house. How he should come to be in that situation intrigued me. Furthermore, I was struck by the fact that he referred to me as a "fellow author" rather than as a fellow surgeon; this perhaps indicated how far he had drifted from his surgical past.

I flew to Santa Barbara. Dr. Lewis was moderately tall, possibly about six feet, and very thin — a result no doubt of his enthusiasm for jogging, hiking, and cycling — and was casually dressed in a maroon polo-neck sweater, lightweight beige trousers, white socks, and canvas shoes. He also wore a denim jacket, and certainly looked more like a writer or artist than a surgeon. His hair was curly blond-gray and short, brushed slightly forward over the forehead and temples in a rather artistic way. He had a gray mustache (Figure 18).

Dr. Lewis told me that he had retired at the age of 59 and immediately moved to Santa Barbara, where he began not one but a series
of activities and pastimes to fill his retirement. He had been married
since 1946, but when I met him he had been divorced for three years.
To be married for so long and then to divorce during one's retirement
seemed odd to me, but he explained that when one's children leave
home, the partners in a marriage find that they can each do what
they want and they tend to grow apart. He had three children and
seven grandchildren.

His guest-house apartment was situated in one of the suburbs of
Santa Barbara. It was small and cramped. I presumed that he rented it,
since the white-painted walls were rather grubby and the rather faded
green carpet was of poor quality. It was clear that he lived the existence of an elderly "bachelor" in relatively run-down circumstances.
The scene was of a gentleman who had fallen on hard times. The
apartment had one bedroom, one main room, a kitchen, and a bathroom. The main room was divided into a small area where there was
a television and a sofa, and another area that looked more like a study
or office. Here he had a table on which sat his personal computer,
a nearby filing cabinet, and some old bookcases filled with books.
Another small table, which presumably acted as the dining table, was
flanked by two canvas "director" chairs. On one wall, I noted a very
good oil painting of some Southern Californian buildings, which was
his own work. There were also several framed sketches of his, which,
to my relatively uneducated eye, were not of such good quality.

Since retiring, Dr. Lewis had spent his time painting, sketching,
and writing. He gave me a copy of his unpublished 241-page autobiography, *Time of Life,* which he had typed and photocopied himself.
Divided into five short paperback volumes, one for each period of his
life, the autobiography included sketches by him of certain scenes and
people he referred to in the text. He had also written a large number
of short stories, none of which he had been able to get published, and a
book of poems, which he had again photocopied himself in paperback

form. More recently, he had written a book for the lay public, *So Your Doctor Recommended Surgery,* which was to be commercially published later that year. In it, he discussed alternative methods of treatment and unnecessary operations, and provided guidance to people on whether or not they should go ahead with the recommendations of their surgeons.

On the following day, in a small bookshop, I found two little paperback books written by him. One was *Bicycling Santa Barbara — 12 Great Bicycle Trips with Descriptions, Maps and Elevations.* The other was *Sixty Santa Barbara Churches,* a collection of sketches of churches in the Santa Barbara area, coupled with a few poems written by Lewis, which provide some insight into his attitudes and beliefs. Some poems demonstrate a certain cynicism or a mildly jaundiced view of life.

For example, churches are:

> Sights for marriage,
> Baptism and burial,
> Classrooms for night school,
> And playing fields
> (Cheaper than discos)
> For courtship.

And again:

> These havens for souls,
> Offer the mechanics for absolution,
> With hard pews,
> And music to keep their parishioners,
> Awake until collection time.

## Early Years

John Lewis was born in Waseca, a small town in Minnesota, in 1916, but brought up in Tracy, Minnesota, about 60 miles farther west, where his father was a railroad locomotive engineer with the Chicago

Northwestern Railway. Tracy was a town of only 2,500 people. The young John went to high school there, graduating in a class of 59 students. Of these, only a handful went on to college.

From his autobiography, *Time of Life,* I learned that John Lewis was an only child and, as Norman Shumway (chapter 12), one of Lewis's former trainees, noted, "in a sense [he] remained alone throughout his career." At his small high school, he tried for both the football and basketball teams, finally making the football team; they lost all six of their games. He also recorded that "I didn't get very far with the girls," despite joining various clubs. "I remember in particular the Christian Endeavor of the Presbyterian Church. If not one already, I was soon to be an atheist, but I stuck with Christian Endeavor, which met once a week, because that's where the girls were." Later, he states, "To me, religion was not only irrational, it was unnecessary."

He attended the University of Minnesota. "From home I got encouragement because my father and mother, like many people of that generation, thought the most wonderful thing they could do for their children was [to] provide an education. I chose medicine because this was the only science I could think of at that time. It didn't occur to me that I could become a physicist or chemist. At the University, I got through pre-medicine in two years. I did very well in physics. I sometimes wish I had followed that direction, but I stuck with medicine. I don't regret it in the sense that it was a bad mistake, but I suppose I was attracted more to the scientific features of medicine than the actual practice of caring for sick patients. My family was very pleased that I had chosen medicine. It was a real step up. To my father, being a local locomotive railroad engineer, it was important to become a professional."

At medical school, Lewis wrote a thesis on biostatistics. He graduated in 1941 and had a year of internship in surgery before going into the army. In his autobiography, he comments, "I think I decided to go into surgery because in that specialty you had something definite to do beyond making the diagnosis of an essentially untreatable disease.... I never did too well in the Army. I ended up as a battalion third surgeon in the 3rd Infantry Division. I didn't join them until we reached the River Rhine. We ended up with the highest number of casualties of any division in the American forces, including the Marines. The 3rd Infantry's best known hero, Audie Murphy, was to become Hollywood's leading cowboy after the war."

Being in the army, however, "was mostly a terrible bore and altogether it was a bad experience, and the last thing that I possibly wanted to do was stay in the Army....It was, in a way, a shameful time of life—serving with the most destructive military force in history—while at the same time it was peculiarly gratifying and remarkably intense....After it was over, I believed that our country should stay out of foreign involvement in the future—stay out of war....I became confirmed in what had been a growing distrust of politicians, national leaders, and similar newsmakers....I came out of the Army at Christmas, 1945. I immediately got married and by January or February I was a resident surgeon back in Minneapolis."

I reminded Dr. Lewis that many of those who made big advances in surgery in the 1950s did so at a very young age, certainly relative to surgeons in positions of authority today. I asked him whether the war had some effect in making his generation more mature.

"It probably made you more ambitious because you lost all of that time in the war. I think that the experience of getting shot at provides a kind of training. Who can say? The war was part of the lives of many of us, and any important part of life changes your character, just how is too subtle for me to understand. I should say there was a certain antipathy between the 'draft dodgers' and those who were in the forces. Although it was mostly suppressed, it was not always so. A whole bunch of guys who were my age or younger when I left to go into the army were now more senior in the department. I remember it caused bitterness."

Among the major influences on Lewis during medical school, and particularly afterward, was Owen Wangensteen, the chief of the department of surgery. Although he did not contribute directly to the development of heart surgery, Wangensteen was clearly a key figure in its development since he provided the opportunity and stimulus for innovative research and clinical surgery throughout his 37 years as "benign dictator" and chairman of surgery at the University of Minnesota.

Lewis was not so certain that Wangensteen had the brightest residents to work with. He believed "Wangensteen ended up with the guys who, for some reason or another, either wanted to stay in Minnesota where they grew up or couldn't get a job anywhere else. I'd say he did mighty well with the guys he had."

At the end of his residency, Lewis faced a choice of setting up in private practice or staying on in academic surgery. He chose academia.

"My main objective as a junior member of the staff was to develop a clinical practice, and so that had to have high priority. As a senior resident, you were a dominant figure in the hospital and you had the charity patients to look after, and so had lots of operating. The moment you got on to the faculty, you had nothing. I sure as hell didn't have much of a clinical practice.

"In the lab, I worked on many problems. One time Wangensteen directed me towards the artificial kidney [the dialysis machine], and I was the first person at the University of Minnesota to run the artificial kidney. But he was willing to give you a fair amount of independence in the direction you went, as long as you did *something*. My memory with regard to heart surgery is hazy, but I presume I thought that if I could get things sorted out in the dog lab, then I could go to the cardiologists to get some patients.... I think my interest in hypothermia came mostly, as I remember, when Dick Varco [chapter 7] came back from a meeting and said he had heard Bill Bigelow talking about using hypothermia in experimental cardiac surgery. Internists and pediatricians trusted him [Varco] and so, when I wanted to use hypothermia in a clinical case, I had to get his collaboration."

## Inside the Heart — A World First

At this historic first operation, Lewis was assisted by Dick Varco, Walt Lillehei, and Mansur Taufic, with two surgical residents. Taufic, who had helped Lewis with all of the experimental work in dogs, recalled that the patient withstood the procedure well; there were no complications during or after surgery. For Taufic, "It was somewhat emotional because we knew that we were doing the first case and, naturally, despite the fact that we had very good experience acquired in the dog lab, we had to be somewhat concerned. But we weren't fearful because of our experience in the dog lab. Taking part in it was a great honor."

Lewis recalled, "Our first patient survived. I had feelings of elation and some confidence. We had done it a hell of a lot in the dogs, and there it had worked beautifully. We got into some trouble later when we faced complicated [heart] defects, but fortunately the first one was a simple defect."

Dr. Lewis did not recollect that he felt any sense of a race with other surgeons, such as with Bigelow: "I don't remember that. I thought it was an innovation that was going to be done by somebody, but I can't remember being keenly interested in wanting to be the first or not."

At a follow-up 35 years later, the patient remained in good health, both physically and mentally; she was married and had two children. She was known to be alive 42 years after the operation.

With regard to "innovative" or "experimental" surgery, Lewis's opinion was, "Most doctors I have known were well motivated. They wanted to help; they wanted to do good.... They were concerned with prestige and their personal reputation, but they tried to keep their patients' interests uppermost. My own failures in this regard [in the aggressive use of innovative operations] have been a nagging source of confusion or regret."

## The Move to Northwestern

In 1957 Lewis left the exciting professional environment of Minneapolis to take up an appointment at Northwestern University in Chicago, which, at that time, was far less stimulating.

"The chief was anxious to have most of us move," he recalled.

"He had an ambition to have his men around the country to be known as 'Wangensteen's men.' To some extent he achieved that. That was his objective, so he tried to get me to move before I should have moved, I think. I realized I was slowly being edged out, and I was pleased to get out anyway. It got to the point where I wasn't operating at the University Hospital anymore, just at a local hospital and in the lab."

In his autobiography, Lewis wrote, "In Chicago at Northwestern University, I was their first full-time member of the surgical faculty. The chairman of the department was Loyal Davis, a neurosurgeon who was the father of Nancy Reagan. At least, Nancy was his wife's daughter and she became his adopted daughter.... Since Loyal Davis was about 60, the Chairmanship would open in a few years, and I hoped optimistically that if I got that job I might be able to modernize and improve the department. No one promised me that I would get it, however. The job the Dean offered me had no power and only an Associate Professor's rank."

Lewis's personality may not have enamored him to his new colleagues. Morley Cohen (chapter 7), who was a surgical resident under Lewis in Minneapolis, remembered, "He had a very biting sense of humor. He could say things without a smile, and you weren't sure whether he meant it or not, but later on it was quite clear he obviously was baiting you with it. We had a journal conference once a week of which John was chairman, and he could ask the most devastating questions. He was good, and everybody respected him. You couldn't help but respect him."

Despite some good features of the job, Lewis wrote that he "found serious barriers to a successful academic career at Northwestern. The department lacked the environment favoring the investigation that characterized Minnesota.... I tried to get things going in the cardiac field, but I never developed a strong clinical service.... The other direction I went into somewhat later with a considerable amount of energy was biomedical engineering. My last major effort, which lasted quite a few years, was in computer substitutes for physicians or nurses.

We were some of the earliest people to work in that direction. I thought it was fascinating."

In time, Lewis gave up trying to develop cardiac surgery at Northwestern. "Looking back now from a different perspective, I think I might have done better at Northwestern. I might, for example, have given up the practice of general surgery and limited my practice to cardiac surgery. That way I would have more easily enlisted the help of the other general surgeons who, quite naturally, didn't want to face any more competition in general surgery than they had to.... That was a serious professional mistake. The earlier that I had done this, the better. But I didn't do it at all. I might also have tried harder than I did to find a job at some other medical school."

The great heart transplant pioneer Norman Shumway (chapter 12) clearly thought extremely highly of Lewis, writing that "F. John Lewis truly was a great man who easily met the specifications of genius. In most company he was the brightest, most critical, and certainly the most entertaining." But Dr. Shumway mentioned to me that heart surgery had become a team event, and because Dr. Lewis had trouble delegating to others, he was no good at organizing a team. Also, the second operation that Lewis attempted in Chicago under hypothermia proved to be not a simple atrial septal defect, but a more complicated abnormality known as a sinus venosus defect. Ideally, it requires much longer than six minutes to repair, but time was, of course, a luxury that Lewis didn't have. In closing it rapidly under hypothermia, Lewis narrowed the superior vena cava — the main vessel draining the blood from the upper part of the body — thus causing some obstruction and eventually leading to the death of the patient, who was the child of a leading Chicago banker. This, of course, did Lewis's reputation no good at all, and led to his eventually abandoning heart surgery and limiting his work to general surgery. "He got more and more cocooned off," said Dr. Shumway. "He sort of withdrew from society. Most people bored the daylights out of him. He just couldn't stand idle chatter."

## Disillusion and Early Retirement

Nothing seemed to work out quite as well in Chicago as Lewis had hoped. For example, he was not appointed chairman of the department on Loyal Davis's retirement. Norman Shumway pondered why Lewis had not been successful in this respect. He suggested that Lewis "could not tolerate second-rate individuals or dilettantes in medicine. This lack of tolerance did not help his career, to say the least."

In *Time of Life,* Lewis mentions that in Chicago, for a period of time, he threw himself into sailing activities. He considers, "Maybe I was trying to achieve success in sailing that I was failing to get in my work. Or was I searching for still another way to fail?" These are not the comments of a happy man, certainly not one fulfilling a successful career.

As early as the age of 55, the disillusioned Lewis began to consider quitting surgery, and by the spring of 1977 he had moved to Southern Califonia. He was only 59. During retirement, his interests ranged from writing to drawing, painting, studying, exercising, and piano playing.

Lewis never received any honors — honorary degrees or other formal recognition — for his contributions to cardiac surgery. "No, nothing like that. I don't feel put out," he said. It surprised me that the surgeon who had taken this monumental step forward, even though the concept of hypothermia was not his own, had not received some public recognition, or at least some recognition by the medical community.

Lewis seemed reluctant to contribute reasons why he had taken certain steps in his life. His autobiography is full of introspection, and so I couldn't help but think that he had thought about these problems but perhaps didn't want to talk about them with me. I wondered whether he felt he had any special qualities that made him an innovator or whether he was just in the right place at the right time. Would he have been an innovator if he had been at a different place? "Probably not. I'm not sure. Self-analysis is treacherous. However, I think it was mostly the location and the opportunity. The stimulation and example of Wangensteen was very important. There is nothing more exciting than to work on something to prove that you are unique."

## Reflections

I asked Dr. Lewis whether the demands of his career had affected his home life. He responded, "I had a good marriage and a good family life." One of his married daughters had moved into the country with her husband, "built their own log cabin, provided electricity with solar panels, and planted trees. They have become prominent in the movement to reestablish the chestnut tree in the U.S.A."

"They're happy," I ventured.

"No, they're not happy. Who the hell is happy?" This was perhaps one of the most insightful statements Lewis made during our time together. "My son owns a couple of bicycle shops in Ohio and is a moderately successful businessman. My youngest daughter is a born-again Christian who put her husband through theological college. She is also self-educating her children at home."

I suggested that his two daughters seemed to have done something a little out of the mainstream. Had they gotten that maverick streak from him?

"Maybe. I encouraged that stuff."

If he had his life to live again, would he make any major changes in it?

"I'd live a different one. I've lived this one, and I think I would like to live a different kind of life. I've often thought of physics as the most exciting intellectual field in the world. If I had my time in medicine again, I probably would have retired earlier."

After our conversation that afternoon, we arranged to meet for dinner in my hotel. He arrived—still the artist rather than the surgeon—in a red polo-neck sweater with a dark blue blazer. We spoke about his interest in art and writing. His painting was, according to his autobiography, "like the paintings of most amateurs, not much good. And it didn't seem to get better.... The detached, uncritical enjoyment is great, but when you evaluate your work and feel that others are doing this too, you may wonder if you want to keep doing something in which you are always going to be a duffer. Perhaps this means that we have too long and too often been filled with the idea of insisting on excellence in all we do."

He then turned his hand to writing. "Because of our national hypochondria, I thought there would be a good market for medical pieces, and that my writing might actually help some people....I tried, but after a couple of years of trying, I had only one article published [on tonsillectomy] — and that in a rather obscure magazine. So I turned to writing fiction. Fiction should require less tedious research, or so I thought, and since no one, or at least no one I knew among local writers, was getting his fiction published, failure to publish wouldn't embarrass me."

He seemed very keen on improving his writing and mentioned this several times during the course of the evening. It seemed rather quaint, even touching, that a man in his early 70s should still be keen to improve himself in this way.

His whole life seemed to have been a series of attempts at self-improvement, perhaps suggesting a deep-seated feeling of inadequacy. In his autobiography, he admits "to a chronic interest in schemes for self-improvement." At various stages of his life he undertook a private program of reading the "great books," attended night school for several years to study mathematics, and tried, off and on, to learn to play the piano. "My ambition, which I freely confess to anyone — knowing all the while that I'll never achieve it — is to play and sing popular tunes at some local bar. So far I haven't tried to sing; playing is difficult enough." What a surprising ambition for a man who took such a historic step in surgery!

Lewis did not neglect his physical improvement, either. He was at times an enthusiastic backpacker, jogger, weight-trainer, and cyclist, having cycled over most of California and as far south as the Mexican border.

"I work out with those ingenious [muscle-conditioning] machines three times a week, take showers with the guys, ogle the beautiful women who flock to aerobic dancing classes at the same club, and I keep trying. If I keep it up, maybe I'll be in great shape about the time I have reached the end of my mortal rope—a bizarre, wrinkled, well-muscled specimen."

It is ironic that a man who had kept himself so fit by regular physical activity for most of his life, and who therefore might reasonably expect to live to a great old age, should die from something as simple as an infection that began in the leg.

I was left with the impression of a complex man. It seemed incredible to me that he had performed the first open heart operation in the world and then had drifted away from cardiac surgery within a relatively short period of time. Indeed, his interest in medicine had dissolved long before his retirement. Perhaps, as he commented in his autobiography, he was never suited to a career in surgery. I had the feeling that he regretted to some extent the path his life had taken. In retirement, he had become, possibly by choice, relatively isolated from his family and former interests. He admitted that, at times, he was lonely, but he organized his day to ensure that he had plenty to do, and tried to keep to some sort of timetable.

"I've sometimes thought about living as a hermit, " he told me. "Nonetheless, I enjoy the social life at times. It gives me a chance to show off, and a way to hide from the cruel reality that we all live and die alone."

I left Santa Barbara thinking how sad and disillusioned he seemed, a man whose life had not been fulfilled in the way perhaps it could have been. Lewis's written view of his life was perhaps more positive: "I have lived in a wonderful age with more opportunity and challenge than a person with my background could have expected in any other country at any other time. I doubt if anyone ever feels that his potential is being fully realized, but I have had a good shot at it."

It seems, however, that Norman Shumway agrees with my conclusion, for in his obituary notice of John Lewis, he wrote, "It is regrettable that this incredibly gifted individual never became chairman of an academic department of surgery.... He would never say or admit it, but all these other activities never compensated for his unfulfilled destiny." Shumway then added, "John Lewis died September 20, 1993, in Santa Barbara, not from septicemia, as noted in the obituaries, but from boredom." He was 76 years old.

## HENRY SWAN—THE FIRST SERIES OF OPEN HEART OPERATIONS

Henry Swan (Figure 19), perhaps even more than John Lewis, established heart surgery using hypothermia. Although Lewis preempted him in doing the first case, Swan had soon performed the largest series of such operations in the world.

"I'll meet you at the airport in Denver. You'll recognize me—I'll be wearing a cowboy hat." So wrote 81-year-old Henry Swan to me when I planned to visit him in 1994. This fit the image I had of him from a photograph of the pioneers in heart surgery I had first seen in Dr. Bigelow's home, where Swan appeared tall and well built, with perhaps a rather open and direct attitude toward life. It was quite in keeping with his image for him to wear a Stetson.

As it happened, I had to postpone my visit due to bad weather and, on the day I arrived, I took a taxi from the airport to his home, which was about 30 minutes away on the outskirts of the city. The house was way out in the "bush" on the mountainside, and the taxi had to traverse a mud road in order to reach it. It was beautifully situated close to a lake. I was welcomed at the door by his wife, an artist (who looked the part), and his black Labrador (reminding me of my visit to Dr. Bigelow). The house was old for that part of the country, ranchlike, or at least rural, in design, and filled with books and paintings. Modernist paintings by his wife were interspersed with more traditional art. The house was full of plants and old furniture and, although it looked comfortable to live in, had a slightly run-down appearance. Dr. Swan took me out onto the balcony to admire the spectacular view. It was a gorgeous spring day, and one could see for miles around. He pointed out a house not far away where he had been brought up as a child, and another, even closer, in which his parents had lived in their later years.

Dr. Swan wore checked pants with a beige cardigan, and a shirt with a bolero cowboy tie, a large turquoise rhinestone holding the strings of the tie together. At the age of 81, he didn't look much like the photograph I had seen of him in his younger days when he had been big and powerfully built. Originally six feet two inches, he was now under six feet tall and weighed a mere 140 pounds. Although he still retained a good head of hair, he wore two hearing aids and heavy spectacles. I noted he had paralysis of his right hand. This, he told me, had developed some 11 years previously, when it was thought he might be developing Lou Gehrig's disease (the muscular wasting disease that afflicted the eponymous baseball legend, and is the cause of world-famous astronomer Stephen Hawking's health problems), though a definite diagnosis had never been made. He could hardly use his right arm and, indeed, had been forced to relearn to write with his left hand.

When we began talking, it was clear that Dr, Swan was very deaf and, unless he was looking directly at me, often could not understand what I had said even though I spoke very loudly. Initially, I feared my journey to visit him was going to be rather a waste of time, and certainly heavy-going, since I felt sure he wouldn't be able to remember very much of his career. As the day progressed, however, I realized I was clearly wrong. His memory was excellent, and he proved to be one of the most intellectual and informative of the surgeons I visited in the preparation of this book. He retained an excellent knowledge of the biochemistry of hypothermia, and I departed immensely impressed with his clarity of thought.

## Youth and Education

Over lunch, he told me something of his background. He had been born in Denver in 1913, had lived in the valley we now overlooked, and attended Denver High School. His father, who had clearly been a significant figure in Swan's youth, had been a financial investor and advisor, and had also run the Santa Fe Railroad for some years, saving it from bankruptcy. It was intended that the young Henry Swan should transfer to Phillips Academy in Exeter, Massachusetts, when he was 14, but his father "wisely thought that I was kind of young to go back East," and held him back for a year. "Of course, that was a disadvantage in a way, but it did allow me to grow a year older."

After Exeter, he went to Williams College in western Massachusetts. He chose Williams partly because there was a certain family tradition of attending the college, but also because he fell in love with the place when he visited one of his cousins who was studying there. "I look back on my years at Williams College as years of great joy because life was a lot of fun. I didn't work that hard. Bennington College was only 20 miles away and there were pretty girls around. I found my first wife there. We also had these good sporting events, basketball and tennis. I was president of the Williams Theater, so I fancied myself as a thespian. I don't think I was really any good, but I at least had the fun of being in plays for a couple of years." Having captained the tennis team at Phillips Academy, and having been runner-up in the Junior Colorado Championships, at Williams he found he had to accept the number-three spot as the standard was so high. Despite spending much of his time on other activities, he proved an excellent student, ending as valedictorian of his class.

There was a tradition of medicine on his mother's side of the family, as her brother and father were both doctors, and so from Williams he went on to Harvard Medical School, where his progress was equally spectacular. In the final examination, Swan headed the class of 1939. He admitted that this was "a fabulous achievement, particularly with that particular class," which included several who were destined to become medical luminaries, including the great Harvard surgical investigator Francis Moore.

While at medical school, Robert Gross had a great influence on him. He recalled, "I was terribly impressed with Dr. Gross. In fact, I was in the operating room when he did the first ductus operation. I was so excited. I was hoping to hold a retractor, but I didn't get that close."

By the time he graduated, Swan had decided to go into surgery, particularly pediatric surgery. He took a two-year internship divided between the Brigham and Children's Hospitals in Boston, and had completed just one year when the United States entered World War II in 1941. "So I was made resident on the general service at the Children's Hospital. Almost everybody that was declared nonessential was in uniform. They considered me necessary, and I couldn't leave because that would have left them with no resident at all. I worked 20 hours a day."

Swan then spent three years in the military, his extensive surgical experience in Europe extending from Utah Beach on the day after D-Day to the River Elbe. When he came back from the war, he opened a practice in Denver as a pediatric surgeon. However, very soon he was asked to be the first full-time surgeon at the University Hospital. It was a difficult decision, but he made the move and, in 1950, became professor and head of the department of surgery.

## Denver, Colorado

"When I became full-time at the medical school, the very first thing I did was to establish a research laboratory. I started to investigate aortic surgery [surgery involving the main blood vessel of the body] and aortic grafting using homografts [arteries taken from the deceased]. In patients, I started doing ductus operations and repairing coarctations. I decided I wanted to operate on the heart. I had seen Dwight Harken doing a mitral valvotomy. It's hard for people today to appreciate what it was like at a time when nobody knew what would happen when, for example, you stuck a needle into the heart. Nobody, as yet, had any real vision about these sorts of things."

I asked Dr. Swan how he had become interested in hypothermia.

"Hypothermia starts with Bill Bigelow. In 1950, Bill reported a series of dogs to which he had given an anesthetic and had lowered their body temperature to 30°C (86°F). Several of us in the audience thought that this was interesting. When I was driving my car back to Colorado, I thought to myself, 'You know, 15% of those dogs survived with no circulation for 15 minutes at 30°C. That's remarkable.' Within hours, I was writing letters and getting grants to study hypothermia.

"I did over three hundred dogs before I operated on a human. Of course, I was worried and tense about operating on patients, but I thought that we had gained enough experience in the laboratory to demonstrate we could manage and control hypothermia and its complications. We had learned how to do successful defibrillation [to electrically shock the heart out of an irregular rhythm]. We had learned how to massage the heart. When I undertook the first patient, I thought it was reasonable to go ahead. You're always nervous but, gosh, we thought we were ready.

"To cool the [anesthetized] patient, I put them in a large tank of cold water [Figure 21]. I had this tub of water and then just poured in a bucket of ice. Somebody had to stir the water because, even in icy water, a patient will keep a little envelope of warm air around him so he doesn't cool as well. So somebody with a paddle would stir the water and wash away that warm air. I thought that the quicker we cooled the patient, the better.

"Our objective was to cool to 30°C. We thought that the metabolic rate would decrease by about 60% at 30°C . We weren't sure what the safety limits were, but I thought that the longest safe period of time at 30°C was for sure at six minutes. I had one person just to note what the time was so that, when it got to be close, he would say 'three minutes,' and 'four minutes,' and 'five minutes.' If he got to five minutes, he would say 'ten seconds,' 'five minutes and twenty seconds,' 'five minutes and thirty seconds' in a loud voice so that I could hear it. My scheme was that if it got to be six minutes, I didn't want to go any longer, so I would pull the stitches or whatever I was doing. I would just put clamps on the structures and close the sutures so that I could reperfuse the heart and massage it until it started again. We waited not less than ten minutes before we stopped the heart again. Of course, that seems like an age when you are anxious to get back in there. But we would wait ten minutes."

Dr. Swan recounted to me the detailed calculations he had made to determine that six minutes' hypothermic arrest would be safe and that ten minutes' reperfusion was the ideal. His clinical work had clearly been based on firm scientific principles.

"The minute the operation was completed, we started warming. I have always worried about hypothermia. I always viewed hypothermia as a state that wasn't normal for a man. There must be risks involved. It was better to go as fast as you could, get your business done, and get out of there. As soon as cooling was no longer needed, I wanted them warmed as soon as possible.

"I thought there were theoretical reasons why it would be desirable to warm by central warming [to first warm the heart and the blood in it, and allow the heart to pump the warm blood around the body, thus warming the periphery]. So we decided to place endothermic coils [next to the heart] that would bring heat to the heart and veins, and thus warm the body through the circulation. All the organs everywhere would be uniformly warmed throughout the body.

"Apart from Lewis's effort, I believe I was the first to use hypothermia clinically. I reported on thirteen patients at the American Medical Association meeting in June 1953. I had one death. I always considered this to be the first clinical report of a successful series of open heart operations. This opened the door for open heart surgery. All of a sudden, people realized that you could make an incision in the heart and sew it up, and the heart would do fine. Lewis had done one, and that was all there were in the world.

"After that, in 1953 and 1954, our laboratory had visitors from all over the world. All these people visited to watch what we were doing. Colorado wasn't ready for this sort of innovation. Colorado was never first in experimental procedures or developing new fields. The first medical publication that I wrote as a full-time member of the faculty was the first scientific report that had ever been published from the department of surgery at the University of Colorado. There was none before that. Cardiologists and doctors at that time thought that the best conceivable thing they could do was to protect their patients from the surgeon. That was the most important thing for the cardiologist. We had published a number of papers and were getting more patients from France, Ecuador, and Peru than we were from Denver, Colorado."

How had working in such a demanding field as heart surgery affected his home life?

"It had a significant effect on me. There were so many outside obligations. If you're already working pretty damn hard at home, trying to elevate the status of the department, and writing clinical papers, that wasn't easy, and took long hours. My wife developed different interests. I think my children felt me distant for a long time because I just wasn't around any, and it wasn't until later years that I developed a rapport with them. I think you pay the price for that. I wasn't smart enough to be able to do everything I wanted to do. I think it might have been much better if I had seen more of my family." His first marriage broke up.

## Elusive Hibernation — Lungfish and the North American Squirrel

It was then that Dr. Swan's thoughts followed a similar direction to those of Dr. Bigelow. "Following this experience with hypothermia, we wondered whether there was some way to lower the metabolic rate *without* cooling. That would be a wonderful way to go. One day Charlie Hufnagel [chapter 9] and I were having lunch and a couple of martinis. I said, 'Charlie, I want to find an animal whose metabolism can be lowered without having to change its temperature.' Charlie said, 'What do you know about the lungfish?' I said, 'I don't know a damn thing about them.' He told me they lived in Africa mostly and that they could curl up and go for long periods when there was no water during the dry season, and lower their metabolic rate. They could survive without ever eating or drinking for six to eight months. They did this because their metabolic rate had been suppressed. That suggestion of Charlie Hufnagel was enough for me to get a grant.

"It was then 1964. I took my second wife up the Nile, where we found lungfish and set up a way of supplying them from one of the universities in Tanganyika [now Tanzania] to our laboratory. They could indeed lower their metabolic rate without reducing their temperature. We found out enough to know that it was the brains of the fish that contained the active agent that lowered their metabolic rate. If you injected this substance from the brain into a rat, it would lower the metabolic rate of the rat.

"With problems of supply of the lungfish, I wondered if I couldn't do better using a hibernator. We hit upon the North American squirrel. Here again the brain contained a substance that, when injected into rats, lowered the metabolic rate. I had visions of this substance being so valuable in a number of conditions, not only in cardiac surgery but also in cases of trauma or serious infection where one wished to reduce the metabolic rate. I thought it would be more valuable even than insulin, because it would affect the population at large when they were in a situation where it would be therapeutic to lower their metabolism. Even after many years of work, we were never able to identify the substance. This was one of the failures of my life.

"It's a fascinating field. For example, take the hummingbird that has to be very active and feed quickly during the times of day when it is looking for food. When it rests, its body temperature is lowered by a few degrees. Then pretty soon it is feeding time again, and it warms up, and out it goes. It is an energy-saving mechanism for an animal that is marginally nourished. Hibernators, of course, do it, but there are other animals that lower their metabolic rate even if their temperature is really unchanged. Some lizards can do it."

Some years later, Swan published a book on this topic, *Thermoregulation and Bioenergetics: Patterns for Vertebrate Survival*. It was on the basis of this book and his other work that he was awarded a doctorate in science from his alma mater, Williams College. Bill Bigelow had a high regard for this book, believing "it should be read by anyone embarking on a study of low body temperature and metabolism."

## Collapse of Career

Dr. Swan did not mention to me the circumstances of his leaving the department of surgery of the University of Colorado, and at the time of my interview with him I was unaware that he had been forced to leave prematurely. Tom Starzl, who joined the department in Denver in 1961, states in his book *The Puzzle People* that, "in the 1950s, the Department of Surgery had been one of the most honored and productive in the country under the guidance of Henry Swan, a world leader in cardiac surgery, and Ben Eiseman, his VA Chief. Now there was scorched earth. Swan had been deposed when he was in his early 50s and Eiseman had gone to Kentucky. The preeminence in heart surgery which Colorado had enjoyed for almost a decade was lost overnight."

When I spoke personally with Dr. Starzl, I questioned him further about the circumstances of Dr. Swan's departure from the university. He told me, "I didn't work with Henry, but I came to know him rather well socially. When I went to Denver, he had been gone [from the university] for about a year and a half, but he really embraced me right off the bat as a friend. It was typical of Henry Swan. I liked him. He was a tremendous guy, very generous. He had had a 'deadly feud' with the dean. The salaries at Colorado were very low. I can give you some real hard figures because they are mine. I had a big practice in Chicago and made over $100,000 in fees, in addition to my basic salary. Then I went to Colorado. The highest income I ever made in Colorado was $60,000, and this was when I was chairman. Henry Swan was a very wealthy guy, and didn't care about money *per se,* but in principle he didn't like the idea of having the dean's office pocket this torrent of money that he was generating as a very successful thoracic surgeon.

"Also, Swan had been acting erratically. He had several crashes in private planes, and in one of these sustained a rather severe head injury. He was also having marital problems that were harmful to his reputation. What brought him down eventually was that everybody signed a contract that they would not cash any checks that were issued to them but rather these would go into the dean's fund. Any check made out to you was signed over to the dean's fund, or sent to the faculty practice fund. I think Henry Swan signed a check for a small amount of money, from Blue Cross/Blue Shield, for $250 or something like that. They made a 'hanging crime' out of it. That was the approximate cause of his dismissal as chairman.

"He went over to a private hospital and retained research interests for a number of years, some of which were pretty good, particularly in hypothermia and in lungfish. He spent a lot of time working on them at Colorado State University in Fort Collins. Then later, he developed some preservation fluids. But it [his removal from the chairmanship] terminated his creative life because he had to find funds to finance any research. Although I don't know any real details, I think he left in somewhat of a disgraced position. So I would say that his career was finished at that point, and he never really did anything from 1960 onward. This was shocking in a way because he was one of the youngest chairmen of any department in the United States; I think he was well short of fifty when his career went 'belly up.' Wangensteen created a climate [for advances in surgery] and Blalock created a climate. Henry Swan created a climate, but the circumstances of his leaving the scene were such that he really didn't lead his school the way it occurred in Minneapolis and at Hopkins."

Swan's departure from Denver clearly limited the extent of his contributions, which may well have been more extensive had he remained at a university teaching hospital.

## Opinions

I asked Dr. Swan what qualities were needed in those days to be a pioneer in heart surgery.

"You had to have courage to commit yourself to do things that others hadn't done before, and to think that there were good reasons to do these new things. It was important that you knew the scientific principles. I must confess that I had a rather low opinion of the state of the science at the time, which seemed to me to be almost always wrong. There had to be something else that was right. I tend to be a little skeptical about everything. Don't accept what you're told. I think that's important. Don't accept everything as if it's proven. You have to have a little skepticism but, on the other hand, you have to have a basis for action, and I don't believe it should be based on emotional reasons only. I don't think you should do something just because you have an inner voice that speaks to you. I didn't have any voice that spoke to me like that. I read, learned, and went to the laboratory with goals. I had to have purposes. If you're going out to pioneer something, you have to have an objective. You had to be a little bit hard-shelled because of the criticism you would receive."

I asked him whether he felt he had received enough recognition and rewards for his contributions to surgery.

"I never worried about it one way or another. But every once in awhile I feel that our definitive paper on the first thirteen hypothermic cases hasn't been sufficiently remembered as the major step it was. We also published a technique for preserving segments of cadaveric [deceased] human artery or aorta, which we later used in operations where it was necessary to remove and replace a diseased segment of artery. I don't think anybody had done that before. At the Pan-Pacific Surgical Meeting in Honolulu in 1949 or 1950, I reported replacement of a thoracic aortic aneurysm [weakening and destruction of the wall of the major artery in the body]. I believe, without question, that it was the first aneurysm of the aorta that had been resected with replacement. On the plane back from Honolulu, Mike DeBakey grilled me for about an hour and a half about all aspects of the operation. It was after our report, you will find, that DeBakey's papers began. Nobody ever bothered to mention my case, not even DeBakey."

I gave my thanks to Dr. Swan for his time and, while I was waiting for a taxi to take me to the airport, we looked around his house a little further. I noted that he had a patent certificate (on a method of storing organs) from the U.S. Patent Office, dated 1993, when he would have been 80 years old. I was impressed that he had worked on this project in his 70s, and had pursued it to the point of obtaining a patent. My impression was that he was not interested in any money he might make from it, but only in its intellectual and humanitarian appeal.

My final question to him was whether, if he had his time again, he would go into medicine. He replied that he thought he would. "You see, it was such an exciting period. The 1940s and 1950s were just a crescendo of change in the nature of practice. It was the entry of science and research into medicine. It was a revolution in medical education and in the practice of medicine, particularly surgery. I certainly found it extremely and excitingly interesting. I'm glad I did it."

HYPOTHERMIA REMAINED the major method of enabling surgeons to operate inside the heart until the end of the 1950s. However, few surgeons had the requisite speed, skill, and daring to employ it successfully. Furthermore, it was cumbersome and provided too little time to repair complicated defects. Something further was needed that would allow the surgeon a longer period of time to operate in the heart. That something was a heart-lung machine.

CHAPTER 6

# Far-Fetched Ideas:
# The Concept of the
# Heart-Lung Machine

———

## CLARENCE DENNIS, JOHN GIBBON JR.,
## VIKING BJORK, AND AKE SENNING

ALTHOUGH THERE WERE occasional efforts to develop a machine that would support a patient's circulation, or at least provide partial support, and thus allow the heart to be operated on, it was the work of Clarence Dennis and John Gibbon Jr. that led to the first trials of heart-lung machines. They were very soon followed by the Swedish group of Clarence Crafoord and his associates.

Surprisingly, one of the first people to consider designing a heart-lung machine was Charles Lindbergh, the pioneer aviator. In 1932, Lindbergh had a sister-in-law who had valvular heart disease, probably mitral valve disease. Her cardiologist said it was going to kill her, but, with great vision, added that the tragedy was that if the circulation could be supported while the heart was opened, then the valve could probably be repaired quite easily. Lindbergh contacted Alexis Carrel, the leading research surgeon of his era, who thought it too ambitious to begin work on a heart-lung machine. He suggested they work together on a pump that would maintain a heart in a viable state outside of the body, which they did. However, this was a far cry from designing a machine that could actually support the life of an entire person. It was, in fact, more than another 20 years before attempts were made to support a patient's circulation by a machine that enabled the surgeon to open the heart and correct the lesion inside it.

Although Clarence Dennis was the first to try total bypass of the heart and lungs in a patient, it was John Gibbon who began his research earliest and, ultimately, was the first to succeed.

## CLARENCE DENNIS— SO CLOSE AND YET SO FAR

Clarence Dennis (Figure 22) is something of an oddity in the development of heart surgery in that he was basically a general surgeon—not even a chest surgeon—who, as a research interest, attempted to develop a heart-lung machine. Although he took up this project much later than John Gibbon, he actually had his machine ready for clinical use at an earlier stage. While at the University of Minneapolis, he used the machine in two patients before anyone else had attempted this approach, but unfortunately neither attempt was successful. In this respect, Dennis was very unlucky, because in neither case was the lack of success related to an inherent deficiency in his machine. In the first case (on patient Patty Anderson on April 5, 1951), failure was associated with a mistaken diagnosis, and in the second with human error. He therefore did not receive the accolades that Gibbon subsequently did for his single successful attempt, or that others, such as Lillehei and Kirklin, did for really establishing open heart surgery. Dennis is, therefore, in some ways a sad figure in that he came so close to surgical immortality, only to fail, through no fault of his own, at the last hurdle.

It was not until June 1955, by which time the Swedish group and Kirklin and Lillehei had entered the field, that Dennis successfully used a heart-lung machine to carry out open heart surgery. Nevertheless, Clarence Dennis, who died in 2005 at age 96, will go down in the medical history books as the first man to attempt open heart surgery using a heart-lung machine. In my opinion, therefore, he can rightfully claim a place among the originators of heart surgery, and he demands our great respect despite the fact that he was initially unsuccessful.

There is one anecdote relating to Dennis — told to me in the preparation of this book — that I just have to include. Dennis was evidently a very meticulous, but extremely slow, surgeon — so slow, in fact, that, rather than keeping one eye on the clock, his surgical assistants were said to take a calendar into the operating room with them.

## JOHN GIBBON JR. — THE MAN WITH THE SILVER SPOON

John Gibbon Jr. (Figure 23), or Jack, as he was known, came from a privileged "old money" Philadelphia family. He is the epitome of someone born with the proverbial silver spoon in his mouth. He had what many would believe to be a charmed life. Born into a wealthy "aristocratic" family — a dynasty of surgeons — he grew into a young man with good looks, charm, intelligence, and many other natural gifts. His career was successful in every respect, and he became an immensely highly regarded leader in the profession, liked and respected by almost everybody. Gibbon was rewarded by election to almost every high office open to the surgical hierarchy, including the presidency of several leading surgical societies. He became an establishment figure in surgery — intellectual, distinguished, erudite, admired by all — and received many honors, including the prestigious Lasker Award (in 1968). If it were not for the fact that he seemed to be such a nice person, one might almost develop a sense of resentment that everything seemed to be so easy for him.

Gibbon, who was born in 1903, had an idyllic childhood running wild on the family farm and developed an early interest in literature, especially poetry, graduating from Princeton University in 1923, and from the Jefferson Medical College in 1927. At one stage as a medical student, he seriously contemplated giving up this career in order to devote himself to creative writing, but his father dissuaded him. He was the fifth generation from his family to practice medicine, his father preceding him as professor of surgery at Jefferson and also as president of the American Surgical Association.

After marriage, Gibbon and his family of four children initially divided their time between a townhouse in Philadelphia and a farm in the country. Later, he moved to the farm permanently. He and his wife entertained frequently and graciously. Throughout his life, he was a keen tennis player who also listened to music, read widely, wrote poetry, and painted in watercolors and oils — in other words, something of a "Renaissance man."

John Templeton III, a colleague of Gibbon for many years, first encountered Gibbon when Templeton was a medical student at the University of Pennsylvania. He recalled, "I was extraordinarily impressed with him. To begin with, one's first impression was that he was a very handsome man, and with a winning personality; not overtly familiar, but very friendly. And he had a 'presence'; when he entered the room you knew that someone had come into the room. This, plus his fine brain, made him a very, very impressive person."

Writing in memoriam of John Gibbon in 1973, Rudolph Camishion, who trained under Gibbon and then was his partner in practice for a number of years, wrote, "The contributions of John H. Gibbon Jr. to science and medicine have ensured his greatness. However, for his friends, it is difficult to determine which facet of this gem of a man glistens most radiantly." Praise indeed.

Gibbon would have been the tabloid press's nightmare, the paparazzi's despair, for it is almost impossible to find anyone who has any criticism of him. To a large extent, he seems faultless and unblemished, although, as we shall see later, there may have been at least one small chink in his otherwise perfect armor.

## The Long Night

John Gibbon is credited with the development of the first successfully used heart-lung machine. He began this lifetime work in the 1930s, when he was a junior research fellow at the Massachusetts General Hospital. The story goes that in 1930 he was assigned to keep an eye on a patient who had developed a pulmonary embolus. Blood clots had formed in the veins of the legs or pelvis, and at least one large clot had broken off and traveled in the venous bloodstream to the lungs. The clot could not pass through the small vessels of the lungs, and so obstructed the blood supply to part or all of one or both lungs. (This is the same problem that afflicts people who sit in cramped positions during long air flights, and which has gained considerable publicity in recent years.)

In 1930, the operation of pulmonary embolectomy, by which the blood clot (or embolus) is removed from the lung arteries, was extremely hazardous. It was in the nature of a "smash and grab" procedure, the surgeon working feverishly to clear the clots from the arteries, since this put a further strain on the heart. The operation was accompanied by a very high mortality rate; indeed, no successful operation of this nature had ever been performed in the United States at that time, although a handful of successes had been achieved in Europe, such as three by Clarence Crafoord in 1927 and 1928.

The patient Gibbon was assigned to watch was in a precarious state, teetering on the brink of sudden heart failure since her heart was under great stress as it tried to pump blood through the obstructed arteries to the lungs; furthermore, the heart was itself getting little oxygen, making its difficulties worse. The professor of surgery at Massachusetts General, Edward Churchill, assigned the young Gibbon to watch the patient for signs of deterioration. If further failure in heart function developed, a last-ditch effort would be made to save the patient's life by performing the operation of pulmonary embolectomy; this would involve rapidly opening the chest, cutting into the main artery to the lungs, and trying desperately to fish out the clot.

While watching the woman in the semidarkness of the night, it occurred to Gibbon that her life could be maintained if there was a device to support her circulation while the clot dissolved. To do this, a machine would be required that would take over the work of both her heart and her lungs to ensure the satisfactory circulation of blood (normally provided by the heart) and the adequate exchange of gases, such as oxygen and carbon dioxide (normally provided by the lungs). This experience stimulated Gibbon to subsequently write, "...watching helplessly the patient struggle for life as her blood became darker and her veins more distended, the idea naturally occurred to me that, if it were possible to remove continuously some of the blue blood from the patient's swollen veins, put oxygen into that blood and allow carbon dioxide to escape from it, and then to inject continuously the now-red blood back into the patient's arteries, we might have saved her life.... We would have bypassed the obstructing embolus and performed part of the work of the patient's heart and lungs outside the body."

Early the following morning, the patient suddenly stopped breathing and her pulse was no longer palpable, forcing Dr. Churchill to open her chest and rapidly remove the embolus from the pulmonary artery. Unfortunately, the operation, like all those previously performed in the United States at that time, was unsuccessful, and the patient did not recover.

With this vision in mind, Gibbon determined to develop such a machine—a heart-lung machine. Use of such a machine to perform surgery inside the heart does not appear to have occurred to him at that time; he was solely interested in supporting a patient with a pulmonary embolus. His work toward this aim would be delayed for some years while he returned to the University of Pennsylvania in Philadelphia to complete his surgical training.

He went back to Philadelphia, however, not only with his new idea, but also with a wife. He married Dr. Churchill's laboratory technician, Mary ("Maly") Hopkinson, who became a staunch lifelong co-investigator in his research to develop a heart-lung machine. Maly

Hopkinson must have been an attractive young lady; George Humphreys, who was in the same laboratory as Gibbon at the time, emphasized to me that Gibbon, "like everybody else, fell for Maly but, unlike her response to other young medical people, she responded to him."

In 1934, Gibbon persuaded Dr. Churchill, who was neither enthusiastic nor optimistic about the project, to allow him to return to the Massachusetts General Hospital for a further period of research, where he and his wife concentrated their attention on the development of this device. Gibbon soon realized that the heart-lung machine would require four basic components (Figure 24) — a reservoir to collect venous (blue) blood from the patient; an oxygenator to oxygenate the blood; some method of maintaining the temperature of the blood passing through the device, and thus through the patient; and, finally, an arterial pump to return the oxygenated (pink) blood to the patient. He was fortunate that heparin had recently become available, and so he had a means of preventing clotting of blood in the machine.

A means of providing gas exchange in and out of the blood proved the major challenge. The larger the surface area where blood and oxygen could meet and mix, the greater would be the gas exchange. In this respect, a little turbulence in the blood increased gas exchange. The provision of a pump to circulate the blood back into the patient was not particularly problematic, as there were several commercial pumps available that were suitable for this purpose. However, the device must not cause excessive damage to the patient's red blood cells, and therefore the pump, in particular, had to be gentle.

The oxygenators that were developed by the pioneers can broadly be divided into two types — "filmers" or "bubblers" — with a third design following a little later, the "membrane" oxygenator.

The "filmers" depended on a large interface between blood and oxygen. Gibbon tried various approaches, but eventually used large vertical screens over which a thin layer of blood flowed. Gas exchange occurred because the film of blood was so thin. If the screens were rotated through a trough of flowing blood, they picked up more blood, which could then spread out over the screens. The same effect could be achieved by a drum, a cylinder, or a series of flat discs that revolved through a trough of blood, and for a time Gibbon tested this approach, though he ultimately returned to flat screens.

The "bubblers," as their name implied, consisted simply of bubbling oxygen into a container of blood so that the gas would be picked up by the red blood cells. The problem was that if actual bubbles of oxygen persisted and were carried to the brain of the patient (or research animal), they caused injury to the brain. It is perhaps ironic that, although oxygen is essential to the brain's functioning, actual air bubbles can occlude the small vessels, just as a blood clot can, and result in damage.

Later, "membrane" oxygenators arose from Willem Kolff's work when developing the first dialysis machine (artificial kidney) (chapter 13). Kolff observed that when he passed blood through a length of thin sausage casing, oxygen diffused through the membrane and the blood became pink. Today, with years of refinement, membrane oxygenators have replaced the early filmers or bubblers, but it was these relatively unsophisticated designs that enabled open heart surgery to get underway.

John and Maly Gibbon returned to Boston to work on this idea. Using their first primitive heart-lung machine, in 1935 they were able on occasions to support the circulation of a cat for periods of up to about 30 minutes, during which period the cat's own heart and lungs were not functioning. On the first occasion, they were so excited by this achievement that they danced around the laboratory together. Years later, Gibbon stated that "nothing in my life has duplicated the ecstasy and joy of that dance with Mary around the laboratory."

Given the relatively primitive materials and facilities that were available to them at that time, this was a remarkable achievement, but there was still a long way to go before the machine would be of a size and efficiency sufficient to support the life of a human. After a year's hard work in Boston, Gibbon and his wife returned to Philadelphia, he as a research fellow at the University of Pennsylvania, where the couple continued their studies.

Gibbon's work was interrupted by World War II, which he spent in the U.S. Army as a surgeon in the Pacific. Upon return from the war, he was soon appointed to the chair of surgery at Thomas Jefferson Medical College in Philadelphia, where he embarked again on the development of his machine. His main stroke of luck occurred in the late 1940s when International Business Machines (IBM) became interested in the project. Thomas J. Watson, who was the chairman of the board at IBM, provided expert personnel, in the form of consulting engineers, and the resources of his company to advise and assist in modifying Gibbon's existing machine to one that would support a human circulation. Without this support from IBM, it seems unlikely that Gibbon's machine would have been ready to be used clinically by 1953. Much credit must be given to Watson for his vision and foresight, and for his willingness to commit resources to this project without any prospect or, indeed, desire of financial return for his company.

The Gibbon-IBM heart-lung machine (Figure 25) was a substantial piece of equipment, being more than five feet long and four feet high and reputedly weighing several hundred pounds.

## First Clinical Attempts

At the time he carried out his first open heart surgical procedure, Gibbon was a general surgeon with a major interest in surgery of the lungs, but had relatively little experience of closed heart surgery, such as mitral valvotomy. His first attempt at using the machine was on a 15-month-old girl, who weighed just 11 pounds, in February 1952. Unfortunately, although he expected to find an atrial septal defect, the preoperative diagnosis was incorrect. Before he could ascertain what the problem was (actually a simple ductus that he could have dealt with, of course, without the need for a heart-lung machine), the baby died. This chastening experience impressed on Gibbon the great importance of accurate diagnosis, and stimulated him to investigate subsequent patients by cardiac catheterization before they were subjected to surgery.

His second attempt (on May 6, 1953) was successful, 18 years after his first successful bypass in a cat. His patient, Cecelia Bavolek, was an 18-year-old girl with a simple atrial septal defect (that could, of course, have been closed using the hypothermia technique of Bigelow, Lewis, and Swan). Although the operation took most of the day, the period of time that the heart-lung machine was required to support the circulation was relatively brief. The patient was connected to the apparatus for 45 minutes, but was totally dependent on it for only 26 minutes. Although almost a disaster, because the blood began to clot within the machine before Gibbon had completed the operation, the patient survived, establishing Gibbon as the foremost pioneer in the development of the heart-lung machine. He followed this operation with two further procedures using the machine, both of which were unsuccessful, either through preoperative misdiagnosis or for other reasons.

He then abandoned open heart surgery forever. I shall repeat that statement in case you, the reader, did not take it in. *He then abandoned open heart surgery forever.*

This incredible decision on his part has absolutely amazed me, and many others before me, and has been a topic of discussion among cardiac surgeons for years. Why would a man who, except for the war years, had devoted much of the past 20 years to the development of a heart-lung machine abandon its use after just four operations — only one of which had proved successful? In truth, Gibbon did not state he was abandoning open heart surgery, but he felt that a further period in the research laboratory was essential before attempting more clinical cases. Yet, at the same time, he handed over the development of heart surgery at Jefferson to younger colleagues. I believe that, in his heart of hearts, he knew he would never personally operate on a patient again using the heart-lung machine.

Why did Gibbon give up his lifetime work? Perhaps he thought his work was completed when he achieved this one success. The

Gibbon-IBM machine was then taken over by John Kirklin and the Mayo Clinic group, who, after making further modifications, were the first to use it in a truly successful series of heart operations that began in 1955 (chapter 8).

In 1967, John Gibbon retired from surgery at the age of 63, and subsequently devoted his time to painting and his many other interests. He died in 1973, at the age of 69, while playing tennis. Ironically, he had been experiencing chest pain (angina) upon exercise but refused to seek a medical opinion. Several books have been written about him and his career, and these have been a valuable source of information for me. I never met Gibbon, but I have had the opportunity of speaking with many surgeons who knew him well and/or worked with him, and thus knew of his work firsthand. These included Dr. Bernard Miller, who ran the heart-lung machine for all of Dr. Gibbon's operations; Dr. Robert Finley, who assisted in the operating room at that historic first successful operation; Dr. Anthony Dobell, who also worked with Gibbon at the time this clinical series of operations was being carried out; and Dr. John Templeton III, to whom Gibbon subsequently entrusted the heart surgery program at Jefferson.

## Gibbon and Jefferson Hospital in the 1950s

"Dr. Gibbon was noted for his research," began Dr. Anthony Dobell, "and he also undertook all of the thoracic surgery. He was really a pneumonectomist [lung surgeon], and not many heart operations were carried out at Jefferson. I used to go over to Hahnemann Hospital to watch Charlie Bailey [a fact he kept secret from Gibbon, who did not exactly approve of Bailey, who was considered rather "beyond the pale" by the Philadelphia surgical elite], who was doing much more heart surgery. Somehow I knew that heart surgery was going to come. I knew that Dr. Gibbon had done all of this work with the heart-lung machine but, surprisingly, a lot of the other fellows at Jefferson didn't even know this. His research into the heart-lung machine was almost a separate part of his life from his clinical work.

"He was one of those surgeons, like Churchill and Blalock before him, who believed that surgery was one specialty, and he didn't want to separate off little bits of it. He didn't want to become a cardiac or even a cardiothoracic surgeon. He could encompass everything that was known in surgery. However, it was the end of that era, and his attitude was clearly wrong. Specialization led to enormous progress.

"He was a very busy man who gave excellent clinical care, but I do not think he knew most of his patients terribly well. As a technical surgeon, he had a tendency to make operations very complicated. There were too many movements in his procedures. He was not as good a surgeon as some of his colleagues. Gibbon was more of a cerebral surgeon.

"There wasn't a whole lot of heart surgery at Jefferson. I am not even sure that anyone looked at pathological specimens of hearts to prepare for the open heart surgery. The idea was that we would just open the heart and fix it. We would find the hole and close it. It was pretty naive. I always thought it was extraordinary that they didn't look at pathological specimens before beginning this series of experiments. One of the surgical residents, Bob Johnson, did heart catheterizations. He used a ureteral [a type of urinary bladder] catheter for the procedures. It was totally primitive, but that's the way it was then."

In a published lecture given by Dr. Dobell in 1989, he highlighted the primitive conditions under which this first series of heart operations was performed: "The public wards at Jefferson in this era were modeled after those designed by Florence Nightingale for St. Thomas' Hospital in London, and quite similar to the wards that existed in America from the time of the Civil War. The wards consisted of 40 beds — 20 on each side of a long cavernous chamber; the beds were a specified distance from each other, head to the wall, feet to the central passageway. The nurses' desk at the ward entrance allowed the nurses close access to the sickest patients . . . it was to such a ward that Dr. Gibbon's famous [first] patient, Cecelia, was brought after her operation."

The problem with the early cases Gibbon attempted, Dr. Dobell explained, "was, first, incorrect diagnosis. One of them had a huge ductus that was the cause of an awful lot of blood spurting into the field. The second problem was anesthesia, which was primitive at Jefferson at that time. The routine was that the surgeon himself intubated the patient [passed a breathing tube into the patient's throat] while the patient was awake, and then the nurse anesthetist would administer some pentothal [a sleeping drug]. Some of the cases took a long time. In the first successful case, I think you will find the operation began at 8 A.M. but they didn't go onto the heart-lung machine until about 12 noon. The team hadn't worked together. I am sure that if Bernie Miller or John Templeton [two of Dr. Gibbon's assistants] had done the operation, it would have all been over quickly. Instead, of course, Dr. Gibbon quite rightfully did the operation himself.

"The fact is that the operations were pretty chaotic. The amazing thing is that one patient survived, which was a near-thing because the heart-lung machine clotted up. Towards the end of the pump run, as the pump was no longer oxygenating the patient, Bernie Miller had to leave the operating table, where he was helping Dr. Gibbon, to try to resuscitate the heart-lung machine. The blood was clotting, as they hadn't given enough heparin. It's surprising that she survived. When you think of the Mayo Clinic [chapter 8] or the Minnesota [chapter 7] groups who reviewed pathological specimens and developed superb teamwork so they could do the operations quickly, there is an enormous contrast."

## The Married Couple

Although the research of Gibbon and his wife has become a legend in surgical circles, it is perhaps something of a myth. All credit must go to them for getting the project off the ground, but the contributions of others seem to have been largely overlooked. Although a methodical investigator, according to Dr. Dobell, "Gibbon wasn't a 'gadgeteer' and didn't like to play with tools, and yet that's just what it took to develop a heart-lung machine." In this respect, he received very significant help from others.

Dr. Dobell related, "There is no doubt the Gibbons were very, very close as a couple, and there is no doubt that she was intimately involved with the heart-lung machine from the beginning, but when I worked in the laboratory, I never saw Dr. Gibbon or Mrs. Gibbon. The lab was run by Bernie Miller. But this was much later in the development of the machine. I doubt that she [Maly] had been around in the laboratory in recent years, probably not since he moved to Jefferson. Her help was mostly in Boston and then perhaps at the University of Pennsylvania after Dr. Gibbon came back from the war.

"She was his alter ego in the surgical firmament. Their friends, by and large, were surgeons, the leaders of American surgery. She went with him to every meeting. They were at the center of whatever was going on. He and she loved meeting people, and loved the people they were associating with. Dr. Gibbon was a total liberal and a sort of ecumenical. He just liked everything. Gibbon wasn't a 'buddy, buddy' type of person, although he was a good friend to me, but he talked to me as an equal, which was kind of a funny experience at first. He would ask me what I thought about things, as he did the other residents. We hadn't been brought up to be asked by the chairman of the department what we thought. Mrs. Gibbon had the same outlook as he. They were certainly a team, just like Marie and Pierre Curie. They were always together, but I never got the idea that the heart-lung machine dominated their lives. What dominated their lives was the leadership in surgery. By this, I do not mean he was an ambitious person in that respect. He just liked meeting with others in surgery at that time. I wouldn't have thought he had great ambition. Of course, he achieved the presidency of this and that because he was one of the dominant surgical educators; I don't think it was because he had developed the heart-lung machine.

"His whole family was pretty close. They were very creative. The parties they held were incredible — charades, poems, very quick-witted, very artistic, dancing, ballet dancing, and so on. They were a very creative family."

Why did Dr. Gibbon give up open heart surgery so quickly, I asked Dr. Dobell, particularly as he had spent so many years developing it?

"I think he wanted to show that a patient's life could be supported by the heart-lung machine. I don't think he ever wanted to become a heart surgeon, and so I think he felt he had done what he had set out to do. Of course, he wasn't the 'father of heart surgery,' as he is sometimes billed. Heart surgery didn't take off after his few operations. He didn't do anything that couldn't be done by other techniques at the time, for example, by hypothermia. It was Lillehei and Kirklin who developed heart surgery.... Gibbon wasn't that tough. Lillehei, for example, was very tough and could accept the risks."

George Humphreys, a surgeon who knew Gibbon well, put the matter succinctly: "He wanted the credit, which he got deservedly, in view of the many years he had worked on it. That really satisfied him. That's why he stopped doing it. The others were taking the risks and killing the babies, and he didn't like that."

Willem Kolff (chapter 13), who was also close to Gibbon, agreed that Gibbon "couldn't bear" the deaths, and added that they had upset him so much that "he didn't want to see the machine anymore."

Lael Wertenbaker quotes a rather indignant Dwight Harken on this topic: "All of us who have done firsts and gone on and lost lives and spent a good deal of our own lives to create new things realize what it is like to go through all that. We also know the feeling of triumph as well as the feeling of defeat and we resent it when a man does just one successful case and quits! One patient lives and you *can't* just sit down and say, 'Now I've done it, that's it, that's my contribution.' You are *obliged* to standardize the technique so as to serve others."

Most of those I spoke to believed that Gibbon deserved the great deal of credit he has been given as the developer of the heart-lung machine — but not everybody. Heart transplant pioneer Norman Shumway thought that Gibbon's contribution to open heart surgery was "negligible.... It's kind of a wonderful story. When he saw this patient die of a pulmonary embolus, he was stimulated to think that extracorporeal circulation might have saved her. A lot of people were thinking about artificial oxygenators.... Of course, Gibbon marrying his laboratory technician, and their working together as a family unit, and finally achieving success, is a lovely story, but I don't think it amounts to much."

I asked Dr. Shumway why, then, Gibbon had such a revered position in surgical history. Was it simply because of his social background and connections?

"Yes. He had all that, and he was a very aristocratic character. He had a lot of the aura that Blalock had. He had a lovely, modulated voice. I heard him give a presidential address in 1955. It was a very nice talk, without much meat in it, but elegant. He was part of the aristocracy of surgery in those days."

## Bernie Miller and the Chink in the Armour

I asked Dr. Dobell to tell me something about the other people who worked with Gibbon at that time.

"Bernie Miller was trained as a surgeon at Jefferson in general and thoracic surgery. He was a very, very bright person. He was practicing surgery and running the lab for Dr. Gibbon. He eventually went to Chestnut Hill Hospital in northern Philadelphia and developed a practice in general surgery."

What Dr. Dobell did not tell me, but what is described in Harris Shumacker's book on Gibbon, *A Dream of the Heart,* is that Bernie Miller left Gibbon's laboratory under adverse circumstances. Subsequently, in 2002, I contacted Dr. Miller by telephone and sought out his reminiscences of his time with Dr. Gibbon and, in particular, the circumstances of his leaving Gibbon's team. Here are some excerpts from our discussion:

"I became Dr. Gibbon's research assistant in 1950. I had just started a practice in general surgery and thoracic surgery. I was his research associate for about five years. During that five-year period, I would spend the afternoons and evenings taking care of things in the laboratory, and the mornings doing surgery at Germantown and also at Jefferson. I was in charge of the laboratory and of the design, development, and testing of the first heart-lung machine that was used successfully. I was doing about three experiments in dogs each week.

"IBM gave Dr. Gibbon the support of its laboratories and three engineers. The first machine that IBM built was just a stainless steel version of Dr. Gibbon's original design, with a larger cylinder for greater oxygen to pass through. They finally came up with a machine with two components to it. One component, of course, was the heart-lung machine itself. The second component was a power supply cabinet that permitted the device to operate on batteries in the event of a general electric failure. This was right after the war and this was in everybody's mind. I don't think the development of a machine of that quality could have been done without the help of IBM. The workmanship was absolutely beautiful.

"I did all the experimental work. I made several modifications to the machine. I did all the design work, doing all the work in the lab, and ran the pump in his clinical cases. Gibbon did nothing except attend conferences between us and the engineers. Dr. Gibbon and I got along well for a very long time. He called me in one day, and said, 'BJ, you're doing all the work here. I'm going to make you 'co-investigator.' That thought had never occurred to me. The next day he came in, and said, 'I've thought it over, and I think we will wait for that.' He had probably discussed it with Maly, his wife, who would come in every now and then and assist me operating on the dogs. She was really no contribution at all. The first paper I published with him, he asked me if I wouldn't mind if I included her name. I said, 'Sure.' I was very anxious to get along with him. I didn't care. When we came close to doing the first patient, Gibbon came down to the lab to get used to what was going on. He operated on one dog, unsuccessfully. That's all he did.

"In the first successful case, Gibbon and Allbritten [Frank Allbritten, Gibbon's junior colleague] were doing the surgery, and there was the resident assisting. Had it not been for the automatic controls, which I had designed, she would not have survived. When the blood began to clot, the arterial pump was automatically shut down. That really saved her life."

I asked Dr. Miller how he and his colleagues felt immediately after the first successful case.

"We were pleased with everything, but Dr. Gibbon never gave me or the laboratory people any recognition, you know, for what we had done for him. I know for the first and second cases, Mrs. Gibbon came to the operating room that morning with a number of press releases in the event that the operation would be a successful one. They came prepared to announce this worldwide.

"I want to let you know that I resigned. The reason for that was that a number of people from the Junior Chamber of Commerce who had been aware of my role in the development of the heart-lung machine decided to elect me as one of the ten outstanding young men of the year. That was 1954. I was only 34 years of age. And the press at that time called me the 'co-inventor,' which was wrong. They never had that information. That, of course, ruffled his feathers. It was released in *Time,* and in the newspapers. They were supposed to indicate that I had conducted a lot of the experimental work and the development, so you couldn't call me 'co-inventor.' He [Gibbon] confronted me with Allbritten. Dr. Gibbon and I had had a wonderful relationship during this four or five years. I was very surprised that he should be so upset about this. I think [he took such a stance] at the urging of Dr. Allbritten.... I declined the award of the Junior Chamber of Commerce. But, after that, I couldn't continue, and I resigned. My relationship with Dr. Gibbon was strained. That's why I resigned. After I left, the laboratory really almost ceased to exist in a formal way."

I asked Dr. Miller how badly this incident had affected his future career. Did he take a long time to get over this setback with Gibbon?

"I never really did, because I was knocked out of open heart surgery. I never gave up surgery. I remained in thoracic and vascular surgery, and some of the early cardiac surgery—ductuses and that kind of thing. I had a huge practice in surgery, but I never did surgery that required the heart-lung machine."

In answer to a question of mine, Dr. Miller believed that he did not get the recognition he deserved. From my reading and discussions with others, I am inclined to agree with him. I hope this book will help communicate and establish the important role he played.

## Gibbon's Strengths

It is generally agreed that Gibbon was a superb teacher and a good clinician, and did an excellent job of running his department. According to Robert Finley, "His approach to any problem was that it was a soluble problem. When people asked him something, his usual reply would be, 'Yes, we can do this.' 'I can do this.' 'That can be done.' He would then scramble around and try to figure out how to do it. I think the other thing that stands out was his optimism. He always felt that things would be fine. They would work out. The patient would get better. The problem would be solved. We had made a step in the right direction, and so on. People really liked him because he really liked people. They wanted to talk to him, wanted to tell him about this and that, show him, and hear him. He would say, 'Hey, that's really interesting,' or 'Oh, that's good,' that sort of thing. Encouraging. He was an encouraging, supportive, optimistic person. He was terribly honest about himself. If a patient had a complication, he would say that he had made a mistake. He had exquisite 'integrity'—that is the word I was looking for."

How to conclude the story of John Gibbon? Perhaps in the words of Clarence Crafoord, spoken at a meeting planned to celebrate the 20th anniversary of Gibbon's sole successful case, but which in fact was tempered by the fact that Gibbon had died suddenly a few weeks earlier: "To me he stands out as one of the great figures of our time who eminently deserved the many honors and distinctions bestowed upon him during the latter part of his life. I have strongly supported his nomination as Nobel Prize winner, but as perhaps you know, the Prize is very seldom awarded in recognition for work performed in the fields of clinical medicine or surgery.... I will always remember Jack Gibbon as one of the noblest, most consistently straightforward, honest and loyal friends I have known. I will never cease to admire his intelligence, his spirit of discovery, his great working capacity, and the quality of his leadership."

## VIKING BJORK AND AKE SENNING — THE SECOND SUCCESSFUL OPERATION AND THE SECOND GREAT FEUD

While the development of heart surgery, particularly of open heart surgery, is predominantly a North American story, there were Europeans who were not very far behind in pushing forward in this field. Viking Bjork (Figure 26) and Ake Senning (Figure 27) are two of the few non–North Americans who played a significant role in the development of open heart surgery. Although their names are paired here, as they were the major contributors to the development of the heart-lung machine that Clarence Crafoord (Figure 3) used to perform the first successful open heart operation in Europe — the world's second successful such operation — they were serious rivals throughout life. Their "feud" was not the public debacle of the Bailey-Harken feud, and perhaps did not have the bitterness of the DeBakey-Cooley feud (chapter 13), but it would appear to have been more than just intense competition between two highly ambitious young men.

Their rivalry began at an early age, when they were in Crafoord's department in Stockholm, competing for the position of Crafoord's right-hand man, with Senning becoming the "favored son." Subsequently, after Bjork had taken the chair of surgery in Uppsala and Senning the chair in Zurich, everybody believed there would be a showdown over who would fill Crafoord's place at the Karolinska Institute upon his retirement. In the event, Senning, who was probably

Crafoord's preferred candidate, decided to remain in Zurich, and Bjork was appointed. According to Erik Berglund, who knew both men, Senning was technically extremely good and easy to get on with and, had he applied, would probably have been appointed when Crafoord retired. Bjork, on the other hand, was a more difficult person to work with but was very determined. Thereafter, Bjork's star continued to soar for many years, whereas Senning perhaps faded rather earlier from the international limelight in cardiothoracic surgery. Perhaps, however, this impression of mine is a result of the lower international profile Senning maintained compared with the more outgoing Bjork, who was more noticeably in the surgical public eye.

During my surgical training in the United Kingdom, I heard Bjork speak at several surgical meetings when he was at the height of his career. He was of short-to-medium height, and had dark hair and glasses. His presentations were always clear and rather forceful, and he obviously enjoyed putting across information based on his experience. Bjork was enough of a showman for his lectures to capture his audiences' attention. Throughout his career, he must have been hardworking, since both he personally and his department were always productive. For several years, he was among the leaders in cardiac surgery, with an excellent reputation.

In contrast, Ake Senning was tall and elegant, even debonair; like Gibbon, he was handsome as a young man and distinguished when older, with his tall, straight-backed carriage, well-groomed wavy gray hair, and sartorial elegance. His personality, however, could not have been more different from that of Bjork. Senning was much more reserved, and certainly less of a showman. He was very innovative in his early career when he was Crafoord's chief assistant in Stockholm, where he made several important contributions that enabled successful open heart surgery to get started. After his move to Zurich as chief of cardiothoracic surgery in 1961, he was perhaps rather less innovative, though he continued to introduce new approaches, such as the use of natural human tissue taken from the leg (fascia lata) to fashion new heart valves. Nevertheless, Senning's early innovations alone earned him the right to be included among the pioneers of heart surgery.

## VIKING BJORK

As early as the 1940s, Viking Bjork (Figure 26) was closely involved in the development of a machine that was a predecessor to the heart-lung machine, which he used experimentally to perfuse the brains of dogs. Although not directly involved in the first successful open heart operation in Europe (carried out by Crafoord and Senning in Stockholm), he was responsible for confirming the diagnosis in the first patient; he had previously developed a technique for measuring the pressures within the left ventricle and for taking radiographs (X-rays) to demonstrate its anatomy.

By the early 1950s, the work of Forssmann, Cournand, and Richards had established right heart catheterization — in which the pressures in the right atrium, right ventricle, and lungs could be measured — but there was no method of directly measuring the pressures in the chambers of the left side of the heart. Bjork's technique of "left heart catheterization," to measure the pressures within the left atrium and left ventricle, was a dramatic one — innovative and bold, and not without significant risk. It involved blindly sticking a seven-inch-long (18 cm) needle through the chest wall of the back of the patient until it entered the heart. Amazingly, this seemingly very risky procedure was carried out largely without untoward complication.

He followed this up with another technique in which, with the investigator looking down a long metal tube (a bronchoscope) that had been passed through the mouth into the major airway to the lungs (the trachea), a long needle was passed down the bronchoscope through the wall of the airway into the heart (which is situated just beneath the airway) — another hair-raising approach. In an equally bold technique developed by others, the needle was passed from the root of the neck consecutively through the aorta and pulmonary artery into the left atrium. Subsequently, these techniques were replaced by the current catheter techniques whereby the catheter is introduced into an artery, usually in the groin, pushed up into the aorta, and then into the left side of the heart. By enabling studies of the left side of the heart, Bjork's initial techniques, however, played an important role in the early development of heart surgery.

Bjork subsequently left Stockholm to set up an excellent cardiac surgical program in Uppsala before returning (upon Crafoord's retirement) as professor at the Karolinska Hospital, the leading medical center in Scandinavia. He also contributed significantly toward the design of a mechanical heart valve, the Bjork-Shiley prosthesis, that at one time became the most widely used prosthetic valve in the world.

I spoke with him by telephone one Sunday morning in April 1999, some years after he had retired from surgery. At nearly 80 years old, he tended to meander around the point to some extent, and it was difficult both to interrupt him and to get him to answer questions succintly. It was equally difficult to direct him toward a new subject. Bjork seemed reluctant to give judgment and/or opinion on others, and I noted that his wife (who was clearly sitting in the room with him) cautioned him once or twice about doing so. My impression, from what was admittedly a very brief interaction with him, was of a rather self-centered man who perhaps didn't remember much — or didn't want to remember much — about the work of others. Furthermore, there was a certain lack of humor in his answers.

## Youth and Education

Viking Bjork was born in 1918 in a village called Sunnansjo in the middle of Sweden. His father owned a sawmill and a forest, and the young Viking worked in the sawmill in the summers, and sometimes in the forest. After three years in the local school, his father was not convinced that the education he was receiving was satisfactory. Arrangements were made for a private teacher to teach Viking and three other local children.

According to Bjork, "Because of my dyslexia, it was very hard work for me. But after those three years with the private teacher, I could 'jump over' a year. But then I had to continue the same hard way. I finished school at eighteen. After I finished school in August 1937, the family had a meeting to discuss what I should be. There were a lot of economic problems for the sawmill in those days, and so they discussed what was best for the family. At the end of the discussion, my mother asked me, 'Whatever would you be if you didn't have to take any notice of the economy?' Thinking of my interest in biology and, in particular, in the blood circulation, I said, 'I would like to be a doctor.' With that, she said, 'Well, it's decided.'"

The young Viking Bjork studied at Uppsala University for two and a half years, after which he transferred to Lund University. He observed, "The surgical professor at Lund was new, and a new professor is always interested in teaching, and so I was very fortunate. I finished medical school in 1944."

In 1942, during World War II, Bjork won a scholarship to study the treatment of tuberculosis in Italy, after which he returned to Sweden for further surgical training before accepting another scholarship offered by the British Council.

In the book *One for the Heart,* author Gerald Derloshon recounts the difficulty that Dr. Bjork had in traveling to England during wartime. It was arranged for him to fly in a military DC-3 airplane. The route to London was over Norway, where German anti-aircraft artillery was very active on clear nights. Clear weather prevented the plane from taking off for an entire month. Finally, however, Dr. Bjork reached London safely and rented a room with a "landlady," where he recalled that rationed meat was served only on Sundays. The landlady was evidently suspicious that Dr. Bjork was a spy, mainly because he had been to Italy earlier during the war. I must admit to being surprised that Dr. Bjork had studied in both Italy and England during World War II, with the two countries being on opposite sides, which dramatically demonstrated the neutrality of Sweden in this conflict, compared with most of the rest of Europe.

"I went to London in January 1945," he told me, "and spent fourteen months at the Royal Brompton Hospital. I was a clinical assistant to Russell Brock, but it was his colleague, Clement Price Thomas, who later operated on King George the Sixth [who had lung cancer], who spent more time with me." Brock had not started doing any pulmonary or mitral valve surgery at that stage, and so Bjork spent much of his time at the Royal Brompton Hospital studying cancer of the lung.

Crafoord and his engineer colleague, Emil Andersson, had visited Gibbon's laboratory in 1939 and, stimulated by this, began their work on the heart-lung machine during the war years. Andersson gradually produced an experimental model, which Crafoord entrusted to Bjork for further testing and improvement. On his return to Sweden, this heart-lung machine became the prototype of all subsequent "disc oxygenators," a form of "filmer" oxygenator.

## The Primitive Heart-Lung Machine

"It was soon clear to us that Gibbon was on the wrong track," Bjork explained to me, "because he couldn't get enough blood oxygenated in his rotating cylinder [which was the type of oxygenator that Gibbon was working on at that time, and that preceded his vertical screen oxygenator]. The engineer I worked with, Emil Andersson, has the credit for the solution.... We arranged to have several discs rotating within a pool of blood [Figure 28]. By adding more discs [and thus increasing the surface of blood for oxygen exchange], I could get more blood oxygenated.... For a pump, I used a milking machine. A milking machine must be nice to the cow, so I thought it should be nice to the red blood cells, and it was.... Finally, I perfused for half an hour when I completely stopped the heart. All of the work was in 1947. That first heart-lung machine had a spinning disc oxygenator and two milking machine pumps. Based on my thesis, a firm in America made this heart-lung machine. Dennis in Minnesota, Gerbode in San Francisco, and Melrose in London subsequently all built disc oxygenators.

"Then I got a scholarship to go to America for a year—the Swedish American scholarship. I traveled all over. Senning took over my research place in Stockholm. When I came back in the fall of 1950 from the United States, I was not allowed to use the research lab at the Sabbatsberg [Hospital], so I had to go over to the Karolinska Hospital to do research.

"The problem was that I had some competition. Another boy from the same district as I [referring to Ake Senning—see below] was also a very good and energetic man. He tried to redo my experiments, but he didn't do them as carefully as I, and so he spread the rumor that I must have lied. He said it wasn't true what I had written. After that, people didn't trust me. By 1953, my reputation in research became very bad in Stockholm. He was, in fact, a very good fellow. He said he had proved that the discs would not be useful. Instead, he combined a rotating drum with a bubble oxygenator. With those two, they were able to do the first open heart surgery in Stockholm.

"That was a patient with a myxoma [a benign tumor] in the left atrium. Crafoord did the surgery. I had diagnosed it. I had performed a complete left heart catheterization. I put a needle into the left atrium and injected contrast [in order to demonstrate the anatomy by X-ray pictures]. They were very nice pictures, but the pictures disappeared. I haven't been able to include them in any of my papers. So there were these kinds of complications between two people."

## Later Career

Bjork continued, "During that time, I saw how wonderful it was to be independent. I therefore applied to get the job in Uppsala because, if you're a chief, you can only blame yourself. I opened a new clinic [in Uppsala] in 1958. Then I could work free and get my own oxygenator going. Senning applied to Uppsala, but he had no chance compared to me. They looked very much on the quality of papers produced, and I got that job. I was never angry with him because everyone is different as human beings, and there is nothing to be angry about. We are here for patients, and not for fighting with each other. Senning took the Zurich job. I didn't even ask for it.

"In 1964, when Crafoord had to retire, he was on the board for decisions [regarding his successor]. He tried to get another man [Senning] the job. I told you that, when I was a student, I went to Lund because there was a new professor who was interested in teaching. By this time, he was the dean of the Karolinska Hospital. He was the one who would lead the group in its decisions. He remembered a little article I had written when his student, and decided that they had to look more closely at me. He asked outside professors to give their opinions at the same time as Crafoord. They were definitely on my side. I got the honor of being called chief in Stockholm — just because he remembered that I had written a little article as his student."

During his later career, Bjork played a major role in clinical trials relating to a new valve prosthesis designed by an American engineer named Don Shiley, which for several years was used extensively and very successfully by surgeons throughout the world to replace the aortic and mitral valves. He died in 2009 at age 90.

## AKE SENNING

Ake Senning (Figure 27), Bjork's arch-rival in Stockholm in the early days, followed up on Bjork's early research work and developed a pump-oxygenator that was first used in a patient only a few months after John Gibbon's historic operation in Philadelphia.

I spoke with him by telephone at his home in Zurich in 1998 when he was 83 years old. His memory remained excellent. His answers to my questions were direct and precise, with little elaboration or embellishment, which contrasted markedly with Bjork's rather long-winded answers. As a result, our interview was through rather quickly. At times, I feared I was putting ideas into his head, but it appeared to be the only way to seek out his opinions. He came across as a straightforward man, but with little humor or personality. (Indeed, I had previously sat near him at dinner on one occasion, and he had hardly said a word.) It is clearly difficult to judge someone on the basis of one telephone conversation, but this was my impression. Sadly, I heard of his death in 2000.

## Youth and Education

Senning was born in 1915 in a village, Rativik, not very far from Bjork's birthplace. His father was a veterinarian and his mother a nurse. After schooling locally and in Uppsala, he studied medicine in Uppsala and Stockholm. Although he wished to become an engineer, his mother influenced him to go into medicine. His studies were disrupted for a time, as he developed tuberculosis.

"On the thirtieth of November, 1939," he reminisced, "the Russians bombed Helsinki, without warning. I thought they will come to Sweden, and [because he thought surgeons would be needed] I went to the surgical clinic.... During my surgical training, I came to Crafoord as an assistant in surgery. That's what influenced me to go into thoracic surgery."

## Development of the Heart-Lung Machine

"After some months with Crafoord," Senning continued, "he sent me to the experimental department [in 1948] and told me I had to work on the heart-lung machine. Three years after I started with the whole thing, I got the first dogs to survive. In 1951, Gibbon visited us in Stockholm. We put a dog on the heart-lung machine for one hour. That was the best for those days. He saw this operation, and the next day the dog went to Mrs. Gibbon, and was waving its tail and looked in good condition.

"Initially I had a rotating disc oxygenator. [This was Bjork's oxygenator, but Dr. Senning did not mention this.] I later changed these discs to cylinders because these needed very little blood.... Then we introduced hypothermia so the consumption of oxygen was very much smaller. Then the dogs started to survive. But they died when I opened the left side of the heart. I found out that this was from air emboli [air bubbles that went to the brain and other organs and caused severe injury]. When I introduced temporary ventricular fibrillation [i.e., when he purposely prevented the heart from beating in a coordinated fashion by applying a small electric shock], the heart stood still during the operation, and then the dogs survived [because the heart could not expel the air in it to the brain]. After I had introduced hypothermia and cardiac 'standstill,' the machine was suitable for use in a human."

In these few brief sentences, Dr. Senning had described to me two of his most important innovations that were to have a profound impact on open heart surgery for many years, even today.

The first was his concept of combining cooling the patient with use of the heart-lung machine. The idea of combining these two approaches arose after Senning learned of the benefits of cooling the body from Bigelow. Most of the early researchers in this field, notably Dennis and Gibbon, and many others who followed, determined that the combination of the heart-lung machine and hypothermia would be detrimental to the outcome, rather than beneficial. This was probably related to the fact that the heart-lung machine can be associated with detrimental changes in body chemistry, as can hypothermia. The two together, therefore, might lead to further detrimental changes, thus perhaps complicating the patient's management. On the other hand, the combination can be very beneficial. The art was in obtaining the benefits without the detriments. Senning appears to have been able to do this successfully.

He first placed the anesthetized patient in iced water on a plastic sheet until the body temperature was 30°C (86°F), and only then connected the heart-lung machine. The efficiency of his heart-lung machine was insufficient to meet the oxygen demands of an adult patient at normal body temperature, but it was sufficient if the oxygen needs of the patient were reduced by hypothermia. At the end of the operation, the patient would be rewarmed by warm water. For later operations, the temperature was reduced to 26 to 28°C (79 to 82°F).

The second innovation was his use of inducing arrest of the heart (by inducing ventricular fibrillation) to prevent the serious, often lethal, complication of air bubbles to the brain (air embolism) that marred many of the early open heart operations, and is still a risk today. When the heart is opened while it is beating, any air that enters the left side of the heart will be pumped through the aortic valve into the aorta and up into the arteries supplying the brain, where the large air bubbles damage the brain by preventing blood from reaching it. Senning caused the heart to stop beating by stimulating it with a low electric current that caused the ventricles to fibrillate; i.e., the muscle fibers no longer contracted together, but contracted individually in an uncoordinated and inefficient fashion. Although air would enter the left side of the heart, it could not be pumped out of the heart to the brain because the heart was no longer beating. Before closing the heart, the air would be evacuated, its place to be taken by blood, and the heart would then be started by a larger electrical shock (defibrillation). Unlike the initial small shock that caused the heart to stop contracting in a coordinated fashion (by inducing ventricular fibrillation), the larger shock would overcome or reverse this state and initiate normal beating again. This was a simple but important advance, since air embolism was a major problem in the early days of open heart surgery. Furthermore, since the heart was no longer beating while being fibrillated, but was quiescent, this made the surgery easier for the surgeon.

When I asked Dr. Senning what he considered to be his major contribution to heart surgery, he chose the introduction of ventricular fibrillation to get the heart to stand still to avoid air emboli. He said, "That was a good idea, I thought." Indeed, even Bjork agreed that this was an important contribution, stating that Senning's "thesis was very intelligent."

Later, however, it was found that the induction of ventricular fibrillation, particularly if it was sustained for any length of time, had some detrimental effects on the heart muscle, particularly when the muscle was thickened (or hypertrophic) from the stress of trying to pump blood through an obstructed valve over many years. The state of ventricular fibrillation impaired the blood flow to the heart muscle through the smaller coronary arteries, and this could lead to severe, sometimes fatal, damage to the muscle during the course of the operation. Therefore, ventricular fibrillation had to be used judiciously. Although it proved invaluable in the early days, it was eventually, like so much else in medicine, superseded by something better (chapter 8).

The combination of circulatory support by the heart-lung machine, the protection afforded by total body hypothermia, and electrical cardiac arrest by inducing ventricular fibrillation indicated very advanced thinking for that era, way ahead of Gibbon's comparatively simple concept. Senning and Crafoord were clearly the undoubted masters of the field at that time.

Senning even introduced one further important innovative concept at the time. Whenever he needed to clamp the aorta, and thus prevent flow of blood to the coronary arteries in order to see more clearly what he was doing inside the heart, he would cover the surface of the heart with ice slush, lowering its temperature further, and thus protecting the muscle from the temporary lack of oxygen. Norman Shumway was eventually to popularize this approach, known as "local hypothermia" or "local hypothermic arrest," but it seems that Senning preempted him. Senning was clearly a very innovative man, and, outside of Sweden, has probably not received the recognition he deserves.

I asked Dr. Senning what previous work had been undertaken on heart-lung machines in Europe.

"Crafoord had worked with an oxygenator for the brain. He intended to do pulmonary embolectomies." I believed Dr. Senning was referring to the work in which Bjork had been involved. It was interesting that he referred to this as Crafoord's work without giving any credit to Bjork, and also did not mention that it had any relevance toward the development of a true heart-lung machine. I decided to pursue this point by asking him where he saw Professor Bjork in the Stockholm story. "He worked with the perfusion machine for the brain," he replied. I asked whether, at that stage, they saw this work as a preliminary to open heart surgery. "I think you could say so. It was Crafoord's idea with these rotating discs, and so that was the oxygenator." (In his writings, Dr. Senning referred to the oxygenator as the "Crafoord-Andersson disc oxygenator," omitting any mention of Bjork.)

I followed up by asking whether the oxygenater Dr. Senning worked with was based on this prototype.

"Based on that, we can say. But I started after Bjork. He did not wish to continue. He wished to go to the United States. When I took over, he said, 'In ten years, you will not do it.'"

I asked what he saw as Dr. Bjork's major contribution.

"Honestly, I don't know."

Dr. Senning was obviously reluctant to give any credit to Bjork for his contributions toward the early development of the Swedish heart-lung machine, and so I returned to the story of open heart surgery in Stockholm.

## The First Patients

The first use of the machine was in July 1954, on a woman who, at the time of my discussion with Senning, was still living more than 40 years later. "She is now eighty-nine, I think," said Senning. "She had symptoms of mitral stenosis. She had a big myxoma [a benign or nonmalignant tumor] in the left atrium. With the exception of Gibbon's patient with an atrial septal defect, I think this was the first successful [open heart operation using a heart-lung machine] in the world. William Cleland's team [in London] tried a few cases in 1953, but they all died. I was with Lillehei in March 1954. One month after I left, he did the first case of cross-circulation [chapter 7]. He began to use the bubble oxygenator in October 1955. Kirklin also started in 1955."

In Stockholm's first group of patients, approximately one-third died.

"I think we had a mortality of 35%. The patients we were choosing at that time were Fallots, atrial septal defects, and similar cases.

I think our group in Stockholm eventually did a total of four hundred atrial septal defects [one of the more straightforward operations] with only one patient who had temporary hemiplegia [a transient "stroke," probably from air embolism]. That was our only complication."

These were outstandingly good results for that era.

## The First Implantable Cardiac Pacemaker

One other significant contribution that Senning made to the development of heart surgery was by inserting the first completely implantable pacemaker, in 1958. Previously, electrical leads had been placed in the muscle of the heart and brought out through the skin, where they were attached to an external battery or other device that provided the electrical impulses for pacing. A pacemaker that included a small battery, and could therefore be placed entirely in the body, was developed by Rune Elmqvist in Sweden, and Senning performed this first operation. Although today insertion of a pacemaker is a simple operation, the electrical lead being passed down a vein into the inside of the right ventricle and the pacemaker "box" (battery) being implanted just under the skin, in 1958 it was a much more extensive operation. The chest was opened to expose the heart, the leads sutured directly to the heart muscle, and the "box," containing the battery power supply, was placed under the wall of the abdomen.

Senning's patient on that first occasion, a 43-year-old man named Arne Larsson, had undergone up to a staggering 30 cardiac arrests requiring resuscitation *each day* during the previous few days. As Senning initially did not feel the pacemaker was quite ready for use in humans, it was the patient's wife who cajoled him into performing the operation. Despite replacement of the pacemaker battery on numerous subsequent occasions, the patient was certainly alive 30 years later. A very successful businessman both before and after his operation, he was elected to the presidency of the Swedish Association for Heart and Lung Disease in the 1980s.

From this beginning in 1958, the number of completely implantable pacemakers rose steadily until, by 1981, more than 100,000 were being implanted worldwide each year.

Ake Senning died in 2000, at age 84.

AND SO THESE MEN — Gibbon, Dennis, Crafoord, Bjork, Senning, and several others — provided the background work for the great leap forward that was to take place in 1954 and 1955 through the series of operations performed not only by the Swedish group, but also by the two Minnesota teams led by C. Walton Lillehei (in Minneapolis) (chapter 7) and John Kirklin (in Rochester) (chapter 8). Lillehei's pioneering work, in particular, was one of the boldest surgical steps taken by any surgeon in the long history of medicine.

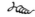

**Figure 1:** Diagram of the normal structure and blood flow though the heart and major blood vessels. "Blue" blood (containing a low level of oxygen) (black arrows) returning from the body passes into a "collecting chamber" (the right atrium), from which it passes through the tricuspid valve into a "pumping chamber" (the right ventricle), which pumps it through the pulmonary valve into the pulmonary artery and thus into the lungs. After picking up oxygen and releasing carbon dioxide in the lungs, "pink" blood (with a high level of oxygen) (gray arrows) returns to the left atrium, then passes through the mitral valve into the left ventricle, from which it is pumped through the aortic valve into the aorta and around the body.

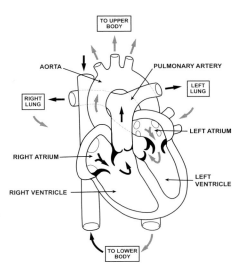

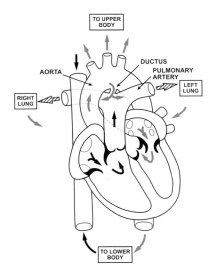

Figure 2: Robert Gross

Figure 3: Clarence Crafoord

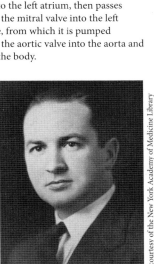

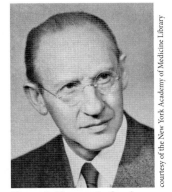

**Figure 4:** Basic structure and blood flow through the heart and major blood vessels in the presence of a patent (persistent) ductus arteriosus (an abnormal connection between the aorta and pulmonary artery). Blood passes from the high-pressure aorta into the low-pressure pulmonary artery, resulting in an abnormally increased blood flow through the lungs. Eventually the lungs become "waterlogged" and/or the left ventricle begins to fail through the extra work it is doing. The operation that Gross carried out to correct the condition involved passing a heavy thread around the ductus and tying it closed (ligation). (Black arrows = "blue" blood, with low oxygen content; gray arrows = "pink" blood, with high oxygen content; striped arrows = mixed blood)

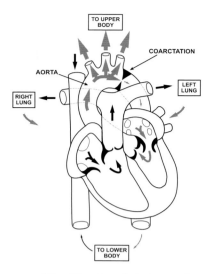

**Figure 5:** Basic structure and blood flow through the heart and major blood vessels in the presence of a coarctation (narrowing or obstruction) of the aorta. The complete or partial obstruction in the aorta leads to a dangerously high blood pressure in the upper part of the body and a poor blood flow to the lower part. Eventually, the high blood pressure in the head leads to rupture of a blood vessel in the brain and/or to failure of the left ventricle through the strain of pumping against the obstruction. The operation performed by Crafoord involves clamping the aorta above and below the narrowed segment (the coarctation), excising this segment, and joining the two cut ends of the aorta with sutures.

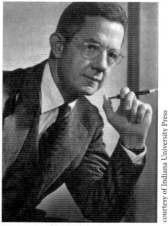

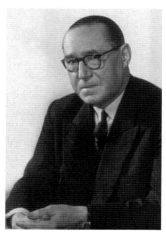

**Figure 6:** Alfred Blalock

**Figure 7:** Russell Brock

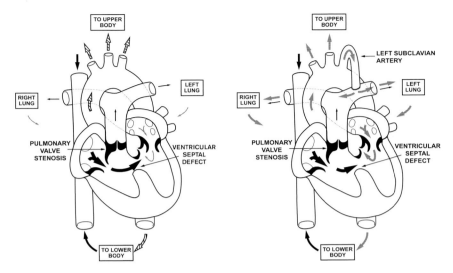

**Figure 8:** (Left) Basic structure and blood flow through the heart and major blood vessels in the presence of Fallot's tetralogy (that includes a ventricular septal defect [VSD] and pulmonary stenosis). The obstruction at the pulmonary valve results in shunting of blood through the VSD. The poor flow of blood to the lungs (because of the narrowing of the pulmonary valve) results in inadequate oxygenation of the blood, with resulting breathlessness on even trivial exercise. (Right) The condition has been "corrected" by a "Blalock" shunt. In Blalock's operation, the left subclavian artery (which normally supplies blood to the left arm) is joined to the left pulmonary artery to increase the blood flow to the lungs (by an "indirect" route). In contrast, Brock pushed a long knife or dilator through the apex of the right ventricle up into the pulmonary artery and split the narrowed valve to increase blood flow to the lungs (by the "direct" route) (not shown).

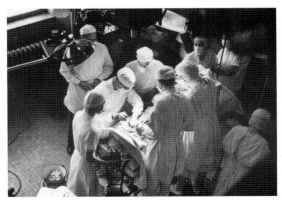

**Figure 9:** Operating room during the first "Blalock-Taussig" operation for Fallot's tetralogy in 1944. Dr. Blalock stands to the left of the operating table, with Vivien Thomas behind him. Dr. Denton Cooley stands opposite Dr. Blalock.

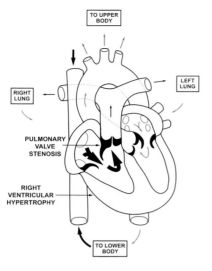

**Figure 10:** Basic structure and blood flow through the heart and major blood vessels in the presence of isolated pulmonary valve stenosis. There is a greatly reduced blood flow to the lungs. The pressure in the right ventricle increases markedly and ultimately leads to failure of the right ventricle. Brock split or dilated the narrowed pulmonary valve, as described in Figure 8.

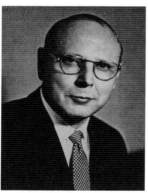

**Figure 11:** Charles Bailey

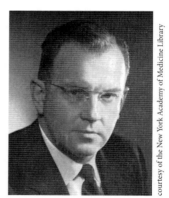

**Figure 12:** Dwight Harken

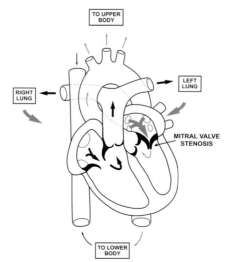

**Figure 13:** Basic structure and blood flow through the heart and major blood vessels in the presence of mitral valve stenosis. Blood cannot pass easily through the narrowed mitral valve, resulting in a "backup" of blood in the left atrium and lungs. The accumulation of blood in the lungs ("congestion") results in severe shortness of breath. In the operation devised by Bailey and Harken, a finger was placed into the left atrium (left collecting chamber) and pushed through the valve to split it. If the finger proved insufficient, a knife was passed along the finger and the valve was cut.

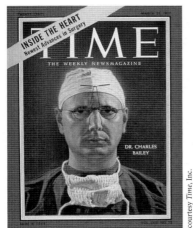
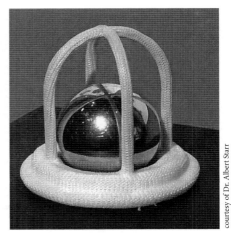

**Figure 14:** In Charles Bailey's opinion, there was a similarity between the structure of the mitral valve (right) and that of a lady's girdle (left). The leaflets of the mitral valve are tethered to the wall of the left ventricle by "chordae" that resemble the garters of a lady's corset. (In the other drawings of the heart, the detailed structure of the mitral valve is not shown.)

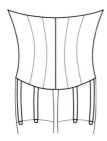

**Figure 15:** Charles Bailey on the cover of *Time* magazine in 1957

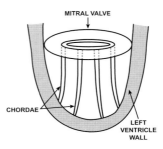

**Figure 16:** An early ball-and-cage valve prosthesis

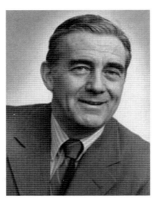

**Figure 17:** Wilfred Bigelow

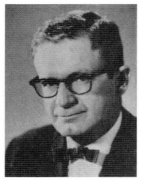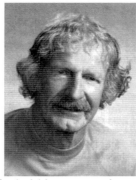

**Figure 18:** John Lewis before (left) and after (right) his retirement from surgical practice

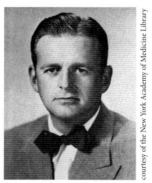

**Figure 19:** Henry Swan

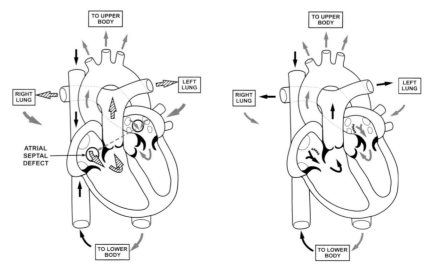

**Figure 20:** Basic structure and blood flow through the heart and major blood vessels in the presence of an atrial septal defect (ASD) before (left) and after (right) its surgical closure. As the procedure could be carried out within a few minutes, this was the most common operation performed with the aid of hypothermia.

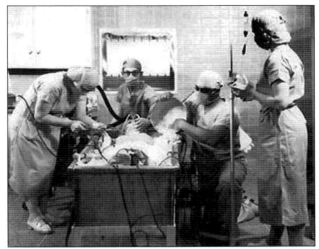

**Figure 21:** An anesthetized patient being cooled in a bath of iced water (to reduce body temperature) before undergoing open heart surgery.

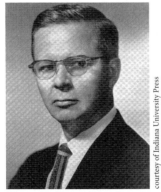

**Figure 22:** Clarence Dennis

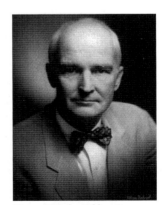

**Figure 23:** John Gibbon Jr.

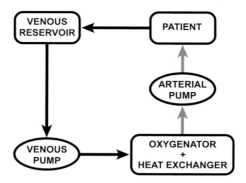

**Figure 24:** Greatly simplified diagram of the basic components of a heart-lung machine. "Blue" blood (with low oxygen content) (black arrows) from the patient is pumped into the oxygenator of the heart-lung machine, where oxygen and carbon dioxide are exchanged. The resulting "pink" blood (with high oxygen content) (gray arrows) is pumped back into the patient to supply the brain and other vital organs while the heart is operated on. The heat exchanger is used to control the temperature of the blood passing through the machine; the blood can be cooled when the surgical procedure begins (to provide protection to the patient's brain), and warmed when it is concluded.

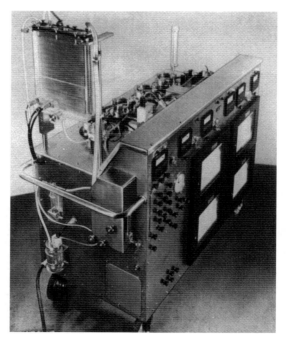

**Figure 25:** An early Gibbon-IBM heart-lung machine. The vertical screen oxygenator is nearest to the camera and the roller pumps are behind it. The oxygenator consisted of a series of vertical screens over which thin films of "blue" blood (from the patient) flowed. The blood's exposure to oxygen enabled it to pick up oxygen. This "pink" blood was then returned to the patient.

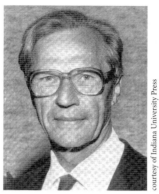

**Figure 26:** Viking Bjork

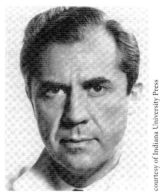

**Figure 27:** Ake Senning

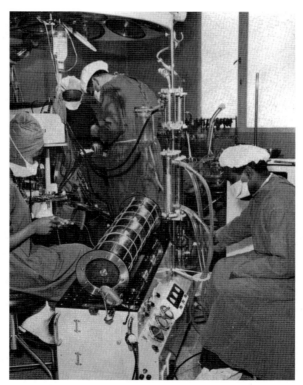

**Figure 28:** An early heart-lung machine incorporating a disc oxygenator (which consists of a series of discs over which a thin film of blood flows, exposing the blood to oxygen).

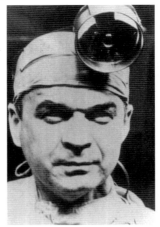

**Figure 29:** Clarence Walton Lillehei

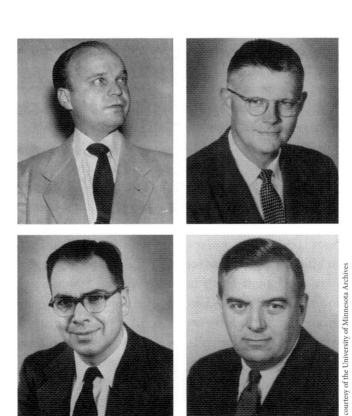

**Figure 30:** The team that developed cross-circulation in the laboratory and used it in a series of patients in the operating room. Clockwise from top left: C. Walton Lillehei, Herbert Warden, Richard Varco, Morley Cohen.

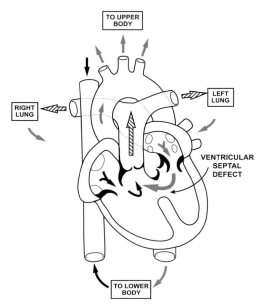

**Figure 31:** Basic structure and blood flow through the heart and major blood vessels in the presence of a ventricular septal defect (VSD). Blood from the high-pressure left ventricle is shunted into the low-pressure right ventricle and then into the lungs, causing increased work for the right ventricle and congestion in the lungs.

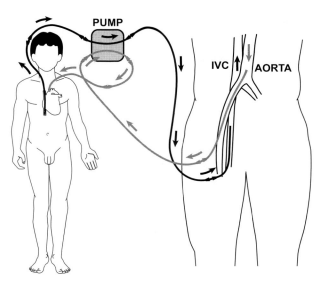

**Figure 32:** Diagram showing blood flow during an operation using cross-circulation. The heart and lungs of the adult "donor" (on the right) acted as the "heart-lung machine" for the child "recipient" (patient - on the left). The "donor" received "blue" blood (with low oxygen content) (black arrows) from the child, oxygenated it as it passed through the lungs, and pumped "pink" blood (with high oxygen content) (gray arrows) back into the child.

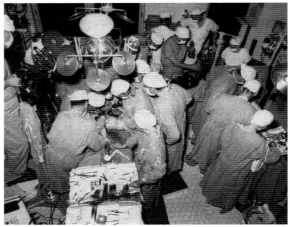

**Figure 33:** Open heart operation at the University of Minnesota involving cross-circulation. The surgical team operating on the patient is on the left, and the team operating on the "donor" is on the right.

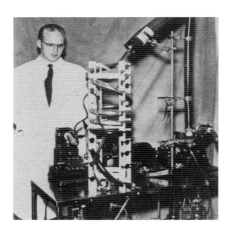

**Figure 34:** Richard DeWall and his early bubble oxygenator. After the blood was oxygenated by the flow of oxygen into it, any remaining bubbles in the blood would rise to the top of the helical tube (as being lighter than blood) and thus would not be pumped back into the patient, where they might cause injury to the brain from "air embolism" (in which air bubbles obstruct the flow of blood in small blood vessels).

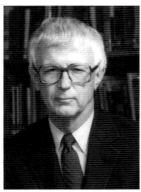

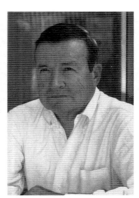

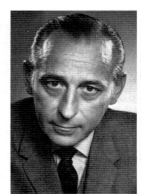

**Figure 35:** John Kirklin

**Figure 36:** Arthur Voorhees

**Figure 37:** Charles Hufnagel

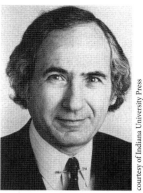

**Figure 38:** Albert Starr

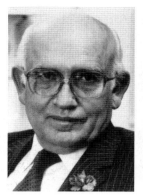

**Figure 39:** Donald Ross

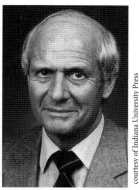

**Figure 40:** Brian Barratt-Boyes

courtesy of Indiana University Press

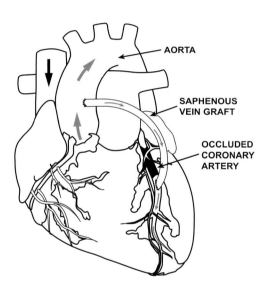

AORTA

SAPHENOUS VEIN GRAFT

OCCLUDED CORONARY ARTERY

**Figure 41:** Drawing of a heart with a coronary artery bypass graft. A vein from the leg has been used to connect the aorta with a coronary artery below the site of a stenosis (narrowing or obstruction), thus bypassing the obstructed segment and bringing blood to the heart muscle beyond the obstruction. When several arteries have obstructions, multiple vein grafts can be inserted. Today, an artery that lies on the inside of the chest wall is frequently used instead of a length of vein.

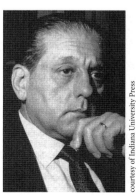

**Figure 42:** A Rene Favaloro

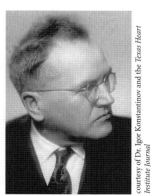

**Figure 43:** Vasilii Kolesov

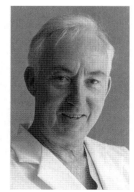

**Figure 44:** Norman Shumway

courtesy of Indiana University Press

courtesy of Dr. Igor Konstantinov and the *Texas Heart Institute Journal*

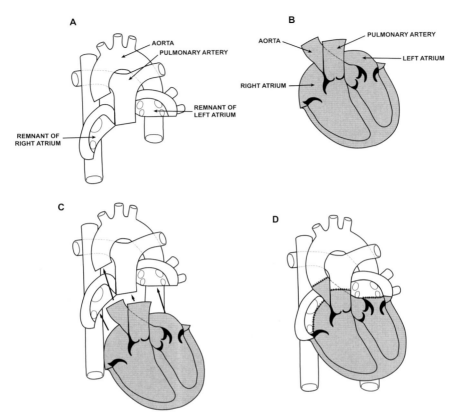

**Figure 45:** The operation of heart transplantation. (A) The structures that remain in the recipient after removal of the diseased ventricles (pumping chambers) and all four heart valves. (B) The donor heart (shaded) that is to be transplanted into the recipient; this basically consists of the two ventricles and all four valves. (C) The donor heart is placed next to the remnants of the recipient heart, so that the various chambers and blood vessels can be sutured to each other. (D) The completed operation.

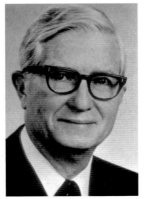

**Figure 46:** James Hardy

**Figure 47:** The operation consent form signed by the patient's next of kin in the first heart transplant ever performed (in 1964), in which a chimpanzee was used as the "donor." The one-paragraph document states that no heart transplant has ever been carried out before, but makes no mention that the "donor" might be a chimpanzee.

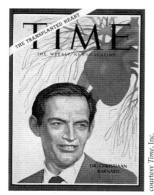

**Figure 48:** Christiaan Barnard on the cover of *Time* magazine in 1967

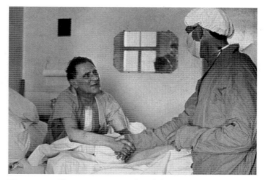

**Figure 49:** Christiaan Barnard with his patient, Louis Washkansky, after the first human-to-human heart transplant, performed in 1967.

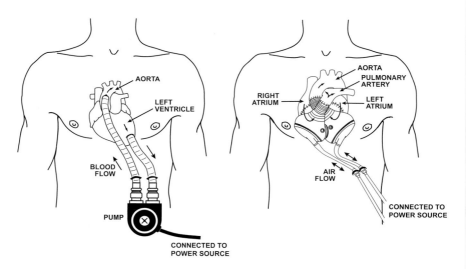

**Figure 50:** Drawings of patients with a left ventricular assist device (LVAD, left) and a total mechanical artificial heart (TAH, right). There are various different designs of ventricular assist devices and total artificial hearts. Although it is the left ventricle that most commonly needs support (by an LVAD), if the right ventricle is also failing, two assist devices can be inserted—to support both the right and left ventricles. With a ventricular assist device, the pump lies outside of the body, whereas with an artificial heart it is implanted within the chest; however, a "driveline" still needs to come out through the chest wall to connect the mechanical heart to a power source.

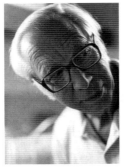

**Figure 51:** Willem Kolff

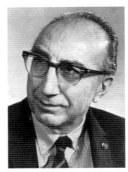

**Figure 52:** Michael DeBakey

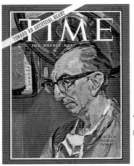

**Figure 53:** Michael DeBakey
on the cover of *Time*
magazine in 1965

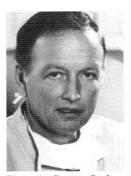

**Figure 54:** Denton Cooley

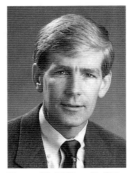

**Figure 55:** William DeVries

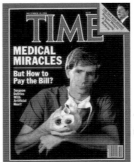

**Figure 56:** William DeVries,
holding a Jarvik artificial
heart, on the cover of *Time*
magazine in 1984

## CHAPTER 7

# Innovation and Risk:
# The Golden Minneapolis Era

————

## C. WALTON LILLEHEI AND RICHARD VARCO

T HE FEW ATTEMPTS and even fewer successes using the heart-lung machine before 1954 were a preliminary to the first series of open heart operations in which the surgery was not restricted to the six minutes or so allowed by hypothermia. It was the group at the University of Minnesota that took this next step forward. Owen Wangensteen had developed an atmosphere in his department conducive to innovation, and it was his protégé, Clarence Walton (Walt) Lillehei (Figure 29), and his several colleagues who, like their predecessor, John Lewis, took full advantage of this environment.

There was a competitive spirit among the younger members of the staff, which Dr. Wangensteen did nothing to discourage. Apart from John Lewis, Clarence Dennis, and Walt Lillehei, another young surgeon, Gil Campbell, was using monkey and dog lungs to oxygenate blood and allow open heart surgery in children, although this was never very successful. Without doubt, the five or six years in Minneapolis from 1951 through 1956 must have been among the most exciting and important ever experienced in the long history of medicine.

This period in Minneapolis, together with the work of Lewis and Swan, demonstrated that innovation in surgery was moving west from the traditional hotbeds of surgery on or near the East Coast of the United States and in Europe.

The technique Walt Lillehei used to move forward was one of the most astounding clinical experiments ever carried out: cross-circulation. Lillehei led a small group of investigators who came up with the idea of using a parent (or other adult) to provide continuous oxygenated blood to support a child while the child was undergoing heart surgery. By joining the two circulations, the parent's heart and lungs could pump and oxygenate the blood for both parent and child. In other words, the parent would be the heart-lung machine for the child. If you planned such an operation today, more than 50 years later, even with our vast experience of heart surgery, it would remain a highly risky procedure. It took a surgeon of great courage to pursue this approach.

## C. WALTON LILLEHEI —
## THE BOLDEST INNOVATOR

Clarence Walton Lillehei (Figures 29 and 30) is, in my opinion and in that of many of the surgeons I interviewed, *the* major figure in the development of open heart surgery. He was certainly the boldest of the surgeons involved in this branch of surgery, initially introducing an operation with a potential 200% mortality — the deaths of both child and parent. Without taking this bold step, and following it up with the development of an inexpensive disposable oxygenator that could be used widely, it is likely that open heart surgery would have taken several more years before it became an established and common surgical procedure.

Denton Cooley (chapter 13), the surgeon who did much to demonstrate that open heart surgery could be carried out on a large scale, has said that surgeons have to be grateful to Walt Lillehei since he "provided the can-opener for the biggest picnic thoracic surgeons will ever know." Not only did the work of Walt Lillehei's group enable open heart surgery to be performed worldwide, but it has also been estimated that he personally trained approximately 140 heart surgeons who spent periods of time with him when he was in his heyday in Minneapolis and, later, New York. Norman Shumway (chapter 12) summed up the opinions of many when he said that, in the mid-1950s, Lillehei "was the greatest surgeon in the world."

Like Charlie Bailey, Walt Lillehei was something of a maverick, and certainly one of the most colorful characters among the surgeons involved in the development of heart surgery. At a young age, he cheated potential death from a malignant tumor, and this may have contributed to his living somewhat dangerously throughout most of the rest of his life. Not only did he live dangerously as a surgeon, taking risks that most others balked at, but his personal life was also one of risk-taking, some would say recklessness. His lifestyle eventually led to the total collapse of his career, from which he never fully recovered, although by the time of his death he had regained much of the professional respect he indubitably deserved. His life was a veritable roller coaster of triumphant highs and humiliating lows.

I had first come across his name when I was a medical student in the late 1950s and early 1960s, when reading the surgical journals in the medical school library. I repeatedly came across the names of Lillehei and Varco, who appeared to be leading members of a team of surgeons in Minneapolis who were performing the most astounding surgery. This was the beginning of true open heart surgery, and their reports of operations for repairing a hole between the two pumping chambers of the heart, i.e., a ventricular septal defect (or VSD) (Figure 31), and for the complete correction of Fallot's tetralogy, i.e., repairing a VSD and opening a narrowed pulmonary valve (Figure 8), in ever-increasing numbers of patients — usually children — raised my eyebrows.

Some years later, when I was a junior faculty member myself, I recognized Dr. Lillehei (from photos I had seen of him) at one or two medical congresses. However, at these congresses he seemed never to be a speaker, or even chairman of a session, and I had the impression that he was a forgotten man. I could not understand why someone who had been such a pioneer in the field had become such a "nonperson." I presumed it was because he no longer did any innovative work. It was only some years later that I learned about his fall from grace as a result of several scandals that had befallen him. These were the years when he was in the medical wilderness. Fortunately, his reputation was rehabilitated, particularly by his former trainees and by his erstwhile competitor, John Kirklin (chapter 8), and in the later years of his life he was able to receive more of the honors and respect that were due to him.

## Wangensteen's Young Men

In the incredibly research-friendly and supportive environment created by Wangensteen at the University of Minnesota, Lillehei and his colleagues were able to establish open heart surgery over the period of a handful of years. The department attracted a wealth of young talent to its surgical training program. Not only had people of the caliber of Lewis and Lillehei passed through it, but they were joined during this highly creative period by outstanding young men, such as Norman Shumway (chapter 12), Christiaan Barnard (chapter 12), Christian Cabrol, and Aldo Castañeda, all of whom went on to make major names for themselves in the field of heart surgery. These were ambitious and gifted young men driven to succeed in the newly developing field of heart surgery.

An example of their motivation and drive is provided by the young Aldo Castañeda, whose enthusiasm for open heart surgery was such that, as a *medical student* in Guatemala — not a country normally associated with medical innovation — he had obtained a simple motor pump, fabricated a helix bubble oxygenator of the DeWall type (see below), performed open heart surgery in dogs, and written a thesis on the topic. This demonstrates immense initiative, and was a clear indicator of Castañeda's potential and a prelude to the significant contributions to pediatric heart surgery that he eventually made.

Dr. Castañeda related to me the story of how he, as a young man, managed to get himself accepted into the Minneapolis surgical training program. It is an amusing story. A congress on pediatrics was being held in Guatemala, at which Castañeda, because of his fluency in both Spanish and English, was asked to provide simultaneous translation of the presentations. A pediatric psychiatrist from Minnesota gave one of the lectures in English, Castañeda translating into Spanish. He did well for awhile, but then the speaker began to relate a long-winded (and possibly not very funny) "Scandinavian joke, which, of course, I didn't understand." As the joke unfolded, Castañeda, in Spanish, informed his audience through their headsets that a joke was being told but that he couldn't understand it, and he could not translate it for them. However, after the obvious punch line, although unintelligible to the translator, Castañeda told everybody through their headsets that they should laugh. They obliged him by laughing heartily. The speaker was extremely impressed that the joke had been translated so well and had proved so successful. After his lecture, he thanked Castañeda profusely, and offered any help he could provide to the young man's career. Castañeda took the opportunity to bring up his keen interest in obtaining training in open heart surgery at Minneapolis. The professor returned to Minneapolis and told Wangensteen, "There's this genius in Guatemala, and I think you should offer him a job."

Bob Frater, although not one of Lillehei's trainees, remembers that Lillehei "was a man with a great fertility of ideas. Ideas came pouring out of him, and he was absolutely open in his discussion of those ideas. He had a willingness to pass these ideas on to somebody else to try and develop them. There wasn't the slightest hint of 'I'd better keep this to myself for awhile until I've got it published so as to boost my bibliography.' You've seen people who are secretive and somehow strangely jealous of a thought they might have had. Thoughts to him were to be spread — anywhere, everywhere.

"I have an immense affection for him. He's an example of what a senior person should be to young people — always available, always within the bounds of common sense. He was so completely willing to lash ideas back and forth, but was not opinionated. He didn't say, 'That's an absurd idea.' He'd say, 'Let's just think about that.' Lillehei was an absolutely marvelous fellow."

## Conversations with Walt Lillehei

When I first met with Walt Lillehei in 1988, he was of medium height and slight built. He wore a rather flamboyant suit with a brightly colored silk lining. Bob Frater described Lillehei's sartorial taste as "quite bizarre; color schemes were all wrong, and very flashy. Half the time, he looked like a bookie from a racetrack." He had a slight but obvious deformity of his neck that resulted from the major surgery for a malignant tumor he had undergone as a young man. I also had the privilege of meeting him on several subsequent occasions; this slight tilt of his head to one side became rather more marked in his later years, and was quite pronounced in the years before his death. He was always warm, affable, and friendly, characteristics that were also noted in the writings of many of his former colleagues and juniors. Although clearly proud of his contributions to medicine, as far as I could detect there was not a hint of pomposity about him, although in his younger days I understand he could show considerable academic arrogance now and again. Dennis Melrose, who developed the first heart-lung machine in the United Kingdom, mentioned to me, "Walt is a little different now, but in those days he had conquered the world and wanted you to be sure and know it."

Throughout life, Lillehei's nice sense of humor would surface every now and again. In an after-dinner speech, at a function in 1987 in Oklahoma City to celebrate the 20th anniversary of the first heart transplant performed by Chris Barnard, one of Dr. Lillehei's trainees, Lillehei said that "Chris readily admits that I taught him everything he knows." He paused, and then slyly added, "But I didn't teach him everything *I* know."

## Young Days

Walt Lillehei was born in 1918 and grew up in Minneapolis. His father was a dentist, and he had two brothers who followed him into medicine. The youngest, Richard, developed an international reputation as a surgeon, particularly in the field of pancreas transplantation, before tragically dying at a relatively young age. All of Lillehei's education was in Minnesota — grade school, high school, undergraduate, and medical school. At the time he graduated from high school, he was only 15 years old.

At the end of his second year at college, he had accumulated the necessary grades to transfer to medical school. He graduated as a doctor at age 21. "Because I had signed up a couple of years earlier in the reserves, after a year of internship I joined the army in June 1942," he told me. "I don't know exactly why I had signed up earlier, except that I wanted to travel. They didn't give you anything for signing up, like they do now, when you get certain privileges or perks. I thought, 'Gee, this war is going on, and I want to miss it?' It sounds pretty strange now, but that was the psychology in my mind. I was in the army a little bit shy of four years."

The young Lillehei was soon shipped to the United Kingdom, and was later involved in the North African, Sicilian, and Italian campaigns. In North Africa, he commanded a Mobile Army Surgical Hospital (MASH) unit in the campaign against German Field Marshal Rommel's Afrika Corps. From Africa, Lillehei participated in the landing and bitter fighting at Anzio, south of Rome, in 1944. After 46 months in the army, he was a lieutenant-colonel and wore a Bronze Star, a Bronze Arrowhead, and a European Theater Ribbon with five battle stars.

## Residency in Minneapolis

In October 1945, at the age of 27, he returned to Minneapolis for formal surgical training, which for all Wangensteen's trainees included a substantial period in the research laboratory. It was during the last few months of his surgical residency in 1950 that Lillehei developed a lymphosarcoma, a notoriously malignant condition, in the glands in his neck. On the day after he completed his residency, Lillehei underwent more than ten hours of radical surgery to his neck and chest to remove all of the lymphatic tissue, and he subsequently received radiation therapy to this area. Wangensteen led the surgical team that operated on his junior colleague, with Richard Varco and John Lewis (Lillehei's close friend) being the thoracic surgical members of the team. Lillehei was forced to take four months off from his work to recover from this therapy, after which Wangensteen appointed him to his staff.

Dr. Lillehei expanded on the state of heart surgery when he joined the staff of the University of Minnesota: "Heart surgery in Minnesota in the late 1940s and early 1950s was essentially for patent ductus and coarctation. Nobody had really extensive experience. Dr. Varco was the principal cardiac surgeon at that time, along with Clarence Dennis. Dr. Varco was also innovating valvulotomy for pulmonary stenosis using inflow stasis [i.e., he was operating on children with narrowed pulmonary valves, though using a slightly different technique from that originally introduced by Brock]. This involved temporarily obstructing the blood returning to the heart [to provide a fairly bloodless operating field], and then opening the pulmonary artery to allow access to the stenosed [narrowed] pulmonary valve, which could then be opened up with a knife [a similar operation to that introduced by Brock]. This was all done at normal body temperature, and therefore had to be carried out very quickly. The heart needed to be restarted within three to four minutes. It was clearly evident to me that, if you could somehow work inside the heart under direct vision, the possibilities were incredible."

Lillehei was present when Clarence Dennis carried out his two operations using his heart-lung machine in 1951. He was impressed by the immense complexity of the machine and already realized that, if open heart surgery were to become common, a much simpler machine needed to be developed

As part of his preparation to embark on open heart surgery, Lillehei went to pathology museums to look at the hearts of patients who had died with congenital heart abnormalities. He found this to be less helpful than he had anticipated, as hearts stored in formalin tend to be stiff and rigid, preventing any assessment of how the abnormality could be corrected. He recalled, "So I put myself on call for about two years with all of the pediatric pathologists. Any death of an infant or child under ten or twelve, regardless of the cause, I would come in for. They were pretty good about calling me. I think one case, a premature baby, had a tetralogy of Fallot. The abnormalities were extremely severe but, in the fresh specimen [as opposed to the specimen preserved in formalin], you could close the ventricular septal defect quite easily—just a couple of stitches. That gave us the confidence to disregard those formalin-fixed specimens, because they were just misleading."

## Morley Cohen

The first of Lillehei's junior colleagues to play a major role was a Canadian, Morley Cohen (Figure 30). He was set the goal of coming up with a means of oxygenating the blood artificially, as would be required in a heart-lung machine.

"Initially, Walt suggested I read about this in journals and try things in the lab, but just keep him informed as to what I'm doing. He would call me once every week or ten days and see if he could come over, or sometimes he would drop in unexpectedly. We had a little nook on the top floor of the science building. He gave me free rein for what I wanted to prioritize. My first idea came from having had fish tanks as a hobby when I was in grades seven and eight and up to high school. They had had fine bubbles in them. I found out very quickly that you can certainly oxygenate blood that way with relatively little trauma, but the problem was getting rid of the bubbles." (The bubbles in the blood caused damage to the brain.)

In contrast to Clarence Dennis and John Gibbon, who tried to maintain a normal blood flow, Cohen began to wonder what was the lowest possible blood flow that was essential to supply the brain in order to keep a patient or experimental animal alive when you stopped and operated on the heart.

"Sometime later, Walt came over to the lab, and said, 'Here is an example of how little blood you need to get an animal to survive for a limited period of time.' He gave me a reprint of a paper from the *British Journal of Surgery* [in 1952] by two men called [Anthony] Andreasen and [Frank] Watson, who, although they hadn't measured anything, had occluded the venae cavae except for the blood that was returning through the azygos vein [i.e., they had prevented the return of blood to the heart from the entire body with the exception of blood returning through one small vein, the azygos vein]. They did this in about twelve dogs or so, and all but one had survived for a period of thirty to 45 minutes at normal body temperature just on the azygos blood flow. So I said, 'How much blood actually is that?' Walt said, 'Why don't we find out?'

"I did a series of experiments where I measured the blood flow in the azygos vein, and it came to somewhere between eight and thirteen cc [milliliters] per kilogram body weight per minute; that is, it was less than 10% of the total body blood flow.

"Herb Warden [Figure 30] joined the lab about six or nine months after I did. Herb's a very good guy, a solid citizen, and a good surgeon. The two of us spent time talking about how we could oxygenate enough blood. At the time, my wife became pregnant with our first child. I can't remember exactly how it came up, but I think I said to her, 'It would be wonderful if we could have an artificial placenta [to oxygenate the blood].' After all, the mother acts as the oxygenator, and pumps oxygenated blood to the fetus. She laughed, but it occurred to me that if we could use another dog to provide the small amounts of blood that were needed [as determined by the azygos flow studies], then things would be much improved over the methods that we had been using."

The idea that Cohen and Warden came up with was simple. By connecting the two blood circulations, one large dog would become the heart-lung machine for the other, smaller, dog (Figure 32). The "donor" dog's heart would pump blood around both animals, and the "donor" dog's lungs would oxygenate that blood. This would enable the "recipient" dog's heart to be stopped entirely and would allow any defect in that heart to be operated on under almost perfect conditions. In itself, the idea of cross-circulation was not new, as it had been a laboratory technique for physiological studies since 1890, but it had never before been conceived as a means of enabling operations to be performed inside the heart.

Cohen continued, "I explained the idea to Lillehei, and he said, 'Go ahead, but be sure that you're not trying to take any shortcuts.' So we tried it, and it worked. We ran a series of about sixty animals. Most of them were long-term survivors. Then we autopsied them, and looked at all the organs. As far as we could detect, everything seemed to be okay. We were encouraged by this, and by the simplicity of it.

"From the summer of 1953 until the following spring, Walt used to come over about once a week on a Friday afternoon. Utilizing this technique in the lab, he did numerous procedures inside the heart. We all found it very stimulating, particularly because we could show that one could work within the heart with safety. The beauty of it was that it was so very simple. Walt said, 'I really think we're ready to get permission to try this clinically.' He went to discuss it with Dr. Wangensteen, who asked him to document our experience, and then gave his approval."

This meant, of course, that if a child with a heart abnormality were to be operated on, its blood circulation would need to be maintained by a larger human, most probably one of the child's parents. By any stretch of the imagination, some risk to the parent, as well as to the child, was involved. It would be a bold step to take.

## The First Operations Using Cross-Circulation
The first historic operation using cross-circulation took place on March 26, 1954, when Lillehei was only 35 years old. There was

considerable feeling at the University Hospital that it shouldn't take place and the planning for it should be stopped.

According to Vincent Gott, a surgical resident who was in the operating room on that day, "The resistance was mainly from hospital administration. It is my understanding that the day before Walt was to do that first case, the hospital administrator said, 'No, you're not going to do it.' I think the hospital administration was concerned about the malpractice [medicolegal] aspects of it. Walt then went by Dr. Wangensteen's office to tell him he was ready to go ahead tomorrow. Wangensteen was out, but on the afternoon before they did that first case he sent Walt a little note that said, 'By all means go ahead, OHW.'"

That simple little note took on legendary significance to the young researchers in Minneapolis; for them it symbolized the faith Wangensteen had in them and his extraordinary willingness to support them in their research.

The first operation was on a one-year-old boy named Gregory Glidden, whose father, Lyman, acted as his "heart-lung machine." Dr. Gott explained, "There were Walt and Dr. Varco [Figure 30], of course. Walt took the lead, but Varco was there as his first assistant for all those early cases. Varco was a master technician. He was always encouraging Walt. He was there all through that first year of cross-circulation, and certainly the next two years, as I remember, with the bubble oxygenator. At that first case, Morley Cohen [who was then back on the clinical service] and Herb Warden prepared the femoral artery and femoral vein [to connect the donor circulation to that of the recipient]" (Figure 33).

Cohen remembers being "a little apprehensive. My hopes were that everything would go well. I wasn't apprehensive about it not being feasible. I thought we had proved that pretty well in the lab, unless there was something totally unperceived that might occur in the clinical case that didn't occur in the lab. They all went technically well, except one, where there was an error on the part of someone who pressurized an IV bottle and either left it or forgot about it; the patient developed air embolism." (In order to speed up the delivery of fluid to the "donor" parent, the anesthesiologist was pumping blood into the donor and inadvertently pumped in some air, injuring the parent's brain.)

(Two members of Blalock's Johns Hopkins surgical team, Henry Bahnson and Tom Starzl, happened to be in the visitor's gallery watching that operation. Dr. Starzl told me that they could see the air traveling down the infusion line toward the patient, but, because there was no sound communication system between them and those in the operating room, they were unable to attract the attention of any of the operating room staff to abort the impending disaster.)

Richard DeWall, a surgical fellow who was in the operating room on that occasion, added, "I think she was able to get back to a functioning lifestyle of a sort, but there was some permanent damage. It was a tragedy. This was not a basic fault of the perfusion cross-circulation system. It was human error. Whenever you do anything, of course, you're at risk from human error."

Dr. Lillehei mentioned to me that he had spoken to the unfortunate woman and her family and had encouraged her to sue him and the hospital in order to obtain some money to help her rehabilitation. Instead of negotiating directly with the hospital, which Dr. Lillehei told me would have been willing to settle with her for a reasonable sum, she hired a lawyer. He persuaded her to sue for a sum so large that the hospital felt unable to agree. The case therefore came to court, which found *against* the claimant, presumably because she had been made fully aware that there would be risks involved, and the poor woman ended up empty-handed. This story was confirmed to me by Norman Shumway, who offered it as an example of "Lillehei's humanity." Lillehei, of course, received severe criticism for this mishap, being branded "a criminal" by a few.

However, this mishap did not stop the cross-circulation work. It proved a very exciting period for young men such as DeWall. He recalled, "It was a tremendous emotional experience. There was an influx of surgical people from all over the world. To get acquainted with world-famous surgical figures on this basis, to work in the laboratory and show people what you were doing and what you were trying to achieve — to be able to serve as a teacher — was quite flattering for a young fellow at my stage. I was only 26 or 27. The visitors proved very interested students."

A total of 45 operations were performed using cross-circulation; 28 children, most or all with heart defects that could not have been corrected by any other surgical approach (such as hypothermia), survived. The longest time any of them was supported by their "donor" was 40 minutes. Despite the fact that it saved the lives of these 28 children, there was considerable criticism from other physicians and surgeons for carrying out such a risky procedure.

## Lillehei's Strengths

I asked Dr. Cohen what Lillehei's real strengths were. How could he be summed up?

"If Dr. Lillehei set his mind to something, he would pursue it relentlessly. He was very committed to an idea. He worked on in the face of adversity. He wasn't daunted by the fact that things didn't go well. Some surgeons would become depressed, but with Walt, although he may have been a little bit set back emotionally, it never showed. His ability to muster his energies and focus was just unbelievable.

"I wouldn't say that he was technically of the quality of Richard Varco, but he was technically average or above average for surgeons working in this field. He foresaw problems, and could keep himself out of them. Also, he didn't lose his cool. If things didn't go well in the operating room and we were having problems with patients, Walt didn't say, 'I think we've done all we can,' or 'Call so-and-so and see what he can do about this situation; I'm getting nowhere'; he would just keep working at it."

The cross-circulation work undoubtedly enabled open heart surgery to get off the ground, and therefore was of immense importance in the history of medicine. However, any operation with a potential 200% mortality was going to find it hard to become widely accepted.

Just as Lillehei realized that Clarence Dennis's complex heart-lung machine was not the ultimate answer to the problem, he also realized that cross-circulation did not provide the definitive solution. Cross-circulation, he believed, would not be taken up by surgeons around the world. This proved to be the case, although it seems remarkable to me that there are no reports of other surgical centers using this approach for the repair of cardiac defects. Presumably, hypothermia sufficed for some, and the general feeling was that the other defects would have to wait for the heart-lung machine to be perfected; the risks involved with cross-circulation were simply too great for most surgeons to accept. Richard DeWall and John Kirklin (chapter 8), however, believed that other groups may well have performed at least one unsuccessful case but never announced or published their results.

In 1955, DeWall developed a very simple bubble oxygenator, which enabled Lillehei to discontinue cross-circulation as a means of performing open heart surgery and replace it with the DeWall heart-lung machine. Lillehei, Cohen, Warden, and Varco's great contributions in initiating heart surgery with cross-circulation, however, were recognized by the award of the Lasker Prize to them in 1955. Cohen and Warden went on to successful careers as cardiac surgeons in Canada and the United States, respectively.

## Richard DeWall — The $50 Breakthrough

Richard DeWall (Figure 34) was born in 1926 in the western prairies of Minnesota, and grew up and went to school there. He graduated from high school a little young, and was able to get in almost a year at the University of Minnesota before he was drafted into World War II. After developing rheumatic fever at boot camp, he spent several months recovering. After the war was over, he was discharged from the service with a heart murmur of mitral valve regurgitation, indicating a leaky mitral valve resulting from rheumatic fever.

He returned to the university and graduated in medicine. After a short period in family practice, he became interested in going into surgery but was not accepted into the surgical training program. "There was stiff competition," he explained. "I was competing with a great number of extremely talented veterans who had spent maybe three to five years in the military and were very conscientious. I had not been a stellar student during medical school. John [Lewis] didn't think I was the quality he needed for the surgery residency program at that time, and wouldn't take me on."

However, he was given the opportunity of working in Lillehei's laboratory. "It was a very modest position. I was paid as an animal attendant. I wasn't paid as a resident or even recognized as a resident. I was just there to learn some laboratory medicine. Actually, I was probably pretty well off compared to many of the residents, because a lab technician received about four times [in salary] what the residents were making.

"After several months of working with the cross-circulation, Walt suggested that I turn my attention to see if I could develop an artificial oxygenator. Walt's clinical experience with cross-circulation and low-volume perfusion was an invaluable basis for understanding perfusion physiology, but I didn't really know in what direction to go. There was no obvious direction at that time. Of course, there was Gibbon's work—his one clinical success in 1953 followed by a number of unfortunate failures. The Mayo Clinic had taken over the Gibbon machine and was trying to make it functional, which they ultimately did. I tried to develop some concepts of an oxygenator system, and went through a number of false starts, as you could expect. In Clarence Dennis's experiments, he had had problems with air bubbles, and Walt was afraid that bubbles would be a big problem. Because of this bugaboo about bubbles, I focused on 'filming' systems, which weren't terribly successful. Of course, I was familiar with Bjork's rotating disc oxygenator.

"Then Walt wondered whether I could use some plastic hose, for no other reason than he had a friend who made vinyl plastic hose, which was used in the mayonnaise industry to pump food products. So I got some of this one-inch-diameter polyvinyl chloride plastic hose and began fooling around with it, thinking of ways to prevent bubbles forming. I ran a few experiments with the dogs, and I noticed that, in the process of getting blood down the incline plane into the reservoir at the bottom [of the long tube], any foaming or bubbles were trapped. Blood with bubbles would rise to the surface, and the heavier blood [without the bubbles] would slide underneath. Obviously, blood with air in it has a lesser density than whole blood. So, on that basis, you had a good 'bubble trap.' I think the first length of hose may have been almost 74 inches long, and I used it as a vertical tube. But it is kind of clumsy when you have a six-feet-long tube, so it was easier to wind it in a coil and make it more compact [Figure 34]. I was able to de-bubble by the use of anti-foam, but the incline plane, the coil, helped trap the rest of the bubbles." (Not only did DeWall use "mayonnaise" plastic tubing, he also trapped air bubbles with stainless-steel indus-trial sponges, from which he had to clean off machine oil, soaked with anti-foam. It was clearly a "homemade" oxygenator.)

"The pump I used was an old pump that they had used in the physiology lab, a SigmaMotor pump, which was the pump we used for the cross-circulation. [This pump had several little metal "fingers" that progressively massaged the tubing, thus propelling the blood forward.] The first ten dogs did extremely well. They were walking around the next day. I told Walt, and he became excited about it. He began to watch the experiments. The dogs I was operating on were selected to be the size of a child — 25 to 30 pounds at the most. Using the so-called azygos flow principle, I asked what was the minimum amount of blood I could flow through the oxygenator for a half-hour, and yet still get a normal-functioning dog."

DeWall solved the problems within little more than a year. According to Morley Cohen, "What impressed Lillehei was the fact that we were going to be using something that was so simple. The *less* complicated it is, the *more* likely you'll get away with it. The more complicated it is — too many people, too much equipment, too much monitoring — the less likely it will work."

The other significant point that was important in popularizing the DeWall oxygenator was the fact that it was so inexpensive to make — on the order of $50, whereas the Gibbon IBM heart-lung machine was reported to cost in the region of $50,000. It had one other big advantage that tends to be overlooked. Because it was so simple and so cheap, it was disposable. After use, you threw it out and built another, whereas the Gibbon oxygenator was taken apart and laboriously cleaned for its next use. No matter how well the various parts were cleaned in those days, some "toxins" (foreign proteins) remained, and could cause significant complications, such as fever and low blood pressure, in the patient on whom it was next used (chapter 8). It was safer to use a completely new and sterile oxygenator each time, as in DeWall's design.

## The First Operations Using the Bubble Oxygenator

DeWall continued his story. "The first patient on whom we used the bubble oxygenator [three-year-old Jimmy Robichaud on May 13, 1955], as I recall, was a very borderline candidate with transposition or Eisenmenger's [both very high-risk conditions]. We got through the surgery fine, but the patient died in the postoperative period. There didn't appear to be any special problem with the machine. This was followed by seven patients with standard ventricular septal defects, et cetera, who survived [the first on July 12, 1955]. They all did very well, and so everybody was riding pretty high.

"I often think what role luck plays in our future because the next six patients died, if I recall correctly. It wasn't anything we could identify with the perfusion. But after six deaths in a row, we really had to stop and sit back and wonder what was going on. There were so many variable factors that we had to learn to deal with — patient selection, the patient's condition, surgical problems, perfusion problems, and so on. I remember patients where we just couldn't get their hearts beating. In retrospect, they were probably severely hypokalemic [i.e., they had low levels of potassium in the blood, which is now known to prevent the heart contracting regularly]. But that is hindsight. This kind of understanding of the physiology associated with perfusion came along later. We said we would try one more. We tried a seventh, who lived, and from that time on everything went very well."

The DeWall oxygenator is considered a landmark development in the advance of heart surgery; it enabled surgeons in quite small hospitals with limited resources to embark upon open heart surgery. A couple of units of blood were required to prime the machine, which was a small amount in those days. In contrast, the Gibbon machine required about eight or ten liters.

Whereas hundreds of surgeons had visited Minneapolis to see cross-circulation in use, and yet none went home and used it, the same surgeons returned to see the DeWall oxygenator in use, and many went home to initiate open heart surgery programs.

Vincent Gott made a significant modification to the DeWall oxygenator by designing it as a bag (rather than as a helical tube) — the plastic sheet oxygenator. The patent rights were purchased by the Travenol company, which produced these oxygenators commercially for many years.

After making this immense contribution to the development of heart surgery, in the form of the first simple oxygenator that could be used on a large scale — for which, by the way, he was recognized as one of the ten outstanding young men by the U.S. Junior Chamber of Commerce in 1957, the very same award that had earlier caused the controversy over Bernie Miller — Richard DeWall, the lowly "animal attendant" who John Lewis initially did not think was of the caliber to be a surgical resident, went on to complete his surgical training. (His story is therefore a salutary lesson to all of us who at first do not succeed in achieving our goal.) He subsequently joined the staff of a hospital in Chicago, and later became a staff cardiac surgeon in Dayton, Ohio, where he played an important role in setting up a new medical school at Wright State University.

There is one more amusing anecdote that I have to add to Richard DeWall's story. Dr. James Hardy (chapter 12) told me that he was once on the membership committee of the prestigious American

Association for Thoracic Surgery when DeWall's name came up for consideration for membership. A member of the committee said, rather disparagingly, "So he invented the bubble oxygenator, but what's he done since?" It reminded Hardy of a cartoon in the *New Yorker* of cavemen sitting on stones outside a cave, with one of them saying, "So he invented fire, but what's he done since?"

## Heart Block and the Cardiac Pacemaker

Vincent Gott took over DeWall's place in the laboratory, where the excitement continued.

He recollected, "I guess it was 1955 when Walt asked me if I would like to go into his lab, and I said, 'Yes.' I was in his lab for about a year and a half, and it was a fantastic experience. We were always trying new things. Dr. Lillehei would welcome ideas, and he would send down ideas, and yet when you look at the work that came out of his lab, there were some very significant things that came from his own residents.

"As I remember it — sometime in 1956, I guess, when I was in the lab — heart block was a principal cause of death in the patients with ventricular septal defects [VSDs] and in the Fallot's tetralogy patients. We just lost those patients flat out from heart block. I say 'we,' I mean Dr. Lillehei. I wasn't on the [operating] team at that time."

In this condition of "heart block," the heart beats too slowly to support the circulation. It is caused by damage to the conducting fibers (or "nerves") in the heart along which the electrical impulses that maintain the heart rate are transmitted. The main conducting fibers pass very close to the edge of a ventricular septal defect (a hole between the two pumping chambers) (Figure 31), and, in closing this hole, a stitch could damage these fibers. Sometimes this injury was permanent, leading to permanent heart block, but at other times it was only temporary, the heart rate eventually returning to normal. In these cases, if the heart rate could somehow be maintained until recovery, the patient had a good chance of long-term survival.

"Then Isuprel rectal suppositories became available, and probably there was a 50% survival rate. [Isuprel, or isoproterenol, is a drug that speeds up the heart, but it was not always successful in heart block.] I can remember very distinctly that, sometime in the fall of 1956, we were at a 'Morbidity and Mortality' conference on a Saturday morning. A baby was being presented who had died of heart block. Sitting behind me was the professor of physiology, Jack Johnson. I remember Jack Johnson saying, 'My gosh, we have been stimulating frogs' hearts [electrically] in the laboratory for 25 years. Why don't you put a wire in the heart and get a Grass stimulator and stimulate it?'" (It would seem that, although this was 1956, the Minneapolis team was not aware of the pioneering work of Bigelow's group that began in 1949 and was first presented at a surgical meeting in 1950.)

According to Dr. Gott, some days later he went to the laboratory alone to carry out this experiment. However, William Weirich, a new recruit to the lab, remembered that he and Gott went *immediately* after the conference to the lab, anesthetized a dog, and opened the chest and heart. They put a suture where they thought the conducting fibers would be situated and caused heart block, just as Lillehei did inadvertently in his little patients. They attached a wire electrode to the heart and connected it to the Grass stimulator, and paced it at 80 to 100 beats per minute.

This story by Gott and Weirich, though it differs in detail, is remarkable for two reasons: first in that, with the exception of the work of Bigelow and Zoll, it was one of the first attempts to electrically stimulate a mammalian heart for clinical purposes, and second in the speed at which this advance was made. The young doctors, Weirich and Gott, participated in the discussion at the conference on a Saturday morning and heard the comments of the physiologist. If Weirich's version is correct, that very same day they went to the dog lab and carried out the experiment, which proved the initial effort in a therapeutic approach that was very soon translated into clinical practice. That was how simple (from an administrative perspective) research was in those days. Today, with the need to submit detailed written proposals to an institution's "animal care and use committee" before any work can begin, it is far more complex and time-consuming.

In the early days of heart surgery, the success of cardiac pacing was dependent, of course, on the patient eventually recovering a normal heart rate of his or her own, since in those days you couldn't pace the heart forever. Whether the patient's own heart rate would eventually recover would be found out only by a trial of "pacing."

In true Lillehei fashion, the Weirich-Gott method of pacing the heart was very soon put into clinical practice. According to Dr. Gott, "I guess it was probably a month or so later that Dr. Lillehei had a patient in the operating room with heart block. He called for the wire. It was put in, and the Grass stimulator was used. That patient survived. That first case was January 30, 1957. There were about eighteen cases after that, and all but one of those patients survived.

"One of the problems was that, in order to move the patient from the operating room to the intensive care unit, we had to have a 200-feet-long cord for the Grass stimulator. Dr. Lillehei had the idea of a portable pacemaker. He at first approached an electronic engineer who did the regular maintenance on some of the hospital equipment, and he turned Walt down. Then Walt approached Earl Bakken, who also did some of the maintenance, but was also mainly working in the physiology lab maintaining the monitoring equipment. It was Earl, of course, who came up with the portable pacemaker. As you may know, the American Engineering Society [National Society of Professional Engineers] determined that that particular concept, and then the implantable pacemaker, was one of the ten outstanding engineering developments of the past fifty years — along with the transistor, the moon landing, and things like that. The development of the portable pacemaker by Lillehei and Bakken was considered at least as significant. Bakken developed it to make it commercially available. This was the kickoff for the origin of the Medtronic company by Earl Bakken. A commercial pacemaker that could be sold to other centers was available within about six months."

Ake Senning, who was later to become the first surgeon to implant a fully implantable pacemaker, visited Minneapolis during 1957 and watched Lillehei suture the electrodes to a child's heart, and pace the heart. He later wrote that he considered this innovation "the beginning of the era of clinical pacing."

When Vincent Gott finished his training in Minnesota in 1960, he joined the faculty of the University of Wisconsin for five years, and then moved from Madison to Johns Hopkins Hospital in 1965 as chairman of cardiothoracic surgery.

After his sabbatical year in Minneapolis, William Weirich returned to the University of California in San Francisco, but after a few years became disenchanted with the academic surgical life and went into private surgical practice in a rural community. He eventually closed his office and took a surgical position in Saudi Arabia, which he described as one of the highlights of his life.

## The Remarkable Story of Earl Bakken's Medtronic Company

The story of the late Earl Bakken is remarkable. Like Lillehei, Bakken was born in Minneapolis (in 1924) of Norwegian heritage. As a child, he was reputedly always tinkering with any electrical equipment or wiring he could find. At school, he took care of the public address system, the movie projector, and so on. As the man who designed the first portable cardiac pacemaker, it is interesting to learn that his favorite childhood science-fiction film was *Frankenstein*.

After war service as a radar instructor, he took a degree in electrical engineering at the University of Minnesota. Through his wife, who was a medical technologist, he became acquainted with physicians and increasingly was asked to repair hospital equipment. At the time Lillehei consulted him with the request to make a portable pacemaker, Bakken and his brother-in-law were working from a 600-square-feet garage, taking on repair jobs of medical equipment as well as televisions and the like.

In their first month in business in 1949, they had grossed $8. After developing the first wearable external cardiac pacemaker in 1957, the company they had formed, Medtronic, went on to manufacture one of the first reliable long-term implantable pacing systems, in 1960. By 1963, Medtronic was generating annual sales of almost $1 million, and by 1975 of $100 million. Its yearly revenues had increased to $1 billion by 1991 and to $4 billion by 1999, by which time it employed 20,000 people worldwide. Today, with annual revenues in excess of $13 billion, Medtronic is the world's leading medical technology company. It is one of the great success stories of the early days of medical bioengineering.

## Coping with a Patient's Death

I pointed out to Dr. Lillehei that one of the things that Chris Barnard admired most about him and his colleagues at the time they were developing open heart surgery was the courage they had to keep going when they were having a "bad run." My understanding was that even when they were experiencing a series of operative or postoperative deaths, Dr. Lillehei persisted because he knew what he was doing was right. I asked him how he had coped with the deaths at the time.

"That is a good observation because persistence was an important consideration, but it wasn't always easy. At times, after a particularly frustrating experience, I was almost ready to quit. After a good night's sleep, and maybe a few belts in the local bar, the next morning you felt much better. And I had a great group of colleagues. Usually, we could come up with a solution — perhaps not always the right solution, but something we should have done or should not have done, or could do differently in the next case. Then we went on. One success, of course, rejuvenated you, so to speak, and you could go on. I must say persistence was an important quality. I never understood how a guy like Gibbon could start working in the 1930s and make a lot of progress, and then suddenly quit because of failures. But he did. I later read that, at one time before going into medicine, he wanted to be a poet. Poets are maybe more sensitive than surgeons."

Lillehei's mention of "a few belts in the local bar" may not be as facetious as it may sound. His powers to "party" were legendary among the staff in Minneapolis. For example, Aldo Castañeda commented, "He worked very hard, partied very hard, almost every day, and had the constitution of an ox. He would end rounds about ten P.M. every day, and then he would usually go with some of the guys and have some drinks. The next day, the guy was just there. Amazing! How he did it, I don't know. My observation was that he was fundamentally a very shy individual, and he needed alcohol in a way to come out of his shell and become social." Others felt Lillehei's fairly regular alcohol intake helped him cope emotionally with the deaths of his patients. Dr. Castañeda described it as "an escape valve of an inner life that one didn't see from the outside."

Dr. Castañeda believed that a surgeon in that era had to be totally convinced that the ultimate goal (of making open heart surgery safe and routine) justified the deaths. He described it as requiring "a certain touch of 'immorality'.... You had to be absolutely convinced internally that you were right and that everybody else was wrong. Walt had that, but he was not a person to discuss this kind of personal stuff. Those guys were tough. They kept it to themselves, very close."

## Disappointment

When Wangensteen retired in 1967, Lillehei, the jewel in the Minneapolis crown, would have liked to have been appointed chairman of the department. Deeply disappointed when he was not so appointed, he accepted a position as chairman at New York Hospital–Cornell Medical Center in New York. There are many great admirers of Lillehei who felt that he was not suited to be a chairman. Aldo Castañeda commented that Lillehei "was not involved at all in the department as a surgical structure. He was totally out of it. Even the cleaning lady in Minnesota could have told them that Walt was not a very good candidate [as chairman of a department]. You could walk into his office, and there were these piles of old records. His desk was full of death certificates that hadn't been signed for months."

John Najarian, the incoming chairman, an expert in organ transplantation rather than in heart surgery, asked Lillehei to stay a year to see how things worked out, but within a few months Lillehei accepted the post in New York. The equipment in Lillehei's lab had been purchased by National Institutes of Health funds and, according to Dr. Najarian, should have stayed in Minneapolis. However, one Sunday, Lillehei cleaned out the lab completely and left a red rose in the middle of the empty room. He took everything with him to New York. Cornell eventually reimbursed Minneapolis for some of the equipment.

## Move to New York

To put it mildly, Lillehei's time in New York did not work out well. Norman Shumway later wrote that Lillehei's tenure of his professorship there "made the French Revolution look like a church ice cream social." Mistakes were made on both sides — by Cornell and by Lillehei, whose personal situation was probably not helped by the fact that his wife and children did not accompany him to New York, as it was felt wise for the children to continue their education in Minneapolis. According to Bob Frater, Lillehei's "appointment to New York Hospital was a total disaster. Lillehei's personal life sort of collapsed, although his wife stuck with him until he died; she is a marvelous woman."

Lillehei, always a man who enjoyed a few drinks and a good party, went wild in the "Big Apple." He hung out in bars, and drank even more heavily than usual. To make his job at New York Hospital easier, he had been given the use of a penthouse apartment, in which he threw lavish parties for hospital staff and other "friends," often female, he accumulated in New York City. His wife was quoted as remarking, "I don't mind the fact that he had lady friends there, it was the class of the lady friends I objected to."

According to Frater, "the final disaster was when he was supposed to be operating in New York, but he was in Chicago, and the patient died on the table. And the foolishness of it was almost humorous. His secretary was called, 'It's time for Dr. Lillehei to come to the operating room.' She knew he was in Chicago to give a talk. Presumably somebody had scheduled the case, but he had forgotten that he was supposed to be operating that day. Most people have a little book [to keep track of such commitments], but Walt wasn't that organized. She called him there, got him at his hotel, and said, 'You've got a case this morning.' He said, 'Tell them to wait for me. I'll be there. I'll catch the next plane.' It was three or four hours later that he finally got there, by which time the resident had gone ahead with the case, and the patient had died. That was what [the administration] had been waiting for, and so they got him out."

Stories of this final straw that brought down Lillehei vary. According to John Najarian, Lillehei was going to operate on a relative of the dean of the medical school. The dean went to watch the operation and, although the patient had already been attached to the heart-lung machine by the surgical resident, Lillehei was nowhere to be seen; he turned up much later.

By July 1970, although he was allowed to remain as a surgeon on the staff, Lillehei was removed from his role as department chairman and chief of surgery. He was only 51. But worse was still to come.

## The Internal Revenue Service Investigation and Trial

In 1972, a grand jury in St. Paul, Minnesota, indicted Lillehei on charges of evading $125,100 in U.S. income taxes, a very considerable amount of money at that time. If he were found guilty, he could have faced up to 25 years in prison. Lillehei, who his biographer, Wayne Miller, calls the "legendary procrastinator," had been late — often years late — in filing his income tax returns to the IRS for many years. A special agent was put onto his case who, by delving into Lillehei's personal affairs, found that he had been "leading something of a secret life — a life that included mistresses and even a Las Vegas call girl."

His trial began in January 1973. He was accused of not reporting his income from many different sources, and of claiming parties, gifts to girlfriends, and a call girl as tax-deductible expenses. Veterinary bills for his pets, dance lessons, and tuition were all billed as tax-deductible expenses. One hundred sixty-four witnesses were called by the prosecution, including girlfriends to whom he had given expensive gifts, and 16 by the defense. More than 6,000 exhibits were entered into evidence. According to Frater, "a check for 'secretarial duties' was made out to a person who appeared on the stand; she was an obvious tart. It was a sad, sad tale."

In his defense, Lillehei admitted that his billing system had been lamentable, and his filing system had been one of index cards in a shoe box; in other words, his financial affairs were in chaos through his own neglect, bad judgment, carelessness, and procrastination, but not, his lawyer claimed, from fraud. However, some of his index cards were found to have been altered, for which Lillehei was unable to provide any explanation.

The chaos of his financial affairs was confirmed to me by Bob Frater: "When he died, there were a couple of rooms in his house totally filled with papers. The St. Jude company people helped his wife, Kaye, sort the stuff. They allegedly came across $100,000 in cash in one place or another amongst all these damn papers. The story has probably grown in the telling, but the point is that he was just chaotic."

Wangensteen and Varco testified on Lillehei's behalf. His lawyer attempted to paint a picture of a man overwhelmed by his surgical work and without the time to spend on his personal affairs. The trial took 21 days. The jury found him guilty on all counts. The judge, however, could not bring himself to imprison Lillehei, stating that he recognized, "You have this great talent that should be of use to society." The judge felt that imprisonment would either destroy that ability or render it useless for a period of time. He therefore fined Lillehei the maximum $50,000 and ordered him to serve six months' community service.

New York Hospital–Cornell Medical Center ordered him to leave by the end of the year, even though they honored his contract through the end of 1974. After December 1973, Lillehei never performed another open heart operation. He was developing cataracts, possibly as a result of the irradiation he had been subjected to for his lymphosarcoma, and decided that he would not operate again even though he was only 55 years old. The American College of Surgeons suspended Lillehei indefinitely, and the State of Minnesota revoked his license to practice medicine there until completion of his community service. Lillehei found it difficult to find a hospital that would allow him to serve his community service but, finally, through Wangensteen's good auspices, one was found in Brooklyn.

I asked Vincent Gott whether the problems Lillehei had experienced in later life changed the attitudes of former members of his team. He responded, "It didn't change my opinion of him at all, nor did it any of his people. Frankly, I don't think there was one millimeter of immoral fiber in the man. He enjoyed life to the full; he worked hard and played hard. He obviously pushed things to the limits, but he treated the patients just like he treated us. The fact that he had some problems later at Cornell certainly didn't change our opinions. We had a great affection for him."

At the early age of 55, Lillehei found himself in the surgical wilderness — an outcast in a field to which he had contributed so much. For more than ten years, he remained a pariah to many in surgery. He continued to publish a few surgical papers but was rarely invited to lecture in the United States, although he was still invited abroad. It was John Kirklin who, in 1979 in an address as president of the American Association for Thoracic Surgery, began Lillehei's rehabilitation in the eyes of his colleagues. It took some 10 to 15 years before his reputation was rehabilitated.

In this respect, Lillehei was also helped by an appointment as medical director of a small Minneapolis company that made a mechanical valve, the St. Jude prosthesis, to which he contributed significantly through his surgical experience. Bob Frater, who was appointed medical director of St. Jude after Lillehei's death, explained that "St. Jude gave him the position of medical director when he was essentially on the ground. He did that job most responsibly. When visiting surgeons came to St. Jude's, he would be able to give them a talk and discuss operative aspects with them in a way that would indicate he was still practicing cardiac surgery, although he hadn't been for a good long time by then. He kept up with new advances. He was a valuable advisor on new projects. He never stopped thinking. He was just a unique personality."

Ultimately, in addition to the money he had earned as a busy surgeon, Lillehei made a lot of money through royalties on prosthetic valves in whose design he had been involved, and from investing in the stock market in the 1940s and 1950s. According to Frater, "When he died, he left $15 million. That was from royalties on the St. Jude valve."

After his death in 1999, Walt Lillehei's widow donated $10 million from his estate to the department of cardiothoracic surgery at the University of Minnesota.

## RICHARD VARCO — THE STABILIZER

There was one other key member of the Minneapolis team in the 1950s whose name crops up repeatedly: Richard Varco (Figure 30). Varco seemed an omnipresent figure in the early clinical development of open heart surgery. He assisted John Lewis with the first-ever successful operation performed under direct vision inside the hypothermic heart. With Clarence Dennis, he performed the first two pioneering, but unsuccessful, attempts with use of the heart-lung machine. He subsequently shared the operative procedures with Walt Lillehei in the daring cross-circulation operations, and then equally shared them in the first series of operations performed with the bubble oxygenator. So Richard Varco played a significant role in the development of open heart surgery. Although not the innovator that Lillehei proved to be, he was an important figure in that he brought to the Minneapolis surgical teams his operative experience and superb skills. Described by several as a surgeon with unmatched technical ability, he provided technical expertise, experience, and stability in the Minneapolis operating rooms of that era.

John Kirklin was convinced that "nobody can underestimate the importance of Dick Varco in that Minneapolis development.... He is brilliant. He is one of the most brilliant people who ever walked the streets of cardiac surgery. He is absolutely brilliant. He was a superb technical surgeon. I know everybody always refers to him as the 'stabilizer' of the Minneapolis team. When they got into trouble in the operating room, it was Varco who got them out of it—that's what a 'stabilizer' means. He was a superb surgeon and a totally different individual than Walt. That's probably why they did so well together. The other people over there would know better than I, but, from my point of view, Varco wasn't particularly interested in innovation. He was interested in other things. I think he could have done whatever he wanted. I just happen to be a tremendous admirer."

When I met Dr. Varco in the medical school in Minneapolis in October 1991, I found a short and very substantially overweight man. He wore gray-green baggy flannel trousers, a sports jacket, a rather heavy-cloth blue shirt with collar unbuttoned, and his tie slack around the neck; he had a rather untidy appearance. He was affable, but I sensed he was a little doubtful about the interview initially. By its end, however, he was clearly enjoying himself and had valued the opportunity to discuss his early work. He was quick-thinking and articulate. His answers to my questions were precise and, at times, even lyrical, and required little subsequent editing.

## Early Days

Dick Varco was born in the town of Fairview in eastern Montana in 1912, and went to a school where the first six grades were in one room. His father was a merchant, and his mother was a homemaker. He had no brothers or sisters (although he later had no fewer than nine children of his own). When his mother died, he moved with his father to Minneapolis, where he attended Twin Cities High School, and went on to the University of Minnesota.

"I enjoyed college life to a very high degree," he remembered. "I was introduced to a different scale of social and sports activity. Life was easy on campus. I was by no means a student leader, either from a political or, certainly, from an academic point of view. I was just a student going along with the tide. The reason I went into medicine was because, in the course of the freshman orientation week, I found that I had no interest in engineering or dentistry. So it was a choice between law and medicine. I made the wise choice of going to the law orientation lecture, and came away thinking that medicine could scarcely be anything but better, and so I entered myself as a premed.

"I graduated in 1936. The next day, I started an internship. In those days, most of the internships were rotating internships through a wide variety of specialties in medicine. That's what I did. I then went through Dr. Wangensteen's surgical residency program over the next seven or eight years.

"I spent much more time in the research lab than in [clinical] medicine. In fact, for some time I was an instructor in physiology, headed towards a career in physiology, because I enjoyed the opportunity of providing the technical knowledge of a surgeon to the physiology laboratory staff. People should be aware that the costs of research were much different from today. To give you some idea, in my off-duty hours, if I had any, if one of the other services wanted a preparation, I would shave a dog, take care of it, do the operation, take the stitches out, and do everything else for 25 cents an hour, and I was very happy to get it.

"At the time I took over as senior resident in surgery, I had very little surgical experience in the operating room with regard to patients. The reason was because I had spent such a long time in the research laboratory. Because of people leaving for the war, I was an intensely busy person. Many of the staff had departed with the military hospital, and so we were very short-handed for a long period of time. I completed the senior residency and then went on to the faculty, and then the people started coming back from the war.

"Cross-circulation gave us a period longer than controlled hypothermia, but was short of what we could see we were going to need. With these operations, once we went beyond brief periods of time, we were treading on the edge of safety. We needed extra time to repair more complicated lesions. We were motivated by the precariousness of our position. The heart-lung machine was not only getting ready, but it was a very attractive idea."

Dr. Varco then told me how incredulous he was when Gibbon stopped his work on the heart-lung machine. "I have no idea how a person can expend as much time, emotion and money, and have had so much support from his family, from society, and from his associates—everything argued as cogently as possible to pursue it—and I have no awareness from intuition, or from personal experience or gossip, as to why he stopped. I have no indication at all." Nevertheless, he felt that Gibbon had developed a "new concept in medicine which has benefited tens of millions of people, and he deserves the credit he hasn't received from several sources.

"Most of us were caught up in the competition with John Kirklin, who was doing a tremendous job in the Mayo Clinic series [chapter 8]. We weren't opponents. In fact, we talked with each other and got ideas from each other. We were eager to get ahead and, of course, we were eager for him to get ahead. There was competition, but it was healthy competition. It was a very friendly, open, generous, understanding, let's-get-at-it type of association. There are few persons more in my admiration than John Kirklin for the job he did."

## The Lillehei-Varco Team

"For some time Walt and I worked as a team, and then Dr. Wangensteen decided we should work as separate units. What his reason was I never understood because Walt and I worked well as a team. I think working together lent to the accumulation of a larger volume of knowledge and to a greater capacity for problem-solving. Since we were trying new procedures in the sense of operating on lesions that hadn't been operated on before, we were in need of all the new knowledge or sum total of knowledge that we could amass. We worked well together. There was no conflict of egos of any sort, which, under the circumstances, was perhaps a bit surprising. Walt and I got along extremely well.

"Initially, I had considerably more experience with heart operations than did Walt. Walt was a fast learner, and learned everything there was to learn. But there are things that could best be done from one side of the operating table or the other. We could divide up the surgery and do whatever was easier from one side of the table or the other. This would save time as well as maintain good exposure. I view it as one of the really wonderful experiences in my life to have worked with Walt Lillehei in such an utterly congenial fashion for all of the time we did."

Dennis Melrose remembers visiting Minneapolis and watching Lillehei and Varco operating together: "Varco was a very great support to Lillehei. When they operated together, it was impossible to see who was doing what, as there were four hands working in unity. It was extremely interesting to watch."

I asked Aldo Castañeda, who worked in Minneapolis from 1958 to 1972, to comment on the relationship between Lillehei and Varco. He said, "It was a peculiar relationship because Varco was fond of Walt, but they didn't see eye to eye on many things — attitudes, techniques, training habits, and discipline, and so on. They were very, very different people. But they admired each other. Walt told me that he wanted Varco around because he helped him from a technical point of view."

According to Dr. Varco, "All the people I worked with avoided any callousness that lent itself to accepting a death as 'just another death.' On the contrary, we tried hard and worked longer hours than necessary. In fact, with the first fifty patients — maybe a few more or a few less, but approximately that number—Walt and I, one or the other, was with the patient or in the room next to him for the entire night after the operation. Every hour, either Walt or I was in the intensive care unit or next to it for every patient. He would take part of the night, and I would take part of the night. So work helped to a very great degree, as did intense analysis of why you might have succeeded if you had done this or that. We tried extremely diligently to obtain consent for autopsy, and succeeded because we had a good rapport with the parents of the children who were our patients. In my opinion, there is no underestimating the value of an autopsy in evaluating what might have been done or in determining that there was nothing that could have been done to improve the outcome. So reviewing the record on a moment-to-moment basis, being adjacent to or in the intensive care unit, and the follow-up of those who succumbed all helped carry you through the period of charting new water."

Dr. Varco admitted that Lillehei had not been a great organizer, but believed he could have been a successful chairman of the department if he had been provided with the necessary administrative help. "He could have brought in people to do the organizational work. He could have had bean-counters up to his eyebrows, but the point is that he had the inspiration and the ability to get people excited, to work diligently and carefully for him, and to be very confident in preparing material for him. It's just that his surgical activities occupied so much of his time that he was perpetually putting this or that thing aside 'for the moment.' Make no mistake about it, Walt was an outstanding leader. In addition, though, he did require—and it was part of the problem that developed—an organizer. He required a person who could be his aide-de-camp, his secretary-general, not just his secretary. The person had to have more power than that of a secretary. He needed a principal office executive, but that is the type of person he didn't have. It's a shame, because the right person doing the job would have taken care of that aspect of Walt's career very well. I was very much against his going. In fact, I remember telling him, 'Walt, don't do it. Stay. It will work out better. You've got a lot of people here who are on your side. We support you, you support us.' When he left, it made a lot of difference to us. No question about it."

At the end of our interview, Dr. Varco escorted me to the main entrance of the building in which we had met, greeting one or two people on the way. I observed him closely. To someone who did not know of his achievements, he would not have looked in any way distinguished. His clothes were rather ill-fitting and of relatively poor quality. His bulky frame shuffled along ahead of me. Without wishing to be in any way disrespectful of someone who, in my opinion, rates extremely high in surgical history, I felt he could easily have been mistaken for the janitor. Appearances can obviously be very deceptive.

Dr. Varco died in 2004, at age 91.

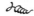

# CHAPTER 8

# The Iceman Cometh: Establishing the Heart-Lung Machine

_____

## JOHN KIRKLIN

Following the pioneering work of Gibbon and those others outlined in chapter 6, the group at the Mayo Clinic, headed by John Kirklin (Figure 35), took on the Gibbon heart-lung machine, developed it further, and performed the first series of open heart operations using this device, beginning in 1955. This series overlapped with Lillehei's cross-circulation work and with the introduction of the DeWall oxygenator. The Mayo Clinic had the financial and personnel resources to take on what was an onerous task, as the Gibbon machine was expensive and complex. John Kirklin was not perhaps a true innovator in the mold of Bigelow, Lillehei, or Hufnagel, but rather a developer. Nevertheless, through this series of operations, he made a major contribution toward establishing open heart surgery. Without doubt, this was an important series of operations, and great credit must go to his group for this work.

John Osborn, who was a contributor to the development of open heart surgery, commented on the advantages of the Mayo-Gibbon heart-lung machine over the DeWall-Lillehei machine: "When Lillehei was using DeWall's bubble oxygenator, he would give lectures at meetings and say, 'This bubble oxygenator cost $7.' He compared it with the Gibbon machine, which cost $50,000 or so. It was a derogatory comparison. But very slowly over the next few months, it became apparent that the Mayo Clinic could do cases Lillehei couldn't do because they could run the heart-lung machine for a longer period. The $50,000 machine was really better. I've always admired Kirklin's character, hearing these comparisons made without ever getting mad."

With Crafoord, Senning, and Lillehei, Kirklin therefore stands as the earliest pioneer in the successful use of the heart-lung machine to operate inside the human heart in a series of operations. He was extremely highly regarded by the other surgical pioneers with whom I spoke. He continued operating until he was 71 years old, helping to establish heart surgery on a scientific footing. With Sir Brian Barratt-Boyes (chapter 10), he co-authored a monumental tome for cardiac surgeons, *Cardiac Surgery,* which provided a most comprehensive review of the entire field.

## University of Alabama Medical Center

I met with Dr. Kirklin in Birmingham, Alabama, in May 1991. The University of Alabama Medical Center was a hodgepodge of buildings, some old, some relatively modern, but none looking very up-to-date. Furthermore, the buildings were not as well maintained as I had expected. The day was, however, rather cloudy and overcast, and I therefore probably obtained a worse impression of the complex than I would have in bright sunshine. The building in which Dr. Kirklin's office was situated had an unimposing entrance, the foyer being nothing more than a small empty hall with very old elevators. The inside of the building appeared no better maintained than the outside.

Dr. Kirklin's office suite doubled as the editorial office of the *Journal of Thoracic and Cardiovascular Surgery,* as well as the base for his own research group. The suite was filled with large computers, which took up almost entire rooms, clearly representing his major interest at the time, which was the statistical assessment of the results of various types of cardiac operations. Dr. Kirklin's personal office was medium-sized and practical. It didn't seem to reflect any personality of its incumbent, although cynics might say that, in a way, perhaps it did; from what I had heard about Dr. Kirklin, I had always thought of him as a rather "gray" man without much personality — certainly not in the Charlie Bailey or Walt Lillehei mold. In many ways, his offices reflected this grayness. Although Dr. Kirklin's personal office was in reasonable shape, of all the office complexes I had been to in the course of preparing this book, this group of buildings was the least attractive and the most run-down.

I am not sure why I expected the buildings of the university to be new and plush, rather like those in the Houston medical complex (chapter 13), but I did. Perhaps this was because I had believed the rumor that had been rife when Dr. Kirklin moved from the prestigious and well-established Mayo Clinic to the then almost-unknown University of Alabama at Birmingham in 1966. At that time, the rumor was that the university had been prepared to put an immense amount of money into his department if he accepted the post of chairman. During the course of my interview with him, I learned that this was not true.

John Kirklin gave the appearance of being a small man, slim though not unduly short; indeed, he was about five feet ten but with a narrow frame. He had gray-white hair, which he combed forward over his forehead without a parting in a rather "ancient Roman" style (Figure 35). His delicate features made up a relatively unimposing face, which was dominated by large glasses that, together with his small frame, made him look anything but athletic; the terms "boffin" or, if they did not have slightly derogatory connotations, "nerd" or "geek" would come to mind. He was dressed in a plain white shirt, tie, and pants — all very nondescript. There was certainly nothing flamboyant about him or his surroundings.

When I had initially written to Kirklin about my project, it was clear he was not keen to participate; he responded with a short letter, stating that he did not have time to be interviewed. Some months later, however, a further approach from me persuaded him to do so. On the day we met, he proved friendly, courteous, and interested in the project. I had anticipated that he might be a very closed and reserved person, reluctant to talk about himself or others. I found this true to a certain extent, since he was generally noncommittal in his comments about other surgeons unless he could be laudatory, but he was fairly open about himself. Indeed, he proved more approachable and considerably more open in his replies than I had expected.

## Student Days

Kirklin was born in Muncie, Indiana, in 1917. His father, a radiologist, was invited to join the staff of the Mayo Clinic in about 1926, where he became head of the department of diagnostic radiology. So the young John Kirklin grew up in Rochester, Minnesota, where he went to high school, proceeding to college at the University of Minnesota from 1934 to 1938, where he majored in psychology, graduating Phi Beta Kappa, and was reportedly first in a large class. He was the student manager of the football team for four years. At that time, the University of Minnesota football team was arguably the greatest in the country, being national champions for three years. He traveled with the team, and enjoyed every minute.

He then went to Harvard Medical School, to which he applied mainly because it was said to be hard to get into. Dr. Kirklin told me, "We all arrived at the Harvard Medical School in the fall of 1938, not very many months after Dr. Robert Gross had first successfully closed a ductus. I think there were 110 guys who were all going to be cardiac surgeons. That was especially so after Dr. Gross came to lecture to us, because he was certainly the public's image of a surgeon — good-looking, immaculately dressed, very quiet; he never had much to say. He had a certain aura about him. Besides all that, this guy had done this world-famous operation when he was just a resident."

In an interview Dr. Kirklin gave to Dr. William Roberts, editor of the *American Journal of Cardiology,* published in 1998, he noted that "my father did not bring his work home. There was not much talk about medicine around the house." He also mentioned that he did not grow up in a "particularly intellectual environment." His childhood coincided with the Depression years, but his father "shielded me from that world." Since the young Kirklin never took much interest in his father's work, I asked him what had influenced him to apply to medical school.

He responded, "I'm not sure. When I was at college, I had in mind becoming a biochemist. I didn't really plan on being a doctor at that point. Even though I came from this fabulous medical environment [presumably referring to his life around the Mayo Clinic], I really didn't decide until I was a senior that I was going to go to medical school."

He did well as a medical student: "I was in the top small group. At Harvard, I got the award for being the number-one person, graduating magna cum laude." When I asked him whether he had to work hard to achieve this success, he replied, "I think you have to work hard to a certain amount, but it was easy." There was a slight degree of smugness about this statement, or at least an absence of the humility that one expects from the highly gifted. Although they may find it easy, the highly gifted don't usually admit to it so readily, or at least they preface what they say with something like, "I was very fortunate in that I did find it relatively easy." Dr. Kirklin made no effort to excuse his academic prowess.

## Surgical Training

In medical school, Dr. Kirklin said that nearly all the students in the class thought they were going to be cardiac surgeons. I asked what made him persist in that aim while all or most of the others changed their minds.

He said, "It was obviously exciting. Cardiac surgery didn't amount to much at the time, but there seemed a real likelihood that a lot of things could be accomplished. By the time I finished medical school, World War II was on, so everything got held up for all of us. I had an internship at the University of Pennsylvania for nine months, then went to the Mayo Clinic for another nine months, and then into the army, where I was a neurosurgeon—I hadn't done enough surgery to qualify to be a general surgeon. After the invasion of Normandy, the army had very many head injuries and they were already air-evacuating them back to the United States. So they took a bunch of us and, in three months, made us neurosurgeons. We dealt mostly with peripheral nerve injuries. I enjoyed that and did a lot of operations. I was in a U.S. Army hospital in Springfield, Missouri, but it was a neurosurgical center. We had about 2,500 neurosurgical patients at any one time." Dr. Kirklin spent a total of 27 months in the army.

"Robert Gross's article on coarctation and Blalock's article [on the shunt procedure for patients with Fallot's tetralogy] came out when I was in the army. So I arranged to take some army patients to Boston, where I went to see Dr. Gross and asked him if I could spend some time with him. I went back to the Mayo Clinic to finish my general surgical training, and then went to the Children's Hospital in Boston for six months in 1948. Since I had known Dr. Gross a little in medical school, I understood him.

"While I was there in 1948, I and another guy, who eventually dropped out of cardiac surgery, kept notebooks on all the operations we could do if we ever got inside the heart. It was in that same year, maybe, that Dr. Gibbon made his first postwar presentation—at a forum of the American College of Surgeons. Gibbon reported fifteen dogs with maybe four survivors or thereabouts. I can almost play that presentation back in my mind as a movie. I remember it very well. Gibbon said, 'Those results may sound bad to you, but we're encouraged and we think that we're making progress.' But nobody was very interested in heart-lung machines—absolutely not.

"I joined the faculty of the Mayo Clinic in 1950. We began to develop cardiac surgery there. I had been interested in it for a long time. Then Bigelow's work on hypothermia began to get great attention. And then there were two wonderful entrepreneurs, Henry Swan and John Lewis, who developed the field, especially Henry, who was charming, skillful, and very aggressive in his charming way. So the whole world was galloping towards hypothermia. Nobody much bothered with Gibbon. Those early hypothermia operations were extraordinarily important because they attracted everybody's imagination. They made open heart surgery a reality. Lewis and Swan were extremely important as individuals. They were both very stimulating and interesting people; cardiac surgery got off to a good start with interesting people. They were a different kind of people from Charlie Bailey or even from Dwight Harken. Bailey and Harken were not only of the 'closed' era, but they were of a totally different era. They were *pre*–World War II guys, whereas all the rest of us were *post*-War people. All of us had been in the army doing something else. I think there's a very big difference, but I'm not sure I can define it easily. Maybe youth had something to do with it."

## The Mayo Clinic

Dr. Kirklin continued, "In 1950, the Mayo Clinic was an absolutely marvelous place. I walked into a hornets' nest of intellectual activity, and was really lucky."

Very early in 1951, Dr. Kirklin had a patient who died after closed heart surgery. With his colleagues, he examined the heart. "We said we weren't going to be able to do anything with something like that unless we could get inside the heart and have some time to do a lot of work. Hypothermia, of course, gave you 10 to 12 minutes at the best. So I never really got diverted into hypothermia because I didn't think it was going to be flexible enough to allow us to do what we wanted to do. After that case, a small group of three or four of us decided we were going to get into the pump-oxygenator [i.e., heart-lung machine] business. At that time, there were three places we could visit to see what was going on in this field. One was in Toronto where

Bill Mustard was using monkey lungs, one was in Philadelphia with Dr. Gibbon, and one was to a fellow named [Forest] Dewey Dodrill in Detroit. Dodrill was very active at that time and, as you might predict, his pump-oxygenator was a little bit like a car engine because General Motors had built it for him. Dr. Gibbon's machine looked a little bit like an IBM computer.

"After we got home from visiting these three centers, we thought for several months and decided there was no reason why Gibbon's machine would not work. His machine was a result of ten years of engineering and development. We thought, why the hell don't we just build a Gibbon machine? Dr. Gibbon and IBM were a little bit reluctant, but they finally gave us the drawings to the machine, and the engineering shop at the Mayo Clinic began to build it. I had to do a lot of convincing at the Mayo Clinic to get them to build this thing.

"We didn't try to reproduce it exactly. We modified it some, and we kept modifying it after we started to use it. By modern standards it was a pretty simple machine but, by standards at that time, it was complicated. It probably took us something like two years from building the machine until we felt ready to use it clinically. We were working in the laboratory all of that time.

"As our development was about to be completed, Walt [Lillehei] did his first cross-circulation case. When everybody picked up the morning paper and read about Lillehei's great case in Minneapolis, I had a lot of telephone calls from my colleagues wondering why we were going about it in such a complicated way with such a big machine when 'those guys over in Minneapolis just hooked up another person.' But it didn't take much imagination to realize that the cross-circulation approach wasn't going to survive. It only allowed small patients to be operated on, and allowed only a very limited amount of time for the procedure to be completed. It never caught on, but I bet you there were a number of places in the United States that did one case. You'll never know, because those surgeons are mostly dead or will deny it. But a lot of people got ready to do it. Absolutely. Just like a bunch of sheep."

## The Clinical Trial

He continued, "Anyway, this little group of us decided we were going to do eight clinical cases in 1955. I think we decided it around the first of the year, because by then we had done ten consecutive dogs, with 30 minutes of bypass, and had lost only one of them. That seemed to mean something to us. So we did a few dogs in the operating room with the nurses. We scheduled eight cases. We told the parents of the eight children we selected that we didn't know how this was going to work and that there was another option, cross-circulation. None of the parents were very interested in serving as a donor. We had decided — all of us — that we would do the eight cases even if the first seven died, unless we learned something that said this approach was not feasible. [In fact, four of the eight patients died.] We were going to do those eight cases and then go back to the lab. We went back to the lab, but we were never able to turn off the clinical work. We began on March 22, 1955. The first case was a five-year-old girl [Linda Stout] with a big ventricular septal defect; she lived."

## A Resident Reminisces

Bob Frater was a resident at the Mayo Clinic in 1955, and described to me his first experience of seeing the heart-lung machine in clinical use, an experience that convinced him that cardiac surgery was what he wanted to do as a career: "Having been spending my time working up medical patients for the urologists, I went into an operating room in October 1955, on a Saturday afternoon, just to see an operating room again. There was this surrealistic scene with John Kirklin operating on an infant with tetralogy.... It was a tall stainless-steel machine, blood trickling down the screens, with pumps directing the blood both to and away from the patient.... The patient didn't survive, but it was a revelation to me. They started open heart surgery in March 1955, and so this would have been about the thirtieth case or so."

Dr. Frater later joined Kirklin's team, and he recounted to me how relatively primitive the operating conditions were compared with today. "This was a machine that you ran standing up. It was waist high. We used normothermia [i.e., they maintained the patient at normal body temperature] for the very simple reason that we didn't have a heat exchanger. We *couldn't* cool the patient. The blood came from donors whose blood had been drawn at six o'clock in the morning, so it was all fresh blood.... The anesthesia was very light — nitrous oxide at 50% and oxygen, and curare to paralyze them. The patients would have memories of the operation; they would ask questions about it afterwards. Even in 1957 we didn't have any of the monitoring that is regarded as normal today. We did not have an arterial pressure line, just a cuff on the arm. We did not have an electrocardiogram (EKG) screen in the operating room; we read the rhythm by the beat of the heart.... We didn't have a decent way of pacing the heart except by placing plates on the chest and sending a shock through the whole body."

Monitoring of the patient after the operation was also very basic. "All of our needles were reused in those days. Our patients didn't stay on respirators after surgery; they were extubated on the operating table for the very simple reason that we didn't have a decent respirator. We were working with an incredible intensity. We were constantly coming upon *solutions* we didn't understand. We realized we were doing something quite extraordinary. The excitement and exhilaration! We were skating on thin ice all the time. Suddenly, something would go wrong with the patient, and you wouldn't know why.

"The first patients who had open heart surgery at the Mayo Clinic had a doctor sitting with them throughout the night in a private room. The nurses didn't really do anything much; they were there, but they didn't have any routine to follow such a patient. So the patients would depend on the residents. One of my colleagues once came out of a room with his face white, and said, 'I've just killed somebody. I've just electrocuted somebody.' I said, 'What happened?' He said, 'I was doing the afternoon EKG, turned the machine on, and the patient convulsed, his heart stopped, and he died.' That was before the days of proper grounding of the EKG machines. My colleague had electrocuted the patient.

"I hope I have given you some feeling for the excitement that we had, and the intensity of the experience. You had to be working at a heightened level of sensitivity to try and understand. You had to be so acute to try to think of what was going on, looking after the patient postoperatively. You didn't have half the tools you have today. You just had to be constantly aware of what the possibilities were, and try to bring every bit of primitive 19th-century physiology that you had at your command to try and understand what you were doing. We were way ahead of the cardiologists. They hadn't thought of three-fourths of the things that we were thinking."

When I asked Bob Frater what were Kirklin's strengths at that time, he replied, "Organization — completely methodical organization. Everything was done by numbers. Everything was written down to an intense degree. Each step was written down somewhere. The manuals he developed later — great big thick manuals — they all start with, 'Put the patient on the operating table.' He had a very precise style of operating. He was not a natural surgeon. He didn't make things up as he went along. If he encountered something that he hadn't prepared for, he would find it very difficult indeed. There was a basin of water in the corner of the room to which he would go; he would put his hands in the basin and hang his head and think for a minute or two in the middle of an operation. If it wasn't in the book, Kirklin didn't know what the hell to do."

But, in Frater's opinion, this very methodical planning was essential for the time.

"Absolutely essential. Vital. We, of course, had visitors all the time. I can think of people who came through the Mayo Clinic on flying visits so they could do open heart surgery back at their home base. A good portion of the people had very poor results because they tried to learn very quickly. The number of surgeons who thought they could fly just by buying a machine and taking it back home with them was enormous. The disaster stories of those days are legion. They would watch Lillehei, who was a remarkable character, immensely inventive, but not organized, and then they saw Kirklin work; if you followed his methods, you would at least do quite well."

Kirklin clearly had a highly organized and disciplined approach to life. Dr. Frater added, "Even with hobbies and pastimes, he approached them with the same extreme methodological intensity."

Although Kirklin was perhaps not a true innovator, he refined other people's ideas and established them successfully. "That's very important," commented Al Starr (chapter 9). "This man took some pretty crude ideas and gave them substance, which is a very precise and rational approach to surgery. It is really important."

## Lillehei and Others

I asked Dr. Kirklin when, in relation to his own work with the heart-lung machine, the Minneapolis group started the clinical work with the bubble oxygenator.

"It was four to six months later. Experimentally, I'm sure a long time before that. One of the things that I'm really very proud of in that era is that Walt and I never got to throwing eggs at each other. We may have had our own opinions about each other and what each was doing, but we were each free to come to the other's workshops. We did talk at meetings — and argued, of course. We had very different views about a lot of things but, in looking back at that era, I can honestly say I think we didn't engage in throwing eggs at each other. We weren't really good friends, but we were certainly not enemies, even though we were highly competitive. I would help his wife look for him at four o'clock in the morning at meetings and so on [an aside directed to the well-known fact that Lillehei would party until late into the night — or, more accurately, early into the morning]. For a year or two, the only place in the world you could get an open heart operation was in Minnesota." (This statement was not strictly accurate, though very largely true.)

Dr. Kirklin also commented on Lillehei's unfailing optimism that they would eventually learn to deal successfully with the complex congenital heart defects they found themselves inadequately prepared to correct at that time.

## The Move to Birmingham

I then directed the conversation toward Dr. Kirklin's decision to move in 1966, at the age of 49, from the world-famous Mayo Clinic, where he was chairman of surgery, to the then relatively unknown medical center at Birmingham. I remembered that when I was a house surgeon (intern) with Russell Brock and Donald Ross in London in the mid-1960s, they had been surprised to hear that Kirklin had chosen to relocate, because everything had been going so very well for him at the Mayo Clinic.

"I don't mean this for the effect, but there was never a sensation that I enjoyed having the world at my feet, as you might say I did at the Mayo Clinic. One thing bothered me, and that was visitors coming through, saying, 'You know, we could do it this way too, if we just had the money that the Mayo Clinic has.' I didn't think that was really true. I confess that one of the motives I had in moving was to find out if that *was* true — if that sort of work could only be done at the Mayo Clinic.

"The second thing that angered me was when I would go to a meeting and hear, for example, a surgeon from the University of Somewhere report his gastrectomy results, with a mortality twice or three times what it was at the Mayo Clinic. He would always say, 'But this is because we have to train residents.' I totally rebelled at the idea that you would have people doing an operation that you knew was going to increase the mortality two or three times, and you would condone it. Those things just kind of sat in the back of my mind, but I'm not sure that they would have really pushed me into doing something.

"I had been offered the job at Stanford in about 1963 or 1964, but I don't know I was quite yet of a mood to do it. When they asked me to come down here [to Birmingham], I really came to look only as a courtesy. Apart from a couple of good cardiologists, for all practical purposes there was nothing here. When I got home, I got a map and a compass, and drew a circle of five hundred miles around Birmingham. There wasn't a really competitive cardiac surgical program anywhere. So I thought I could generate enough money to have a program here that would work. If it didn't work, it would be *my* fault because there was nothing here to obstruct me. I wanted to see if it required the Mayo Clinic to have a first-class cardiac surgical program.

"So for all those reasons, I chose to leave the Mayo Clinic. You know when you're young, you're very self-confident. It would scare me to death to think about doing it now." Dr. Kirklin agreed he was trying to prove something to himself.

Bob Frater's opinion on Dr. Kirklin's decision to move was that "the University of Alabama was looking for a great figure, whereas Kirklin was looking for academic recognition.... The Mayo Clinic was a clinical institution, but not then a medical school, and Kirklin believed he would suddenly start having an immense academic output, which, in fact, proved to be the case."

I mentioned to Dr. Kirklin that, at the time, rumor had it that the University of Alabama was prepared to contribute vast sums of money to build up his unit. Was that true?

"Everybody thought that must be the case. Otherwise, why in the world would he have done it? There is no semblance of truth in that. I think the city, not the university, made a decision that it wanted to turn its back on the past [referring to its civil rights problems] and move into a new era. I think there was a feeling in Birmingham, and maybe a little bit around the state, that they had had enough of the previous era and would like a new era of growth in a good way — less U.S. Steel and more medical center kind of things, and so forth. But the university didn't have any money to do anything special. When I came down here, I didn't have any special financial advantages. We generated money by doing cardiac surgery."

However, having made the move, Kirklin frequently wondered whether he had made the correct decision. "About a thousand times.

The first couple of years here, I wasn't sure where my salary was coming from. And you couldn't believe how bad the physical environment was — the toilets, for example: you could hardly walk by them, let alone go in them. It was unbelievable. I felt personally and financially insecure. I wasn't sure that the program was going to succeed. But by 1970, with some excellent young colleagues, we were growing by leaps and bounds. Then, I guess, I probably began not to think so much about the Mayo Clinic. It was a hard place to leave — cradle-to-grave security, professional, personal, and everything."

Under Kirklin's direction, not only as chairman of the department of surgery and director of the division of cardiovascular surgery but also as chief of the medical staff, the University of Alabama at Birmingham soon became well known throughout the world. In surgeon-scientist John Norman's words, "Kirklin's approach was meticulous, scientific, controlled, disciplined, and systematic. He took Alabama from ground zero to a premier university surgical service whose graduates, or whose work, became internationally known."

Much of Kirklin's success in Birmingham must be attributed to his personal hard work. He recounts how he would get up at 4:30 A.M., work at home on a book or paper, arrive at the hospital at 7 A.M. and operate until 1 or 2 P.M., after which he would deal with administrative and research matters, getting home at 7:30 or 8 P.M.

Terence English, who spent a year with Kirklin in Alabama during his training, remembers that "his Saturday morning Grand Rounds in Birmingham were amazing — the ability of one man to chair a meeting and really get something educational out of every opportunity. The 'Death Conferences' that followed the Grand Rounds were wonderful. He would always chair them. He went over the death, and would say, 'What particular time was an error of judgment, an error of execution, made that related to this patient's death?' He would pursue that until he was satisfied that he had found out the answer. Kirklin's attitude to death of the patient was quite different from other surgeons at the time. He said, 'You know, death should not be part of this business.'

If you did everything right, you made the right diagnosis, you did the operation perfectly, you looked after the patient afterwards, you would never have a death. This was one of his great contributions. I think he influenced many British surgeons like that."

It would seem that Kirklin was an adherent to the surgical aphorism "There should be no 'hope' in surgery." Absolutely nothing should be left to chance.

"He was an extraordinary man," continued English, "who had a great influence way beyond the Mayo Clinic and Alabama. The respect in which he was held meant that, at meetings, he could be absolutely devastating, but that was what was needed at the time, I think. But a very cold man, and a very difficult person. He was very professional to his patients; he always sat down at their bedside, took an extensive history, and did a very good examination. But he wasn't somebody who patients would warm to."

In an article heart surgeon Larry Stephenson wrote (published in the *Journal of Cardiac Surgery*), reminiscing about his time as a surgical resident under Kirklin, he detailed the resident schedule at Alabama at that time: "Routine morning rounds started at 4:00 A.M. We had to call him at home to go over his patients at exactly 6:00 A.M. If we called a few minutes early, he would hang up the phone and we had to call back at exactly 6. If you called a few minutes late, he would hang up and you were in trouble.... I suspect the phone treatment was to let you know he wanted things done his way, *exactly his way!*.... At night, when you were on call in the hospital, you had to call him at home for even relatively minor problems related to his patients — 'no unilateral decisions' — he would tell us repeatedly.... Oftentimes you were so tired that you were almost in a numb state. But Dr. Kirklin did not like to see you looking tired. You always had to be shaved before he showed up in the morning, and you could not look sloppy either.... When you called him at home about a problem which you were required to do, of course he was not very happy to learn of the problem, and this made it all the more unpleasant for you.

The more you called him that night, the worse it got for you, but you did have to call him."

Larry Stephenson also provided information on the "blue book," a book in which Dr. Kirklin had detailed *exactly* how he wanted his patients to be managed. "It was basically a well-organized recipe book on the way Dr. Kirklin did business, so to speak, on his service.... Even though you now had a 'cookbook', so to speak, on how to handle many patient situations, this in no way excused you from the 'no uni-lateral decisions' rule or law."

Stephenson also recorded an incident in the operating room where one of the residents was clearly irritating Kirklin by constantly making suggestions for the management of a patient who was doing very poorly on the operating table. After seemingly infinite patience, "Kirklin looked at the resident and said, 'Claude, let me tell you a little story. There was this old gunfighter who had killed a lot of men, and he was just sick of gunfighting and didn't want to fight anymore. He came to this town, and there was a young punk there who was bother-ing him and trying to provoke him into a fight, but the old gunfighter tried to avoid fighting the young punk. Finally, the young punk, who was trying to make a name for himself, aggravated the old gunfighter so much that the two of them went out into the street and drew their guns.' Kirklin then said, 'Claude, do you know what happened next?' Claude said, 'No, Dr. Kirklin. What?' And he said, 'Well, the old gun-fighter got his gun out first and shot the young punk right through the heart. Do you understand the significance of that story, Claude?'"

## The Qualities Needed to Be a Pioneer Surgeon

"I think it's recovery ability," was Dr. Kirklin's opinion. "Maybe it's a different word for the same thing, but the number of nights that I went home and cried are more than I would like to recount to you. Somehow, the next day, I would recover. I think it's the ability to recover. After all, there is a very fine line between courage and reck-lessness. In the surgical world, recklessness is not very well rewarded, you know. Maybe Walt and everybody I know each responded in a different way, but I believe they went through the same emotions that I felt, and recovered quickly. You don't take six months off because you had a catastrophe yesterday. You may take a day off. Those who couldn't recover quickly decided to opt out."

Dennis Melrose put forward one explanation as to why Kirklin could cope with the deaths he encountered: "I always found John Kirklin so cerebral that he could probably analyze the situation and decide he had made all the right decisions, but that it just hadn't worked. I saw him once attempt to close an atrial septal defect using Gross's 'well' technique in a patient with pulmonary hypertension. [The "well" technique was a surgical approach used by Robert Gross before heart-lung machines had been developed.] The blood kept rising into the well, and it was obvious the defect couldn't be completely closed, and so he left it open. He calmly said that 'the patient will die this afternoon,' and indeed that's what happened. He was at the forefront, and was still learning things. He could do that, and yet work again the next day."

It was perhaps this reputation for ice-cold logic and lack of emotion that caused one surgeon I interviewed, Robert Bartlett, to refer to Dr. Kirklin as "the iceman." And yet Dr. Bartlett also recalled being fascinated by an after-dinner talk Kirklin gave to the residents at the Brigham Hospital. His opening remark was, "Surgeons are people who cry in movies." Bartlett explained: "What he meant was that we are dealing with patients, either in the operating room, office, or clinic; we have to be in charge, absolutely in control, and have to be emotionless and just technically very good. His point was that you have to be that way if you're going to be a good surgeon. But if you get sentimental in a movie and cry, don't worry about it — don't be embarrassed about it."

But despite his "iceman" professional reputation, his "recovery ability" sometimes failed him. Kirklin, like most of the other surgeons embarking on open heart surgery in that era, was far from immune to the emotional impact of a patient's death. Bob Frater remembered, "If he had a bad result, it would be intensely upsetting to him. We had five deaths in one week — not actually on the [operating] table, but later on the same day. On the Friday, he disappeared. He actually had a patient on the table, and he just didn't turn up. We called him, and his wife said, 'He took off in his car last night, and I don't know where he went.' We just woke the patient, and said, 'Dr. Kirklin got sick and we will have to do you next week.' He came back on Monday without any acknowledgment of having been missing on Friday. He disappeared several times. It didn't happen once, it happened several times."

I asked Dr. Kirklin whether his huge commitment to cardiac surgery had affected his personal life. Did his family "suffer" in any way?

"Sure. No doubt."

Was that commitment worth it?

"Sure." (Although this was clearly an honest reply, I felt that it was perhaps a little too quick, and he had too much of a smile on his face. There was no hint of regret or self-recrimination for not spending enough time with his family.) "It's mundane to say it, of course, but my wife [to whom he was married in 1943] held our family together. You have to be lucky to have survived as well as I survived because it was a terrible life. I can't tell you how many Saturday nights I would call my wife, and say, 'I can't go to the party tonight. I've just got to stay here [at the hospital].' I would get home late at night and be gone early in the morning. I suppose my kids suffered some. I always set aside some time, but I surely wasn't as much with them as I really should have been. I think it's tough."

(Although one of Dr. Kirklin's sons is now a distinguished cardiac surgeon in his own right, another son had problems as a young man. Some years after I spoke with Dr. Kirklin, he was quoted as saying, "Perhaps when you ask if I was a good father, probably not.")

## Precision
When I had finished interviewing Dr. Kirklin, he asked me if I would like a bite to eat. We went through to the adjacent room — his small

library—where there was a small table on which his secretary had set down two cardboard picnic boxes, one on each side of the table. I was brought a Coke and he was brought a coffee, both in paper cups. We opened our boxes and found inside two identical sandwiches of salad and turkey. We sat directly facing each other, eating the sandwiches, as if following instructions in Dr. Kirklin's "blue book" that every resident was given, detailing how to respond to every situation he or she might encounter. I felt we were subjects in a David Hockney painting. It all seemed so precise and organized, and it reminded me of Dr. Kirklin and his work, which has always been highly organized and highly precise. Many of his papers have been absolutely loaded with statistics, sometimes seemingly—to me at least—almost to the point that the statistics became more important than the message, although this was clearly not the case. It seemed very typical of him that we should sit in such a formal and precise manner to eat our lunch.

In an interview published in the *American Journal of Cardiology* in 1998, the editor, William Roberts, picked up on Dr. Kirklin's striving for precision in all he did. He quotes Dr. Kirklin as saying, "The precision I think is the key to everything—in your head, your hands, and everything." When Dr. Roberts asked him, "Would you say that the desire to put precision and science into everything you do has been maybe your outstanding contribution?" Dr. Kirklin replied, "I hope so. I sincerely hope so."

Bob Frater agreed that Kirklin's contribution had been to make cardiac surgery precise and scientific: "What he started with [Eugene] Blackstone was the notion of statistical analysis, which has had its pluses, but also its negatives. It remains the essential way we try to work. We try to get reliable evidence, and try to make everything we do based on reliable evidence."

This organization and need for perfection and precision could at times be carried to an extreme. Frater remembers that Kirklin "worked out the position of the operating table that he wanted relative to the heart-lung machine, and relative to the side wall of the operating room. He took a tape measure and moved the table a certain distance from the side wall. Then he measured the distance from the head of the table to the other wall, and he shifted the table by a couple of inches. Then he went back and checked that he hadn't altered the distance from the side wall. It was something that drove us absolutely nuts because we could see no point in it at all. Everything had to be *just* right. He was *too* rigid. He would do something in a particular way; it would have to be done *just* that way and no other way. Then he realized it wasn't working right, and he worked out a new way to do it, and the new way would then become the gospel. It was as though the previous way had never existed. You don't have free innovation under those circumstances, but you have disciplined performance. If Kirklin hadn't been there, systematizing cardiac surgery, I think cardiac surgery would have had more difficulty getting ahead."

The desire for precision and discipline made Kirklin not an easy boss for his juniors. "He was very difficult to work with," said Frater. "Certain people would have a terrible time with him. We were on rounds, and he said to one of the residents, 'Is the patient on digitalis?' 'Yes, sir, I think so.' 'What do you mean you *think* so?' 'Yes, the patient is on digitalis.' 'What's the dose?' 'I believe it's 0.25.' 'What do you mean you *believe* it's 0.25? Is it 0.25 or isn't it 0.25? And when did the patient have the last dose?' 'Well, sir, I think it was seven o'clock.' What do you mean you *think* it was seven o'clock? Was it seven o'clock or wasn't it seven o'clock?' The fellow would immediately run to the toilet and vomit because he would be so churned up by what he had been through. The atmosphere could be incredibly tense. If things were tough, you could make a suggestion. If you made it properly, and persisted in it, and had a reason for it, he would listen to what you were saying. 'Yeah, alright. Let's do it that way.' He actually had a genuine interest in educating us."

Over lunch, I mentioned to Dr. Kirklin that he had a reputation as being a demanding boss. With good humor, he immediately thanked me for being so kind in choosing the word "demanding," and said that at times he realized he had been "impossible." He thought that to be demanding was acceptable, but to be impossible was not. During operations, he had frequently been "impossible" due to his own frustration at not being able to do the operation as well as he would have liked. He did not believe he was "impossible" outside of the operating room, where he maintained he had been no more "difficult" to work with than most others. He told me he slowly developed an increasing awareness of how difficult he was to work with in this respect and, during the later years of his career, he had made an effort to improve. His readiness to accept this fault was one of his good points, I thought, in contrast to the hint of a slight lack of humility he had demonstrated earlier during our conversation.

Kirklin's professional achievements have been so monumental that he has every right to feel highly satisfied, perhaps even smug, about the success of his professional life. For, in the words of William Roberts, written in 1998, "John Kirklin is the greatest scientific cardiac surgeon of this century and his contributions will continue to be influential many decades after he is gone."

Dr. Kirklin died in 2004, at age 86.


## REFINEMENTS

The work of the two Minnesota groups, headed by Lillehei and Kirklin, demonstrated that operations inside the heart could be carried out successfully. Naturally, improvements and refinements to the use of the heart-lung machine continued to be contributed over many years by several groups. Here, I shall mention just three.

### Dennis Melrose — "Metabolic Arrest" of the Heart

The early developers of heart-lung machines included Dennis Melrose in London. The development of his machine enabled successful open heart surgery to take place in the United Kingdom fairly early, following soon after the initial efforts in the United States and Sweden.

Although he never completed his training as a surgeon, but remained a research physiologist, Dennis Melrose deserves mention among the pioneers of heart surgery.

Of equal, if not more, importance to his work on the heart-lung machine was his introduction of the concept of stopping the heart during open heart operations by "metabolic arrest." He initiated this by injecting a solution containing a high level of potassium into the root of the aorta, which was then carried down the coronary arteries to the heart muscle. A high level of potassium arrests the heart immediately, by "paralyzing" the muscle cells, providing excellent conditions for surgery inside the heart. It is obviously easier to operate on a motionless heart than it is on one that continues to beat. It also has the same safety advantage of Senning's ventricular fibrillation in that a motionless open heart cannot pump air into the brain.

This approach caught on rapidly in the United States, more so than in Europe. Initially, the doses of potassium used were rather too high and led to damage to the heart muscle, and so this form of obtaining elective cardiac arrest went out of fashion for some time. However, during the 1970s it formed the basis for further experimentation and the introduction of more balanced solutions that are now used routinely not only to stop the heart during open heart surgery, but also to stop and protect donor hearts being transported for purposes of transplantation. Metabolic arrest of the heart with a potassium-based or potassium-like solution is greatly preferred to electrical ventricular fibrillation for open heart operations today.

Potassium arrest is now almost always combined with local hypothermia. The potassium solution is cooled in the refrigerator to 4°C (39°F) before its infusion into the coronary circulation, and thus the heart's oxygen demands are immediately considerably reduced both because it stops beating (from the paralyzing effect of the potassium) and because it is cooled (to reduce its metabolic requirements even further). During open heart surgery, the motionless heart is often intermittently or continuously bathed in cold saline to maintain a low demand for oxygen. If the heart is to be transported for subsequent transplantation, it is transported packed in ice, again to minimize energy requirements.

## John Osborn — Filtering and Cleaning

John Osborn was another physician who developed one of the early heart-lung machines, which enabled San Francisco surgeon Frank Gerbode to become the first surgeon to perform open heart surgery on the West Coast. In the early days, about half the adult patients in whom the heart-lung machine was used were clearly mentally confused for a few days afterward. About a quarter of them were *very* psychotic for the first three or four days, and had tremors and halting speech. A fair number never completely recovered. The cause was uncertain. Osborn began to wonder whether the confusion was due to very small blood clots (microemboli) that formed in the machine and lodged in the brain of the patient. When fiberglass filters became available, he began using them to filter the blood returning from the heart-lung machine to the patient. He recounted his experience to me:

"In the first patient, when I came in the next morning, he was lying in bed arguing with his wife over some finances at home. I had never seen that before on the first morning after surgery. Usually, these guys were 'flat' — they were really sick. What is more, he seemed to be winning the argument. So I knew something was different. I secretly set up a clinical trial. I didn't dare tell anybody. By random numbers, in some patients I used filters; in the others, I did not. I got up to about thirty patients. Then all of the nurses came in to see me. I remember it so well because some of them were crying. 'Dr. Osborn, we don't know what you're doing, but we know you're doing something. Half the patients are better than they have ever been, and the other half are just as sick as ever. Whatever you're doing, you've got to stop it. Do it for *all* the patients.'

"I went back to my data to see if I had a [statistically] significant difference between the two groups, and there *was* a significant difference. So I stopped, and used filtration in all of them. After that, postoperative psychosis just disappeared."

Osborn then turned his attention to another problem that was very common in those days. After the operation, many patients were either feverish or developed a condition known as "pump lung." The lungs filled with fluid, and, despite being put on a ventilator, the patient might gradually die through lack of oxygen. Osborn considered these complications might be related to a lack of complete cleanliness of the heart-lung machine.

"It was very hard to clean heart-lung machines. The evidence for this was that three times I designed and built a totally new oxygenator. In each case, the first animal did very well; the second animal was very sick, but survived, the third animal died, and all the subsequent animals died. This happened three times in a row with quite different machines. It took that long for me to realize this wasn't just coincidence. The reason it wasn't coincidence was that the first time, the oxygenator was clean. The second time it was *almost* clean; it was never clean again. But nobody at the time recognized it.

"By hindsight, the trouble was a reaction from the 'dirty' surfaces of 'filming' oxygenators. One of the best tests was to smell the oxygenator beforehand. You smelled the inside of it. If there was a bad smell, that patient was going to get 'pump lung.' If it smelled totally clean and chemical, then the patient wouldn't get it. This was a cleaning problem. It wasn't the only cause, but it was a major cause. It was the reason why, for short perfusions, bubble oxygenators did much better than the 'filmers' because they didn't have this problem. But for long perfusions, a 'filmer' was preferable to a 'bubbler,' but it would have to be clean."

The cause was contaminating foreign protein on the surface of the oxygenator, probably from its previous use. In other words, the oxygenator was not completely clean, even though it might be technically "sterile" (i.e., no bacteria or other microorganisms were present). Increasing attention to chemical cleaning of the parts of the heart-lung machine that came into contact with the patient's blood, or by using disposable parts, eventually resolved the problem.

## Nazih Zuhdi — Sugar Water

As a young doctor, relatively newly arrived in the United States from Lebanon, Nazih Zuhdi had the opportunity to work first with Arthur Voorhees, when he was developing synthetic vascular grafts at Columbia University (chapter 9), then with Clarence Dennis on the development of his heart-lung machine in New York, and finally with C. Walton Lillehei in the early days of open heart surgery in Minneapolis. He therefore personally experienced many of the advances in heart surgery.

When he left Minneapolis to develop cardiac surgery in private practice in Oklahoma City, he pursued experimental research for several years. His first innovation was to use stored (or banked) blood, rather than fresh blood, to prime the heart-lung machine. This greatly simplified the logistics of carrying out open heart operations. Before this innovation, it had been necessary to call in large numbers of volunteer blood donors — sometimes up to 20 of them — on the day of the surgery. The use of stored blood made the logistics so much simpler, but still a large volume of blood was needed to "prime" the pump.

Zuhdi then had the vision to perceive open heart surgery being performed without the need for any blood at all. He primed the heart-lung machine with a simple sugar solution (5% dextrose) rather than with blood, and found that diluting the cellular constituents of the blood was actually beneficial to the patient since the flow of "thinned" blood through the tissues was improved. At the end of the operation, the presence of the sugar in the blood stimulated the patient to pass increased amounts of urine — as it does in diabetic patients — thus concentrating the blood once again, and returning the red blood cell content to normal.

This contribution may be perceived as being a relatively minor refinement, but it was, in fact, a very significant contribution to the development of open heart surgery since it enabled this form of surgery to be performed much more readily and inexpensively, and thus on a much wider scale than hitherto. If whole blood had been necessary for every open heart operation, this would have placed immense strain on the blood banks around the Western world, and would have hindered the widespread dissemination of open heart surgery techniques. Just as DeWall's simple and inexpensive oxygenator brought open heart surgery within the reach of cardiothoracic surgeons worldwide, so did priming the machine with 5% dextrose make this form of surgery even more accessible, particularly if the operation needed to be performed in an emergency.

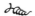

## CHAPTER 9

# Bionic Men:
# Artificial Materials
# and Mechanical Valves

———

## ARTHUR VOORHEES, CHARLES HUFNAGEL,
## AND ALBERT STARR

W ITH ACCESS TO the inside of the heart now assured by the heart-lung machine, surgeons began to suffer the frustration of not being able to deal with many of the conditions they wanted to treat. They could close a hole between the chambers of the heart and they could relieve a narrowed valve by incising or dilating it, but they could not as yet do much else. The congenital abnormalities that infants were born with — the holes in the septum (ASDs, VSDs), valve obstructions (e.g., pulmonary stenosis), and so on — were by no means as common as the conditions people could acquire from disease as they grew older.

Rheumatic fever left many of those affected with leaking valves or valves that were so tightly narrowed and heavily calcified that nothing short of replacing them would be of benefit to the patient. Surgeons therefore turned their attention to searching for materials and metals that could be used to design artificial valves, so-called prosthetic valves. But before this advance was made, the search for synthetic materials that might be used to replace diseased blood vessels had taken place, and it is this development we shall explore first. Although not first used in the heart, these materials soon became useful to patch a hole in the heart or reconstruct a major blood vessel arising from the heart. Initially, however, they were used some distance from the heart to replace segments of the major blood vessel in the body, the aorta.

The wall of a diseased aorta, if affected by the degenerative condition of arteriosclerosis or other cause, can slowly weaken. As a consequence of the high pressure from the blood inside the vessel, the wall can steadily distend, becoming what is known as an aneurysm. Eventually, the aorta may burst, which may be rapidly fatal. Alternatively, the disease process can lead to narrowing of the lumen of the aorta until it is virtually obstructed, preventing adequate blood flow to the legs. It was arteriosclerosis of the aorta that was first attacked by those interested in replacing a blood vessel by a vascular prosthesis.

## ARTHUR VOORHEES —
## ARTIFICIAL BLOOD VESSELS

Arthur Voorhees (Figure 36) is something of an anomaly in the company of most of the other surgeons included in this book in that he was never a cardiac surgeon. He warrants inclusion by the fact that he, almost single-handedly, devised the first cloth graft that was the forerunner of the multitude of prosthetic grafts that are currently used today to replace major blood vessels. As similar materials were subsequently used inside the heart to close defects such as ventricular septal defects, Voorhees's work has had a major impact on the development of this branch of surgery. Although Michael DeBakey and Denton Cooley are usually recognized as the "fathers" of aortic surgery, and their role in expanding and establishing this field must not be minimized, it was Arthur Voorhees who made the initial major innovative contribution.

I met Dr. Voorhees on a rather overcast, but not too cold, day in October 1988. I traveled from Boston by bus to the far western edge of Massachusetts, where he met me in his silver Mercedes. We had a light lunch at a small rustic café; he clearly enjoyed the ice cream with caramel sauce. His large poodle stayed in the car.

In appearance, Dr. Voorhees was an undistinguished little man, not at all imposing. He was short, of average weight, and his straight hair was cut short with a little tuft sticking up at the back. He had a ruddy face with rosy cheeks, deep brown eyes, and a cherubic smile. When he smiled, he occasionally fluttered his eyelids. Indeed, there was a certain sense of innocence and artlessness about him. He proved pleasant, quiet, and fairly articulate.

## The Quaker Community

Arthur Voorhees was born in 1921, and grew up in a community of great affluence not far from Philadelphia, although his own family was less than affluent. While neither of his parents was a Quaker, they lived in a Quaker community in Moorestown, New Jersey, which was, he told me, "extremely socially conscious, not in the sense of high society, but about the underprivileged, the black man, the individuals who they felt for one reason or another were disenfranchised in the community. The difference between public education and education at the Friends [Quaker] school which I attended was vast. We are talking about a school that probably was a match for any English 'public' [i.e., private] school in the intensity, the skill, and the caring of the teaching program.

"I think that I actually came to medicine more through the route of being interested in what you could do for a patient than through the other routes, such as biological curiosity, the challenge of the discipline itself, or the prestige and plaudits that you would get from your fellow man because it's a 'noble profession.' It was for that reason that I started thinking seriously about a career in medicine while I was still in high school. My great-grandfather had been a horse-and-buggy country doctor in Alabama. I had no direct contact with him, but he was lionized in my mother's mind, and she in turn passed on the folklore to me. Later, when I was in my teens, I started working during the summer as a chore boy around a camp, cutting wood, building log cabins, and helping guests. The organization was owned by a rather prominent cardiologist from New York. He tried to interest me in medicine."

At Columbia College of Physicians and Surgeons in New York, Voorhees's role models were surgeons, because he was impressed with their ability to teach. He was able to understand what they were doing because they were talking to him in a mechanical way as opposed to a linguistic way, in which he was deficient. He had been told he was dyslexic.

He continued, "The most important role model for me was Arthur Blakemore. As a surgeon, he was a maverick. He was willing to tackle the most god-awful things. He made his reputation because he was willing to take on operations that no one else would attempt. This came from his courage rather than from his outstanding skills. Anything that was large, deadly, or frightening, he would tackle. He would embark upon procedures that would last sometimes ten, twelve, fifteen hours. I was terribly intrigued, not because of what he did, but because he had the courage of being inventive. He just had a restless, imaginative, challenging mind."

Dr. Voorhees graduated from medical school in 1946. After investigating certain blood coagulation problems with Blakemore in the laboratory, he accepted a research fellowship in vascular surgery at Presbyterian Hospital in New York City.

## Inspiration — The Cloth Graft

"Everybody was coming back from the war and trying their hands at anastomosing [joining] blood vessels. The Ethicon company people were devising these minute, fine silk sutures. There were a whole lot of things coalescing about that time, including the widespread use of antibiotics. It was a very, very exciting period. In the laboratory, I was surrounded by a group of fellows who were working on homografts [blood vessels taken at autopsy from the dead]. The homograft was thought to be the answer for replacing blood vessels. But there was no way that they were going to be able to get enough homografts to meet the demand. So tubes made out of glass and plastics and exotic metals — platinum and the like — were tested to replace blood vessels, but all failed."

During the course of this research, "it suddenly dawned on me that maybe we could make a blood vessel prosthesis out of cloth. At least I could sew it in because sutures would go through cloth material as well as they would go through the aorta. The mere fact that I knew that my colleagues were working on a means of preserving homografts to be used as arterial grafts probably put it into my mind at the time.

"I went to Blake [Blakemore] that very afternoon, and said, 'Hey, Blake, could this work?' I was just talking out loud. In true fashion, he said, 'I don't know. Why don't you try it?' We had some pieces of silk material in our operating room that we called China silk. It was junky stuff, but smooth, and looked like a silk handkerchief. I simply put it into the aortic wall in a few dogs. This would have been January or February 1947. The first one I put in, the dog just literally bled to death. The silk just wept blood all the way through [i.e., blood poured out between the weave of the cloth]. In the second case, I simply compressed the proximal aorta with a finger [thus preventing the blood flow into the region with the cloth prosthesis] and allowed the prosthesis to fill retrograde [i.e., fill with blood under low pressure]. The bleeding did not go on uncontrollably. The graft would swell up and you could see the blood oozing from the surface of the cloth, but it wasn't spouting out in tiny jets. It was then that I realized that within a few minutes, clotting would take place in the interstices of the material. [Blood clots would fill and block the holes between the weave of the cloth, thus preventing further bleeding through the cloth.] So that became my technique.

"I made the grafts myself. I borrowed my wife's sewing machine. I would come home at night and make up tubes using little templates — pencils and test tubes, anything that was tubular — in a variety of sizes. Of course, I had difficulty with fraying at the ends. Looking at the cuff of my shirt, I got the idea that, if I simply folded the material back on itself like a French cuff, I would get rid of the fraying problem. That was the way it was for quite awhile, a year or more."

Voorhees then spent two years as an army physiologist in San Antonio, Texas, where Blakemore urged him to continue this research "on the side." He scrounged around and found some old parachutes made of nylon, from which he could make aortic grafts that worked fairly well. After his military service, Voorhees returned to Columbia Presbyterian Hospital in New York City. A colleague who had been working with plastics advised him to investigate the properties of a fiber called Vinyon-N. "'Where do you get it?' I asked. He said, 'You go to Union Carbide and see a man who has been very cooperative as far as my work is concerned. See what he can do for you.'

"So I traipsed down there, and he heard me out. He looked rather puzzled, and said, 'I can't understand anything of what you're doing, but if this can help you, here.' He reached behind his desk, literally, and pulled out a bolt of cloth, and said, 'This is Vinyon. You can have it. We haven't been able to find any use for it. It's so inert that it won't take an aniline dye, and therefore we can't introduce it into the garment industry because we can't dye it. Here, take it.' And that was it. As far as the porosity was concerned, as far as the weight was concerned, it was absolutely perfect. It had the difficulty of being a flat cloth, so you couldn't stretch it out."

Voorhees tested Vinyon successfully in many dogs, and then presented his research at a couple of surgical conferences. "It was very helpful for me because it was an open meeting and everyone was cross-firing questions. It helped me tremendously in designing experiments. That was the first time that Mike DeBakey heard about it. It was published, I think, in 1952."

DeBakey's name was raised specifically because he later took up the idea of cloth grafts to replace major blood vessels, and indeed became the world authority on these procedures. The original idea, however, appears to have come from Voorhees.

## The Italian in the Night

Until this time, all of Voorhees's studies had been in dogs, and he had yet to test his cloth prosthesis in a patient. The opportunity presented itself in 1953.

"One night a man came in with a ruptured abdominal aortic aneurysm. He was in his seventies, of Italian extraction — a great abdominal mass, tender, and in shock [indicating that his blood pressure was dangerously low from hemorrhage]. But he was still alive. We took him to the operating room and opened him up, hoping to get the aorta controlled and put in a homograft, which were being used in this setting. Lo and behold, there was no homograft available in the hospital, and the homograft bank in New York City had none available. Blake said to me, 'I think we had better get one of those tubes of yours.' So I broke scrub, dashed upstairs, and ran a couple of grafts up on the sewing machine. Blake had his finger compressing the aorta. When I came back, we were able to get down to the aorta and put in the prosthesis, which was a simple tube of Vinyon cloth. We used the usual technique, retrograde flow first, prograde flow second. When we allowed prograde flow, in spite of the fact that we had poured fluids and blood into him and done everything imaginable to keep up his peripheral circulatory competence, he just slid immediately into hypotension [low blood pressure], then finally fibrillated [his heart rhythm became irregular and inadequate] and died.

"However, we had had a long enough time to realize that the graft functioned. That would have been 1953. That was the very first. I was a junior assistant resident, and decisions when to use these grafts were Blake's. So I can take no credit for any of that. He was the one who had the courage and the knowledge. All I was doing at this point was being a high-class technician. It was his decision to use them on all subsequent aneurysms.

"Our experience was presented in 1954 to the American Surgical Association as a combined paper on implantation and experimental technology. At that time, the data sort of hit the fan. The evolution of the mechanics of it progressed very quickly. Manufacturers were willing to adapt their machinery to weave or knit or even braid. Others were very willing to develop mandrels over which they could weave these things, so that they could add side branches of one sort or another.

"Vinyon disappeared for a very real reason. It was a good product for vascular grafting, but it would have been entirely too costly to produce it for vascular grafts alone. Dacron came along and had almost the same properties, but it had the advantage of having a broad market in the garment industry. Splitting off a little bit of Dacron to make prostheses [to replace blood vessels] was economically feasible for the manufacturer.

"Within a period of roughly five years, there was a mass explosion of marketability, transportability, easy storage, purity, and a lot of refinements that the fabricators were mainly responsible for. Frankly, I didn't have much interest in it by then. I knew deep down inside of me that it really didn't make any difference as long as certain things were observed. One was that the cloth didn't allow the patient to bleed to death because of great permeability [i.e., the pores in the weave of the material should not be so large that clot could not form in them]. The other was that you didn't make it solid, because no fibroblasts could grow into it [i.e., cells from the body grew along the graft to form a new living lining]. It also had to conform to the topography of the body [i.e., the graft had to be supple so that it could bend where the artery it had replaced had not been straight]. This was 1955. I moved on to another field entirely." Voorhees's surgical interests moved away from vascular surgery to surgery of the liver, a technically demanding discipline in which he built up an international reputation.

I asked him whether he felt he had received the credit he deserved for his contributions to surgery.

"My wife doesn't think so. As far as I am concerned, I do not care. I really don't. I know [what I contributed], and I know that the people who I felt were important to me knew. I didn't care one whit as to whether 'the world' knew. My wife was concerned because she had seen the amount of sacrifice that had gone into doing this — the hours, years that I had to devote. She felt that there should be some reward for that time spent. It made it particularly bitter for her because Mike DeBakey made considerable publicity about it. Not that he was stealing anything. I don't in any way accuse him of that, but he had a publicity machine that would crank out 'DeBakey grafts,' 'DeBakey grafts,' and so forth. Knowing how much time I had spent on it and how it had taken me away from the family, she resented it when she watched and heard somebody else taking superficial credit for it. That bothered her. And internally it bothered me as long as my attention was drawn to it. If it had never come up, it wouldn't have bothered me at all."

Sadly, Dr. Voorhees died of lung disease and metastatic brain cancer in 1992, at the relatively early age of 70.

## CHARLES HUFNAGEL — THE "FORGOTTEN" MAN

In many ways, Charles Hufnagel (Figure 37) is the "forgotten man" in the development of heart surgery. He was more the backroom researcher and experimenter than the aggressive surgeon, and it is perhaps for this reason that he has not received the public recognition that is his due. He had a finger in several of the early pies of heart surgery. In addition to being a clinical surgeon, he was an innovator, a scientist, and a man who was ahead of his time.

Hufnagel initially worked under Robert Gross in developing the surgical correction of coarctation of the aorta, later using segments of healthy cadaveric human blood vessels (homografts) to bridge the gap resulting from resection of a long coarcted (obstructed) segment; this operation can in many ways be considered the precursor for resection (removal) and replacement of aortic aneurysms, since the principles and techniques are similar. He established a method of storing homografts by freezing them to be used later to replace diseased vessels in patients; again, this can be considered the precursor of the use of aortic valve homografts to replace a diseased valve (chapter 10). His contributions included the development, after the lead set by Arthur Voorhees, of foreign materials to replace diseased major arteries, and surgical techniques for inserting them. Almost single-handedly, Hufnagel designed, developed, and inserted the first totally artificial heart valves. He was also one of the first to work on the membrane oxygenators that are currently used today to oxygenate blood as it passes through the heart-lung machine. He even introduced the concept of cooling the patient to protect the spinal cord from injury when its blood supply was to be interrupted for several minutes during surgery on the aorta; this was one of the first clinical applications of hypothermia (and preceded the work of Bigelow, Lewis, and Swan). These are not contributions to be sneezed at. In addition, based on his extensive experience in the animal laboratory, he performed one of the earliest kidney transplants in the world, way back in the late 1940s. Charles Hufnagel, therefore, was one of the major innovators in the field of surgery during the 1940s and 1950s, and is worthy of our attention. His work laid the foundations for many subsequent clinical advances.

I met Dr. Hufnagel in 1989 in his office at the Veterans Administration Hospital in Washington, D.C. He had retired as chairman of the department of cardiothoracic surgery at Georgetown University School of Medicine in Washington some years earlier, and had thereafter transferred his attention to teaching and research at the Veterans Administration Hospital. He was clearly one of those men who would have felt lost without his professional life.

He was a small and very slightly built man by the time of our interview, in his mid-70s, with white thinning hair. I sensed a calm, quiet personality and a quicksilver mind. Although he appeared well enough, and he made no mention of any personal health problems, I later learned that he was suffering from kidney failure and must have been on regular dialysis at the time I met him. Sadly, he died only a few weeks later, at age 73.

## Childhood and Youth

Charles Hufnagel was born in 1916 in Louisville, Kentucky, where his father was a doctor. The family moved to Richmond, Indiana, a town of about 30,000 people, where he grew up. His father tackled any form of surgery in the small community. Charles attended the local school, where by his own admission he was not outstanding, and then progressed to the University of Notre Dame, where he studied premedical subjects and "played a lot of tournament tennis," representing the college. He was the first graduate from Notre Dame ever to get into Harvard Medical School. He finished medical school in 1941, and was appointed as a house officer at the Peter Bent Brigham Hospital in Boston.

Then came the war in December of 1941. It was his intention of joining a Harvard medical unit that was to join the U.S. forces, but before he could do so he developed tuberculosis, probably from performing postmortem examinations on patients with the disease and from taking care of patients undergoing resection of the lung for tuberculosis.

Dr. Hufnagel told me, "I spent a year in the sanatorium in Raybrook, New York. When I got there, I was assigned to admit all of the new patients, which entailed taking a history and doing a physical examination on them. The remainder of the time I was supposed to be resting, but that turned out not to be the case. I actually had a very time-consuming job in the sanatorium taking care of the patients. I would help the thoracic surgeons who came there to operate on their patients. In a sense, it wasn't the major rest that it was supposed to be. Having tuberculosis maybe gave me an understanding that everything is pretty transient. Most of the patients with tuberculosis I took care of died within a couple of years. Drug therapy was on the horizon, but was reserved for people who were really sick. It gave me an awareness of my own vulnerability.

"When I left the sanatorium [although he was later to return for a second period of "rest" when his tuberculosis flared up again] the admonition was that there was one thing I couldn't do, and that was to go back into surgery and pursue the kind of life I had anticipated. It was believed to be too physically demanding. I paid *some* attention to the advice. At that time at the Brigham, a surgical residency was a six-days-a-week job. If you were lucky, every seventh day you got off, but many times you weren't. So I got an appointment as the Cabot Fellow at Harvard as a surgical research fellow, and that really triggered my interest in research. When I had been in the sanatorium, I had made a list of things that I wanted to do in surgery. One of them was to replace the thoracic aorta, one of them was to find a non-biologic substitute for the aorta and the other blood vessels, and the other was to simultaneously pursue the idea of the preservation of blood vessels."

## Early Research

He continued, "In the lab, I began doing kidney transplants and other work similar to that which Alexis Carrel had done — trying to preserve blood vessels, transplantation, and so on. I was also doing work with Bob Gross on coarctation because that was another blood vessel resection which hadn't been successfully accomplished at that time.

"We pioneered the freeze-drying of blood vessels. As early as 1946 I had a blood vessel bank at the Brigham with cadaver blood vessels which were excised aseptically, frozen in liquid in alcohol and dry ice, and then stored in the dry ice icebox. These freeze-dried grafts made it possible to do reconstructive surgery [replacing diseased blood vessels], and many people lived for a long time who wouldn't have lived without them.

"One of the things that really stimulated me was seeing patients with aneurysms admitted. You knew what the matter with the patient was—he had a ruptured aneurysm—but there was nothing you could do about it except sit there and watch him die. That was really a strong impetus towards the use of rigid tubes because nobody at that time had any concept that flexible woven, or clothlike, tubes were feasible. I became interested in finding a new class of materials to be used as arterial substitutes.

"I thought Voorhees and Blakemore did great work in the concept that a material could substitute for an artery, and in demonstrating that it could work. We investigated other fabrics—'Orlon,' 'Dacron,' and 'Teflon.' I gave a paper [at a surgical meeting] on Orlon and Dacron. It was one of the first papers other than Voorhees's paper. We had about the same number of patients as he did, and very good results with Orlon. After I gave this paper, Mike DeBakey stood up to discuss the paper. He said, 'I wonder why a young man like you is wasting his time fiddling with all these different materials and fabrics when we already have a solution to the problem in freeze-dried homografts.' Today, nobody in the world has a larger number of synthetic grafts named after him than DeBakey.

"I tested a whole series of materials to make an artificial valve. We tested bullet shapes, teardrop shapes, ball shapes, diaphragms, and a wide variety of other designs. I came up with the ball-and-cage valve as the best shape [Figure 16]. Ball valves are an ancient idea, but whether they were dynamically best or not had never been tested. I made the first valves by hand in two pieces, cemented them together, and tested the principle."

Dr. Hufnagel confirmed that the artificial valve that Dr. Harken developed was a minor modification of this design, adding, "I think Al Starr got the idea from it too because I had published it." Indeed, Starr gave Hufnagel full credit in this respect.

Hufnagel carried out all of these studies with minimal help: "I had a technician only to take care of the animals. I had a secretary who had been with me for maybe six months. I had taught her how to scrub and how to act as [scrub] nurse [at the experimental surgical operations]. At the first successful implant I did [in a dog], she was the only other person there."

After a productive period of research and with his health improved, Hufnagel completed his surgical training at the Brigham and Children's. "In those days, help was short [because most physicians and surgeons were away at the war] and I got a real broad background and experience in all kinds of surgery."

## The First Kidney Transplant

In 1946, while still a surgical resident, Dr. Hufnagel was asked by the visionary professor of medicine George Thorn to try to help a patient in kidney failure by carrying out a kidney transplant. This was the first kidney transplant in a patient in Boston, and one of the first in the world.

Dr. Hufnagel said, "They wouldn't let us take her [the patient] to the operating room, because they didn't want to have a death in the operating room. So we got the patient transferred to the third floor of the surgical ward and operated there with a couple of gooseneck lamps. We knew the kidney wouldn't survive very long and we didn't want to get into a lot of trouble, and so we connected the kidney to the blood vessels in the arm using Lucite tubes. We kept it warm, wrapped in saline and so on." (The kidney was not even placed under the skin.)

"The kidney put out urine for maybe 48 hours, by which time the patient began to wake up, and her own kidney started to make urine and recover. [The transplanted kidney began to reject, and was later removed.] She died several months later from hepatitis derived from a blood transfusion. That was really the beginning of the Brigham's kidney transplant program. There had been some similar attempts at acute transplantation scattered over the world; in most instances they were under the impression that the kidney transplant was going to be permanent, which wasn't true."

Hufnagel carried out several more kidney transplants while in Boston. He went back into the laboratory for about a year, and refined some of the things he had been working on. "Nobody really wanted the job, and so I was in charge of the whole laboratory.

"When I decided to come to Washington, Dr. Thorn asked me to stay on at the Brigham. He said, 'We would like for you to continue this transplant program.' But there was too much 'heavy weight' above me at the Brigham for me to see a future there. There was Cutler and Gross and Harken and many other people who were all senior to me. My future progress was going to be very slow because of the large number of senior people who were still quite young. So I said I would go someplace where they wanted to really start afresh."

The surgical work in the field of kidney transplantation at the Brigham was subsequently undertaken by Joseph Murray, a trained plastic surgeon. In 1990, after Hufnagel's death, Murray shared the Nobel Prize for Medicine for his pioneering contributions to this field (carried out after Hufnagel's foray into the world of transplantation). If Dr. Hufnagel had been alive in 1990, I wonder whether he would have regretted not accepting George Thorn's offer of staying at the Brigham.

## The Move to Washington, D.C.

Dr. Hufnagel continued, "When I came to Washington [in 1950], the laboratory at Georgetown consisted of an old building that was full of parakeets in cages. The animal caretaker raised parakeets and canaries in there. There was no work going on at all. They had built a couple of new rooms that were empty. The dog cages hadn't been cleaned for ten years. [Dr. Hufnagel scrubbed them himself! He also cleaned and painted the floors and walls.] That was when I decided to come; after I had looked around, I felt there was an opportunity here.

"At that time, I was trying to work on the ball-and-cage valve, perfecting it and trying to make it in two pieces. If you have a ball in the middle of a plastic cage, how are you going to get the ball in there? That was a problem. I had found a little company that made plastic signs in Boston. I explained my problem to the man who ran the company and so we started to work together on it. He kept working with me when I moved down here.

"I put the first valves in humans in 1952 [the first occasion on which a mechanical valve had ever been placed in a human]. Without the availability of the heart-lung machine [that had not been developed then], these were placed in the descending thoracic aorta. These were only placed in patients with aortic valve regurgitation. [The presence of the artificial valve in the descending aorta only partially reduced the effect of the regurgitation, but many of the patients were greatly improved.] To the best of my knowledge, not one of those failed from a mechanical cause. They may have failed from thrombosis or from some other difficulties, but not from the intrinsic design of the valve. I think that is a record that probably still stands and has not been improved upon by any other sort of valve.

"Later we changed the design because the ball made so much noise of methacrylate on methacrylate you could hear it opening and closing quite readily. The valve was placed next to the left main stem bronchus [the major airway of the left lung]. If the patient opened his mouth, he had an air column that came straight up from the valve, and you could hear it easily. [Others have compared the noise emanating from the patient to that of Captain Hook's nemesis in Peter Pan, the crocodile that had swallowed an alarm clock — one could always hear them approaching.] With the mouth closed, the noise was less. We had tested silicone in animals by that time, and so we made a hollow nylon shell, put a coating of silicone on it, and fused it into a single piece [to create the ball of the valve]. That worked very well, and markedly reduced the noise. I think that was in about 1954."

I have been told by other surgeons that one or two patients committed suicide because they could not stand the noise of the original mechanical valve opening and closing something like 100,000 times a day; it played havoc with their nerves. They could clearly hear any irregularity of heart rhythm, particularly when lying in bed trying to get to sleep; this worried some of them unduly. It was said to be the aural equivalent of the Chinese water torture.

"Although I had been putting in homograft aortas for many years, late deterioration occurs. For that reason, I have always believed that the ultimate solution to cardiovascular problems in terms of substitution is a mechanical device with a predictable and determined life. That's why I've been a great advocate of mechanical valves. Maybe we don't yet have the best mechanical valve, but that doesn't mean that it won't be the best solution in the end."

Dr. Hufnagel then outlined to me some of his ideas for the future development of the artificial heart, which he also thought would ultimately become routinely successful. He believed the problems were solvable.

I left his office full of admiration for his innovative mind. Although not perhaps one of the absolute giants of clinical cardiac surgery, here was a man of infinite originality. I place him in the same category as innovators Bill Bigelow, John Gibbon, Dick DeWall, and Arthur Voorhees — "backroom" men who, by their truly innovative work, created a basis on which others could expand. Dr. Hufnagel's contributions showed others what was possible and formed the foundation for myriad improvements and advances that were ultimately to benefit thousands of patients. Those who improve, advance, simplify, and popularize are worthy of great credit, for without them new ideas may not reach the population they can help. But without the true innovators, such as Charles Hufnagel, there would be nothing to improve and popularize.

I also left Dr. Hufnagel with a feeling of admiration for his determination to progress with his career despite setbacks as a young man that would have deterred most. To develop tuberculosis one year into his surgical training program and then, after seemingly recovering, to suffer a recurrence within a short period of time would have made most of us give up the physically and mentally highly demanding training in surgery, particularly in thoracic surgery, as it was in the 1940s and, indeed, still is today. Even though he was given the opportunity to complete his training under less stressful conditions than was usual — by being allowed to work part-time in the laboratory, where the physical demands may be less — nevertheless, he showed great determination and courage. As he had noted himself, most of the patients with him in the sanatorium were dead within two years. It is remarkable that he was able to shake off this dreaded disease and go on to accomplish what he did. Surgery today is richer because Charles Hufnagel was able to cheat death as a young man.

## ALBERT STARR — SERENDIPITY CALLS

Albert Starr's major claim to fame is that he was the first person to fully establish heart valve replacement as a successful surgical procedure. Though not the first to replace a defective valve with a mechanical prosthesis, Al Starr (Figure 38) put valve replacement firmly on the map. In the words of Harris Shumacker, "Although many different valves were designed and marketed, it was the Starr-Edwards prosthesis that brought the insertion of prosthetic valves into everyday clinical practice." With his engineering colleague, Lowell Edwards, Starr developed a prosthetic valve — the Starr-Edwards valve — that functioned satisfactorily over a long period of time. He demonstrated this by carrying out the first series of successful mitral valve replacements. He therefore can be considered the surgeon who truly established valve replacement, which became and remains a common cardiac surgical procedure.

I first came into contact with him in the mid-1970s when he was invited to be the moderator of a course held annually in London for cardiothoracic surgical trainees and junior faculty. I was at that time a registrar (resident) in a London teaching hospital. Dr. Starr made several excellent presentations during the week's course. He was able to draw on his own experience and that of his group in Portland, Oregon, to provide data indicating the risks and complications of the major operations being performed at the time. I was impressed by the organization of his data. It was obvious that he ran a well-organized program in Portland. Apart from his formal lectures, he was asked to comment on many of the other presentations given during the course, and his comments were always intelligent, helpful, and based on hard clinical facts.

At the formal dinner that was the major social event of the course, Dr. Starr proved himself to be an entertaining after-dinner speaker. The one story that has remained in my mind since that occasion, more than 30 years ago, is a story he recounted of his own experience as a patient in need of heart surgery. He had relatively recently developed anginal chest pain and had been investigated by a cardiologist, who found he had significant coronary artery disease. The dilemma arose as to whether he should undergo the relatively new operation of coronary bypass, in which a vein would be taken from his leg and used to bypass the obstructions in his coronary arteries (see chapter 11). Although he was currently carrying out this operation on his patients, there was still a school of thought that recommended diet, exercise, and medication rather than a surgical procedure that carried some risk.

The first question he therefore had to ask himself, he reminisced, was whether he believed the operation was truly superior to medical measures in the treatment of the patient. Since he was recommending the operation to his own patients, he felt that he must surely believe in it, and it would be hypocritical and unethical of him if he did not submit himself to this form of surgical therapy. He therefore decided that he would undergo the operation.

The second question Dr. Starr had to ask himself was whether he should have the operation carried out in his own center in Portland or take himself to another of the country's prestigious cardiac surgical centers, where they perhaps had more experience of this operation. Should he go to the Cleveland Clinic, for example, where this operation had been pioneered a few years previously, or possibly to one of the major surgical centers in Boston or Houston, or to the Mayo Clinic? In other words, should he request a "big name" cardiac surgeon to do the surgery on him? But he had personally trained the junior surgeons at his own center, he reminded himself, and so he should have full confidence in them. He had given them excellent training and they could do the operation well. He therefore concluded that he should show his confidence in them and elect to undergo the operation at his own center.

The third question he had asked himself, however, was the most difficult to answer. Although he had taught his junior colleagues to do the operation well, when it came to operating on him, their boss, did they *want* to do it well? This was the "rub," as Hamlet would have said. Had he made their lives unnecessarily difficult at times? Did they harbor resentment towards him? Were they ambitious for the top job? After much anxious consideration, he believed his relationship with his colleagues was good enough that they probably would try to do the operation to the best of their abilities. He therefore proceeded to undergo coronary artery bypass grafting in his own center, being operated on — successfully — by one of his junior colleagues.

## A Saturday Morning in Oregon

I interviewed Dr. Starr on a Saturday in August 1990, in his office at the medical office building of St. Vincent's Hospital in Portland, Oregon. He was smaller than I remembered him in London some years previously, probably not more than five feet six or seven, and very slightly built, but the aspect of his physique I noticed most was his rather large hands, which seemed out of proportion to the rest of his frame. He had particularly long, slender fingers, typical of those that surgeons are supposed to have and yet frequently do not; I have known several excellent surgeons with short, stubby fingers. He was dressed in a sweat suit, as he was planning to go for a jog immediately after we had completed our interview. He told me he ran four miles a day, which I thought was pretty good for someone in his mid-60s. Downhill and cross-country skiing have also been part of his life.

Throughout the interview he was courteous, and was able to put his thoughts into words very easily and in a well-constructed manner. He recounted the story of his professional career without any embellishment and appeared thoroughly honest in his recollections. He spoke equally well of the accomplishments and talents of those who had been his colleagues and those who had been his competitors.

Dr. Starr had deservedly received honors and rewards for his own achievements, in both the academic and material worlds. We did not discuss the material benefits he had gained from his surgical career, but, unlike most of the other surgeons profiled in this book, I have always presumed that he benefited not only from performing heart surgery but also from the manufacture and sale of the prosthetic valves that he developed with his colleague, Edwards. Apart from his home in Oregon, he owned a home in the ski resort of Sun Valley, Colorado, and, during the course of our conversation, he mentioned other properties and/or business interests.

## First-Generation American

Al Starr was born in New York City in 1926. His father was a manufacturer's representative in the fur industry, and his uncle was a fur designer. His mother was from England and his father was from what became the Soviet Union. They came to this country as young children with their parents, so Starr considered himself to be a first-generation American. He was brought up in a nice section of Brooklyn. At school, where he managed the baseball team, he was influenced greatly by a biology teacher who directed his interests toward science.

He recalled, "I started Columbia College at sixteen. There, I was introduced to what was to me 'another world' of scholarly people whom I had not been exposed to as a youth. There were very few college graduates in my family. I became an 'intellectual,' I guess is what you'd say. In my undergraduate work, I very much enjoyed philosophy, history, and English — the humanities, in general — and physics. I cannot say that I led a totally balanced life. I was focused on this intellectual world. For some reason, I found the academic world intriguing and intoxicating and completely consuming. It was a case of total admiration for the academic world. I was thinking in terms of becoming a physicist. But then

I took some advanced math courses, and realized that it was beyond me. The mathematics involved in molecular physics was special, and I didn't think I was talented enough to do it. But it was very exciting.

"I finished at Columbia College when I was less than eighteen. I completed what was originally a four-year course in less than two years. They had switched to a wartime schedule and so there were three full semesters a year, and time in between where you could take extra credits. Of course, many of my friends from high school were fighting in the Battle of the Bulge at that time. I was very happy to be where I was and to be able to go on to medical school. They also had a 'bonus' system in Columbia where you received extra credit for every 'A-plus' you achieved, and so that was how it was possible to get enough points to graduate in such a short time. I got enormous encouragement from home because my parents put a high premium on education and were always very proud of what I was doing. Many of my cousins were also going to college. The family, having come to this country very poor, was definitely moving up into the middle and upper middle classes.

"So I went on to Columbia Medical School. This was also during the war and, as both the courses at college and medical school were very accelerated, I finished at quite a young age. When I was a student at Columbia, Arthur Blakemore was a surgeon there. I guess I would have to say that he influenced me to some extent because he was always doing 'far-out' things. In my mind, he sort of legitimized taking chances, and doing things that had not been done before. So I got used to the fact that you did not have to conform to a certain standard in medicine. What was in the medical literature was interesting, but it didn't have to govern what you did. Your horizon was as far as your imagination would take you.

"I think I was 22 years old when I went to Johns Hopkins Hospital as an intern in 1949. At that time, I was shaving only two to three times a week, so I really *looked* young as well as *being* young. Professor Blalock would not believe that I was a doctor. He looked at me, and said, 'Starr, you have to show me your diploma.' Blalock's was a rapid-fire clinical service, which influenced me into realizing that it was possible for surgery to be very exciting in the clinical arena. You did not have to spend a lot of time in the lab to feel that you were on the cutting edge of surgery because the operating room was our laboratory. Certainly the operating room was Blalock's laboratory.

"After the internship, I went back to New York to take the general and thoracic surgery programs at Presbyterian Hospital, which is associated with Columbia."

## Go West, Young Man

Dr. Starr recalled, "I always wanted to 'go West' from New York. I had a room in the dormitory at Columbia right on the Hudson River, and my room faced west. I would see the sun setting over New Jersey and know that there was this great big country out there that I had never even seen. I felt a need to leave New York and see what America was really like. I finished my residency and got a job at the Oregon Health Sciences University in 1957. Portland was a small town then, and had few things that were cultural. However, I was ready to sample a new kind of life. I very rapidly became interested in the cattle business and in farming, and I dug into the culture we have out here.

"I came [to Oregon] as a thoracic surgeon and with the charge to develop an open heart surgery team because the local patients were having to go to the University of Minnesota and to the Mayo Clinic. Open heart surgery was just beginning in different centers around the country. But I was not trained in cardiac surgery. Before I came, I therefore spent four weeks visiting centers doing heart surgery — Western Reserve in Cleveland, Minneapolis, and the Mayo. So I got a fast course in cardiac surgery from these guys. They were very gracious and open and free with their ideas, and it was possible in a short period of time to learn one heck of a lot about heart surgery, at least from what was known at that time.

"The first thing we did was go to the animal lab. I bought a heart-lung machine, which was commercially available by then. We began operating on experimental animals. I created atrial septal defects, and then closed them. I arrived here in August 1957, and it was not until the following April that we did our first open heart operation in a patient. During that time, I was going to the clinics where kids were coming to be seen, and getting to learn a little bit about pediatric cardiology from the cardiologists, reading the cardiology literature, and going to cardiology meetings. I felt it was important for a surgeon to know as much cardiology as he could.

"We did our first operation in April 1958. I think it was an atrial septal defect [ASD]. We did some ASDs and pulmonary stenoses. Then, in September of 1958, we invited the press in. By that time, I was sufficiently confident to operate on a little girl with a ventricular septal defect with the press in on it from the very beginning. That was reported in the state newspaper on the front page, and really stopped the traffic of patients to the Mayo Clinic and to the University of Minnesota. Now everyone accepted our service as a provider of open heart surgery in Oregon."

## Enter Lowell Edwards

Dr. Starr continued, "Later in that fall of 1958, while I was sitting in my office, a gentleman named Lowell Edwards came to see me. He had probed around at the medical school to see whom he might work with on some projects. His proposal to me was to work with him in developing an artificial heart. He was at that time in his sixties and retired. He was an electronic engineer by training, but actually a mechanical engineer by trade. He had numerous patents and a very successful career behind him. His most significant invention, and the one that made him a multimillionaire, was one he developed in the early part of World War II. He developed a fuel injection system for rapidly climbing fighter planes. These systems were put into all the fighting aircraft of the Allies. He was a very important figure in aviation history during the war.

"So, with that background, he thought he could build an artificial heart that might be implantable. He had all the financial resources that would be necessary. With the royalty money that was still pouring in from his inventions, he financed a small company that he called the Edwards Development Company. [The company operated in a building that was] a little bigger than a garage, but relatively small — maybe ten thousand square feet — with a machine shop and a few engineers working for him. So he had the facilities to make things real fast, plus he understood the circulation [of blood] pretty well — not the surgical aspects, but the physiological aspects.

"In the course of my conversation with him, I realized that he was quite serious about this project and that he would be a valuable resource for us at the university. I suggested that we work on one valve at a time because I didn't conceive at that time of an artificial heart without valves. Of course, now we can. The question was which valve would we tackle first? I felt the mitral, because in the aortic valve we were using other surgical approaches that were working out pretty well at the time. The question was how to begin on the mitral valve."

The first design, with plastic leaflets, failed because clots formed around it within hours or days. "We reasoned that if we used a ball valve [Figure 16], since the ball is not attached to the orifice, there was a chance that the clot would stop at the orifice and would not involve the ball. Under those circumstances, the valve would function longer and maybe indefinitely."

This mechanical valve was based on Hufnagel's original design, but, with the aid of Lowell Edwards, Starr's valve became much more refined. Starr and Edwards followed Hufnagel's progress very closely but developed many of their own innovations.

"We started using the ball valve in the fall of 1958 and, by the spring of 1960, I had literally a kennel full of dogs with mitral valve replacements. At the same time, I developed good relationships with the cardiologists. The chief of cardiology came to visit the lab and saw all these dogs, and said, 'Al, I think it's time to put one in a patient.'

"When I approached Lowell about putting the prosthesis into patients, he became very concerned because he was now a commercial inventor with deep pockets. He was afraid of the [medicolegal] liability involved with use of the device. There were no Food and Drug Administration guidelines or any FDA involvement in devices. He had a lawyer get involved. I had meetings with the lawyer, and we developed a form of patient consent, which would pass muster even now. We went to the first patient we selected and explained everything. She signed, knowing that she would be the first person to have this valve implanted."

## Clinical Progress

He said, "We did the first operation in a patient named Mary Harris on August 25, 1960. [Dr. Starr was 34 years old at the time.] She wasn't going to live more than five or six days. She came off bypass with a perfect hemodynamic result. We sent her back to the ward in great shape. The professor of medicine listened to her valve and expressed his amazement." But later that evening she died from a massive air embolus. "I had failed to evacuate air from the left atrium. The air went to her brain and caused a massive stroke.

"We scheduled the second patient for the next month, September. He had no problems after surgery and lived quite some time. During the first year of valve replacement, we did quite a few cases. We had early made a decision to anticoagulate all of our patients. In March 1961, we presented this work to the American Surgical Association, which was the most prestigious surgical group in this country.

"We then made a decision to go ahead and develop an aortic valve prosthesis. I was not aware that, in the previous April, Harken had done the first aortic valve replacement with his cage ball valve. When I subsequently learned that, I wrote to Dwight [Harken] and told him I would like to meet him and see what he was doing. He was very kind and showed me his valve. I watched him do a case. What I noticed about his operation was that he didn't have a real good assortment of sized valves. Also, the valves had no sewing ring. He was obsessed with the idea that something would interfere with the motion of the ball. The prosthesis had a double cage, like a birdcage, with lots of different mini-struts to it. It was a complicated operation, and it looked like he did not really have good engineering support for this project.

"I went back to Lowell, and said, 'I think we should go ahead and design an aortic valve prosthesis because I don't think Harken is going to be able to do it. He doesn't have the kind of engineering background to do it. And he doesn't have the concept of the complete one-piece prosthesis, where the surgeon has to do nothing but sew it in. So let's go for it.' In a very short time, we developed the aortic valve prosthesis. By then, Edwards Laboratories had started, in California. [Edwards had moved his company for tax reasons.]

"We continued to have a very active program in the lab. We had no idea whether we were on the right track and so we had a very aggressive program. We tried everything. We tried mechanical methods of non-suture techniques [i.e., fixing the mechanical valve in position without the need for stitches]. We developed the most bizarre-shaped valves, which had some advantages, and tested them in the animal laboratory. Some of them worked. We also tested all kinds of materials. It became a very fast-paced development program. By 1962, I was doing double valve replacement [replacing both the aortic and mitral valves in the patient's heart]. We did our first triple valve replacement in early 1963, I believe [additionally replacing the tricuspid valve].

"By 1963, however, we realized that the current valves were not going to make it. [Late problems were developing in the valves that included the formation of clots around the cage and deformation of the ball so that it no longer moved easily within the cage.] Because we had the earliest experience of these prostheses, we also experienced the earliest complications. The world was very excited about these valves and was using them in large numbers, but Oregon was not a happy place at that time because sooner or later the world would figure out what we already knew.

"So in 1963, we began a frantic search for other approaches. We put in cloth-covered valves in animals to try to avoid the problem of thromboembolism. We began testing other materials to avoid fatty infiltration. We deployed a new valve in 1965. Within two years, we knew we had done the right thing. Since 1965, we have tried many other types of artificial valve, but have never found one that could objectively perform better than what we had then. I think that's true to this day with all the other prosthetic valves. To any significant degree, there is essentially no difference in clinical performance. They all require anticoagulation. By 1965, the field of valvular heart disease was fully explored."

## Personal Life

As with several of the surgeons profiled in this book, the extensive effort required by his work took a toll on Dr. Starr's personal life.

He told me, "I married at 31, just before I came here [to Oregon]. My two children were born during this early phase of working with Edwards. There was a lot of conflict within myself with regard to the relative amounts of time I was spending at work and at home. The marriage eventually came apart. I don't know exactly why, but for me there was a need and drive for productivity to see something happen beyond my own personal happiness. I had to make a mark on something beyond my own personal happiness. If I were to be born to be personally happy and to die, that was not enough. I had to choose one pathway or another, and the pathway I chose was the professional one. In retrospect, now that I am older, that was a mistake. I think marriage doesn't necessarily have to be a distraction. Now I am very happily married to my second wife."

There are some people who, no matter what they achieve, feel they have never made a sufficient contribution, but Dr. Starr is fortunate in not being one of those.

"I feel happy that I have made it. I had that feeling early on. When we did the first [mitral valve replacement] operation, I turned to Mary Ellen O'Reilly, who was my research assistant at the time, and I said, 'Mary Ellen, do you realize what we did this morning?' She smiled, and said, 'Yes.' At that time, that was all I ever really needed to do.

"There was one other time in my life when I felt that, if I had died, it would have been okay. After I had interned at Hopkins and gone back to Columbia, there was the Korean War going on, and I was drafted into the U.S. Army. I was in a Mobile Army Surgical Hospital (MASH) unit for a year. I was put in charge of an abdominal team. That was the best job you could get at a MASH. During that year I did more than one thousand abdominal operations. I remember thinking that, if anything ever happened to me, it was worth having gone through medical school just for that experience. I considered that as having validated all that had come before it. Anything after that was pure gravy."

As I reflected on what I had learned from Albert Starr, I felt that he, perhaps more than any of the other surgeons whom I had interviewed, had been met by one enormous piece of luck when the retired engineer Lowell Edwards walked through the door of his office and volunteered to design an artificial heart *and* fund its development. Starr took this opportunity with both hands and made a great success of it. His own contributions to its development were very considerable. Edwards could not have done it without Starr, just as Starr could not have done it without Edwards. Albert Starr deserves every credit for making the very best of his opportunity. As Louis Pasteur once said, "Chance favors the prepared mind."

## CHAPTER 10

# Life from Death:
# Human Valve Transplants

———

## DONALD ROSS AND
## BRIAN BARRATT-BOYES

I N PARALLEL WITH the developments taking place in the design-ing and testing of mechanical valves, surgeons were continuing to explore the possibilities of using heart valves taken from human donors after death, so-called homograft valves. It was Donald Ross (Figure 39) and Brian Barratt-Boyes (Figure 40) who achieved this goal, which was a technically more difficult surgical procedure than the insertion of a mechanical valve. Both Ross and Barratt-Boyes had natural surgical skills in abundance.

The risk of rejection of the valve was considered small. A valve is little different from a piece of artery, and segments of artery had been inserted in the treatment of coarctation of the aorta for many years without rejection. The notion was that if a cornea (the "window" of the front of the eye), a structure lacking blood vessels, could be trans-planted, then why not a valve? Most aortic valves do not have blood vessels. To some extent, nutrients and oxygen can penetrate the aortic valve directly from the blood.

# DONALD ROSS —
# AT ONE END OF THE WORLD

Donald Ross (Figure 39), one of the few non–North American surgeons to make a significant contribution to the development of heart
surgery, spent his most productive years at Guy's Hospital in London.
When I was a freshman medical student there, he was chief assistant
(senior registrar) to Russell Brock. I first saw Mr. Ross (surgeons in the
United Kingdom being designated "Mr." rather than "Dr." in view of
their historical origins as uneducated barber-surgeons rather than as
university-educated physicians) in the operating room with Brock in
1957. Watching from a windowed dome over the operating table, my
main impression of those operating room scenes was that Ross was
a quiet, stabilizing influence on the more excitable senior surgeon,
Brock. Capped, masked, and gowned, it was clearly impossible to
make out Ross's physical features except to note that he was of short-
to-medium height. When I finally saw him outside of the operating
room, at first sight he was not a particularly handsome person, being
largely bald and wearing heavy glasses. However, he had a certain grace
and quiet confidence about him that was appealing, and his gentle
sense of humor made him likeable and popular.

Ross was soon promoted to become Brock's colleague as the second consultant cardiothoracic surgeon on the staff at Guy's. Some
little time later, he gave up some of his operating sessions at Guy's in
order to take up an appointment as a surgeon to the National Heart
Hospital in London. This move was partly motivated by Ross's feeling
that he was still working in Brock's shadow.

When he was promoted to the position of consultant surgeon,
and particularly when he developed a busy private practice, i.e., operating on fee-paying patients rather than those in the British National
Health Service, Ross developed a taste for well-cut handmade suits,
silk shirts, and expensive ties, and generally exuded an air of success
that added to the aura around him. He moved to a fashionable Nash

Terrace house in Regent's Park and drove himself around town in a large Rolls-Royce. These outward trappings of success were coupled with a demeanor of quiet, relaxed confidence. His surgical opinion was second to none in this field in the United Kingdom, and his technical skills became highly sought after.

However, outside of the operating room or the surgical ward, where he was always very professional, Donald Ross was known as someone who, on occasions, enjoyed a good time. Although certainly not a regular imbiber, such as Lillehei, Ross liked a good party or a social drink with his colleagues and friends. Colleagues who know him well describe him variously as "happy-go-lucky," "delightful," "a great character," or even, very occasionally, "socially irresponsible."

Ross had superb technical skills and was a born innovator. He had obviously developed considerable clinical acumen during his years spent under Brock. He was generally considered the best cardiac surgeon of his generation in the United Kingdom.

## Early Career

More than most, Donald Ross earned his success. After a brilliant career as a medical student at the University of Cape Town, where he was the number-one student in his class — a class which, by the way, included Christiaan Barnard (chapter 12) — he filled the top house appointments (internships) at Groote Schuur Hospital before moving to Great Britain for postgraduate surgical training. After basic training, he joined Brock at Guy's Hospital in 1952, then the "mecca" of cardiothoracic surgery in the United Kingdom — indeed, with Toronto, in the British Commonwealth — as a research fellow. He was responsible for the development of novel methods of hypothermia that Brock used to operate on patients with relatively simple heart defects, such as atrial septal defects.

He then became Brock's senior registrar, and played a significant role in the development of open heart surgery in the United Kingdom. He designed a pump-oxygenator, based on the disc oxygenator design, and without his presence, Brock might have found it difficult to move into the open-heart surgical era. The Guy's-Ross heart-lung machine enabled open heart surgery to get off the ground at Guy's, following soon after the Cleland-Melrose group at London's Hammersmith Hospital. When Ross was promoted to become Brock's colleague in 1958, it was Ross, rather than Brock, who forged ahead with the new surgical techniques that soon became possible.

Donald Ross was, in the opinion of most of his peers, an outstandingly good technical surgeon, although his rival Sir Brian Barratt-Boyes considered him "an average surgeon." He had small, delicate hands that appeared almost double-jointed, so flexible were his fingers. Ross made difficult procedures look easy. He almost always appeared relaxed and "laid back," even during demanding operations, and, in contrast to his senior colleague, Brock, only rarely did he become difficult to work with.

When I had the privilege of working with Donald Ross in the 1963–65 era, open heart surgery was still bedeviled by difficulties. Although the technicalities of the procedures were fairly well worked out by that stage, postoperative bleeding, not associated with technical deficiencies in the surgery, were quite common. We presumed it had something to do with destruction of clotting factors caused by a long period on the heart-lung machine, but in those days it was a mystery as to what these defects were. I can well remember us expending immense efforts toward the end of long operations trying to stop bleeding, which took the form of general oozing from all cut surfaces.

We believed that fresh blood, transfused immediately after being drawn from the donor, was preferable to stored blood. On one occasion, when we were unable to stop bleeding in a patient, as I was of the same blood group, I volunteered as a donor. The senior surgical assistant stuck a needle into a vein in my arm, and blood was pumped directly from me into the patient in a desperate effort to bring about some clot formation. Unfortunately, this last-ditch effort proved unsuccessful, but it demonstrated the lengths to which Donald Ross and other surgeons of that era were prepared to go to try to bring their patients successfully through these operative procedures.

## "Biological" Valves

It was as a medical student in 1962, at one of the outstanding Friday afternoon medical teaching sessions at Guy's, that I learned of Donald Ross's performance of the first homograft valve replacement, shortly after he had performed this procedure (on July 24, 1962). In this operation, he had excised the patient's diseased aortic valve and replaced it with an aortic valve taken from a deceased (cadaveric) human subject. This was a new approach inasmuch that, although homograft valves had been inserted previously in the descending aorta (leaving the diseased native valve intact), no one had used one successfully to actually replace the diseased native valve.

The great advantages of the natural human valve over a mechanical valve are that the blood flow through it is not impeded in any way, for example, by a ball or disc, and, most importantly, clots do not form on it, so the patient does not need to receive anticoagulant drugs. This is particularly important in women of childbearing age and, equally, in the elderly who might be more prone to spontaneous bleeding, such as brain hemorrhage ("stroke"). The great disadvantage is that, no matter how the valve has been prepared or stored, homograft valves tend to deteriorate with time — the tissues become hard or break down — and therefore inevitably require replacement in time, which is not always the case with mechanical valves. With experience, it has become clear that human homograft valves deteriorate more quickly in children and young people than in the elderly, and replacement sometimes proves necessary within a few years. Nevertheless, the homograft valve offers an alternative to the prosthesis that is preferable in selected patients.

Ross further developed the concept of the use of biological (human) valves by using aortic homografts to replace a diseased or abnormal pulmonary valve. The structure of the natural human aortic valve is almost identical to that of the pulmonary valve. In view of the low blood pressure that surrounds the pulmonary valve, mechanical valves are not suitable, as clots form on them and they cease to perform properly. In contrast, a human homograft valve can function very well without the need for anticoagulation.

Ross even developed a complicated operation in which he replaced the diseased aortic valve with the patient's natural healthy pulmonary valve and, in turn, used an aortic homograft valve to replace the pulmonary valve. He had good reasons for this approach, but the concept remains controversial to this day. In view of the technical demands the operation placed on the surgeon, it was not taken up by many others.

His innovations, and those of Brian Barratt-Boyes, in the field of homografts stimulated many other approaches to the "biological" replacement of heart valves. Valves from pigs were used, and valves were fashioned from other tissues obtained from deceased donors, such as the pericardium (the external sac in which the heart resides), the fascia lata (a strong supportive tissue in the leg), and even the dura mater (the external sac in which lies the brain and spinal cord).

Ross's final, but more transient, claim to fame was in performing the first heart transplant in the United Kingdom, on May 3, 1968, an operation of which I had the privilege of being an observer. This was only the 11th human heart transplant ever performed. Perhaps less commendably, Donald Ross also goes down in the medical history books as the first person to transplant a pig heart into a human subject. This operation was also performed in 1968 when he was faced with the difficult situation of having not one, but two patients in adjacent operating rooms whose hearts were not functioning adequately after routine open-heart surgical operations. Both patients faced imminent death since they could not be weaned from the heart-lung machines. No human donor organ was available. As one of Ross's colleagues had been advocating the transplantation of animal hearts for some time, a decision was made to use pig hearts to support the failing human hearts. This decision was made in the absence of any experimental work, which, if it had been carried out, would have indicated this approach was doomed to immediate failure, which indeed it was.

## Personal Story

As young people, Ross's parents had emigrated from the United Kingdom to South Africa "to get away from the misery and horrors of Scotland at the time," and eventually settled in Kimberly (previously the center of diamond mining). Their son, Donald, was born in 1922.

After high school, Donald Ross won a scholarship to study medicine at the University of Cape Town. He began medical school one year ahead of Chris Barnard but, since he spent an extra year completing an additional course that led to a bachelor of science degree, they carried out their clinical studies at the same time and graduated in medicine in the same year (1946). According to Ross, "At that time, education in South Africa was probably as good as any in the world, if not better. The teachers were mainly from the old Scottish schools. All of the basic sciences were wonderfully taught, and the clinical teaching was equally good."

On graduating first in his class, Donald Ross became a houseman (intern), first to the professor of medicine and then to the professor of surgery. He therefore obtained probably the two most competitive and highly sought-after jobs in the hospital. Immediately after completing his house appointments, he traveled to England.

He recalled, "I came to the U.K. to take the Fellowship of the Royal College of Surgeons of England [a qualification similar to the "Boards" in the United States]." After working in Bath, he became assistant to a leading chest surgeon in Bristol, Ronald Belsey. By that time cardiac surgery had taken root; Belsey was doing some Blalock shunt operations and closure of ductuses. "I became fascinated with it, and Belsey said, 'I'll pass you on to Brock.' I got a research appointment at Guy's Hospital in 1952." Brock had already done his first mitral and pulmonary valvotomy operations some years earlier.

## Research at Guy's

"I did eighteen months full-time in the laboratory at Guy's. That was very exciting because what I took up was hypothermia.... I became very excited about it, and made quite a name for myself because a lot of visitors came to see Brock and the work I was doing."

This was at about the same time that the first hypothermia operations were being performed in Minneapolis (by John Lewis) and Denver (by Henry Swan). Ross's contribution was that rather than placing the patient in a bath of cold water or wrapping the patient in a cooling blanket, a blood vessel was cannulated and the blood was cooled externally, and then, after being returned to the body, the cold blood cooled the patient's various organs.

"I then switched over to the clinical program and became Brock's senior registrar. I gradually eased over, still doing research part-time for another year or so. It was a very active research unit. It was a magnet to the world. We were all involved in it. We were interested in everything that was possible. It was while I was in the research laboratory, but after we had introduced hypothermia clinically, that Lillehei first described the DeWall bubble oxygenator."

Ross designed a heart-lung machine that was subsequently used at Guy's for several years until commercially available oxygenators could be purchased.

## The First Aortic Valve Homograft Operation

Ross explained, "Charles Hufnagel had put in the first homograft in the descending aorta, and Gordon Murray [in Toronto] also put valve homografts into the descending aorta, beyond the subclavian artery. They put them into patients with aortic regurgitation. Their work was very successful. In 1952 in the lab, we had inserted homograft valves into the descending aorta. We didn't do any patients by this technique because I thought that, if possible, the homograft valve should be put where it belonged [at the site of the natural aortic valve].

"In patients, we developed aortic valve surgery slowly. At first, we decalcified the valve by picking off the calcium plaques [i.e., when the valve was so diseased that calcium collections or "plaques" had been deposited in its leaflets, making it hard and rigid]. It was in 1962, when I was trying to decalcify a valve in a patient, it fell apart, and so I put in the first clinical homograft valve in the aortic position. We had some stored valves in the hospital for research purposes. So, when this valve came apart during the operation at Guy's, in desperation I inserted one of these freeze-dried valves.

"There wasn't such a thing as a mechanical valve in Britain at the time. This was one year after Starr's first valve replacement. We thought the homograft would keep our patient alive until we could obtain a Starr [mechanical] prosthesis to insert. At first, we were very apprehensive, expecting the homograft to fall apart. We gave the patient steroids and all sorts of things [to prevent possible rejection of the valve]. But three months later, the patient was 'laughing,' and we didn't need to replace it."

Mr. Ross was under the impression that Barratt-Boyes had learned of his work from a New Zealand surgeon who had visited Guy's, and that it was this that had stimulated Barratt-Boyes's own efforts to replace the aortic valve. His relationship with Barratt-Boyes had subsequently become strained, and only in later years did they become in any way amicable. This opinion differs markedly from that of Sir Brian Barratt-Boyes (see below).

In Sir Terence English's opinion, "I think they did their work independently. Then they heard they were each on the same track, and there was a degree of jealousy between them."

Mr. Ross continued, "Homografts took off at that time. Several surgeons became interested, including John Kirklin. However, there are technical difficulties, as opposed to the ease of inserting a mechanical valve. The operation needed a certain amount of skill, and still does, and took a longer time. And the Americans were more mechanically minded. Also, with time, the homografts started deteriorating, as do all biological tissues. The operation really never took off in the U.S."

The quality of Ross's clinical work was far ahead of that of other surgical groups in the United Kingdom at that time. John Wright remembers that, as a trainee, when he moved to the National Heart Hospital from the Royal Brompton Hospital in London, "it was a revelation and a breath of fresh air. I hadn't realized how surgery could actually be done safely and so well. It seemed that I had jumped ahead a few years."

I asked John Wright what Mr. Ross's strengths were.

"Dedication. Ability. Nobody feared Donald [comparing him with Brock]. They loved him. He had the ability to build up a loyal band of supporters and warriors, to build teams, to motivate people, and to fire their enthusiasm, and the technical ability to carry it through. He was a very good teacher. He was meticulous in postoperative care."

Bob Frater, like Ross a University of Cape Town graduate, drew attention to the large number of young surgeons from almost every part of the world who received some of their training under Ross. They learned, however, by watching and assisting, rather than from being formally trained by Ross.

By the late 1960s, Donald Ross's clinical commitments largely overwhelmed his interest in innovation and research. He built up an immense private practice, operating in several private clinics in central London. He resigned from the staff of Guy's to devote more time to the National Heart Hospital and his private practice.

Ross has been honored by many leading surgical societies. Surprisingly, to my mind and that of many others, he was not honored by the Queen with a knighthood or other award that happily befalls some surgeons in Britain. His contributions to surgery, both in the United Kingdom and internationally, have been significant enough that he should have received this recognition. Now in his 80s, he is still living in London.

# SIR BRIAN BARRATT-BOYES — AT THE OTHER END OF THE WORLD

Apart from Christiaan Barnard (chapter 12), Sir Brian Barratt-Boyes (Figure 40) is the only surgeon who worked in the southern hemisphere to be included in this book. Although one or two others were born in countries such as South Africa (Dennis Melrose, Donald Ross) and Argentina (Rene Favaloro), they did their important work in the northern hemisphere.

Sir Brian was early into open heart surgery, as he was one of John Kirklin's trainees at the Mayo Clinic in the 1950s. After returning to New Zealand, where he had been born and educated, he quickly developed a superb open-heart surgery program at Green Lane Hospital in Auckland. As New Zealand was still closely associated with the United Kingdom, he received a knighthood from the Queen in 1971 for his services to medicine. In 1977, he was named the Royal Australasian College of Surgeons' "surgeon of the decade."

Very shortly after Donald Ross, Barratt-Boyes introduced aortic valve replacement using a cadaveric homograft valve (on August 23, 1962). These two surgeons were largely responsible for popularizing this surgical approach as an alternative to mechanical valve prostheses. Barratt-Boyes then went on to modify a technique, initially developed in Japan, for operating on infants and young children using "deep" hypothermia. With this technique, the infant was cooled on the heart-lung machine to extremely low temperatures — much lower than those used by Lewis and Swan for their heart operations using hypothermia in the early 1950s. Then the heart-lung machine was turned off, and the heart was actually stopped while the defect within the heart was repaired. During this period of time, there was, of course, no circulation whatsoever to the brain and other vital organs, but at these cold temperatures the surgeon had something just short of one hour to perform the necessary repair and reconstruction. Barratt-Boyes's unit published outstandingly good results using this technique. These two contributions of homograft replacement of the aortic valve and of deep hypothermic arrest established his position among the pioneers of heart surgery.

I met Sir Brian in Auckland, New Zealand, in early 2002 while visiting as a guest of the Transplantation Society of Australia and New Zealand.

## Young Days

When Barratt-Boyes was only five, his father contracted poliomyelitis; later he had the added misfortune to also contract tuberculosis and, for many years, was an invalid who was kept away from his children so that they did not contract this infectious disease. At school, the young Brian was to some extent bullied because of his good looks and the fact that his family was a little better off than some other families. At first his academic performance was only modest, but when he decided to apply for medical school, it improved and he won several prizes. He began medical school in 1942 at the University of Otago in Dunedin (graduating in 1946), then the only medical school in New Zealand. For some years, he lodged with a clergyman and, in fact, was very active in church activities, having previously considered going into the ministry. He did not take part in many of the usual medical student social events, and he might have been considered something of a prude by his fellow students.

During my short stay in Auckland, after visiting Green Lane Hospital in the morning, I was taken by Sir Brian to a restaurant in the harbor area where we conversed over a lengthy lunch. He was in his late 70s, a slightly built man of short-to-medium height, with a bald head rimmed by gray hair. He had fairly bronzed features with dark brown, penetrating eyes. His posture was a little stooped, and he walked with relatively short steps at a slow pace. Indeed, he looked rather more debilitated than I had anticipated, no doubt a result of his three operations for coronary artery disease, the last being only a couple of years earlier. Surprisingly, he mentioned that he still played tennis, but my impression was that he wouldn't have been able to get around a court very quickly.

Discussing his heart problems with him reminded me that he had visited the Hammersmith Hospital in London when I was senior registrar there in 1975. At that time, the (possibly apocryphal) story going around was that he had shown some X-ray films to a group of eminent cardiologists "of a patient with coronary artery disease who had already undergone one operation to bypass his diseased coronary arteries." My understanding was that the cardiologists' uniform opinion was that the disease of the coronary arteries was so advanced that no further operation could be performed — the patient was deemed "inoperable." Only then did Barratt-Boyes, a heavy smoker, inform them that these films were of his *own* coronary arteries. I can imagine how their opinion must have been a severe psychological blow to him, even though it would appear that they were incorrect since he subsequently underwent two further operative procedures to bring a new blood supply to his heart muscle, and was still alive and active more than 25 years later. (Like Albert Starr, Barratt-Boyes chose one of his junior colleagues, whom he had personally trained, to operate on him.)

Sir Brian was very pleasant, but without a particularly dynamic personality. Although he spoke openly enough, my impression was of a fairly reserved person. He was articulate, speaking with only a mild antipodean accent. He displayed a good memory, and generally had balanced views on the other surgical pioneers we discussed, although at times he was rather more critical and negative about their achievements than I would have anticipated. He had a reputation among some of the other surgeons I interviewed as being slightly arrogant, and this may be because of his willingness to openly criticize his peers. Although retired from surgery, he was still involved in a peripheral way in research on pig valves (aortic valves excised from dead pigs and used to replace human valves) sponsored by the Medtronic company, and from time to time he lectured in various countries on the development of these valves.

He told me, "My father was an accountant and died of tuberculous laryngitis, a dreadful disease. My mother was a remarkable woman. She was dominant in almost everything she did, in a very pleasant, nice way. She had a great influence on her children. She had to work when my father was ill so that we could be educated and go to university. After my father died, she remarried and moved to Canada. When her second husband died, she came back to Auckland. There was no one in medicine in my family. There was, however, a family friend, a spinster, who was a nursing sister [senior nurse], who had an influence on all of us. I think that did have some effect on me. For some reason, I always wanted to be a doctor.

"I always wanted to do surgery. I was very good with my hands, naturally good—for example, at carpentry. I also used to play the piano. I think the reason I was interested in thoracic surgery was because of my father's illness. During my medical school days, they really knew very little about thoracic surgery. It was done, of course, but surgery at medical school was not outstanding in any way. Of course, at that time, cardiac surgery didn't exist. Even when I went to the Mayo Clinic in 1953, it was to do thoracic surgery. Cardiac surgery blossomed during the time I was there."

## The Mayo Clinic

"When I went there, I was already a Fellow of the Royal Australasian College of Surgeons, well-trained in general surgery. John Kirklin was a young guy then, and open heart surgery was just beginning. The Mayo was working desperately to develop it, as was Lillehei in Minneapolis. Kirklin was chosen to do that type of surgery because he was young and outstanding."

Barratt-Boyes had a very high opinion of the Mayo Clinic at that time. He recalled that it was "very well run, with very high clinical standards. Very good too in research—in the forefront of the physiological assessment and pathology of heart disease. The patients were completely and accurately documented at the Mayo Clinic; that was one of the great things about it. All put together, it was a very productive group. We worked out many of the congenital heart conditions that really weren't understood at that time."

He was very much in awe of John Kirklin. "He was a very hard worker. He worked long, long hours, starting at six o'clock in the morning doing rounds, and finishing at 10 P.M. in the operating room. This went on day after day. He was devoted. He was a slow operator, so a lot of it was very tedious from my point of view because I was much quicker at doing things than he was. But his results were very good. We got on very well together."

There were several similarities between Kirklin and Barratt-Boyes. Both were perfectionists, both were considered by some to be self-opinionated and arrogant, both were reluctant to confide in others and had few intimate friends, and both rarely spoke of personal disappointments and unhappiness. Barratt-Boyes was one of the few surgeons who Kirklin genuinely respected, and there were not too many of those.

Bob Frater was also training at the Mayo Clinic during this period and was able to observe Barratt-Boyes during this stage of his career. "Barratt-Boyes was a very serious fellow working very, very hard with Kirklin. I have this image of him working intensely in the typical style of those of us who came from overseas to get extra experience. We felt we just had to get the most out of it. We were very pure, I might say — we didn't think of money. The *opportunity* is what we wanted, the opportunity to work. 'Knowledge' was absolutely essential, and time was limited. That's what Barratt-Boyes was like. He was more advanced in his training than the rest of us; he wasn't there as a trainee, but rather as a postgraduate student. He was working incredibly hard to suck everything he could out of this pool of knowledge that he came across at the Mayo Clinic. Although I never really saw him operate much, from what I hear, he was a technically excellent surgeon." On a personal level, Frater described Barratt-Boyes as "a slightly irascible guy. Brian has always been a very prickly character."

Indeed, he could not have been an easy man to work with. In an obituary in the British newspaper *The Independent,* he is described as "aggressive, autocratic, patriarchal and tough. His peers found him opinionated and intolerant, his juniors found him aloof; bureaucrats found him a formidable opponent; patients found him formal. But he also inspired loyalty, replied personally to children's thank-you letters, and adored being a grandfather."

Barratt-Boyes used to be sent down to Minneapolis as a spy to see what was going on, "because they were a little ahead of us," he told me. "They did the first tetralogy, for example, and other first operations. So we wanted to know how they were doing them, and what was happening there. I was very impressed. Lillehei was a very vigorous guy. Not a fantastic technician. A lot of the credit for their early technical success goes to Richard Varco, who was a very good technician. He used to assist Lillehei. Together, they were an outstanding team."

Kirklin offered Barratt-Boyes a permanent position at the Mayo Clinic, but this was not attractive to him, as he realized he would be entirely subordinate to Kirklin. Developments, changes, and techniques would be dictated largely by Kirklin, and Barratt-Boyes felt there would be a continual conflict of personalities. He was not prepared to settle for second-in-command. Instead, he chose to spend some time in the United Kingdom on a research fellowship in Bristol (where Donald Ross had spent some time a few years previously), the purpose of which was to try to develop open heart surgery there.

## Return to New Zealand

When Barratt-Boyes returned to New Zealand to develop open heart surgery at Green Lane Hospital in Auckland, the then chief, Douglas Robb, stood aside and let his younger colleague take over.

I mentioned that Donald Ross thought that his idea of the homograft valve had been "purloined" by the New Zealanders.

"Not so. I had been thinking about it for some time. It is interesting that Donald should think that, but it is not true. The first I knew about his interest was his preliminary communication [about his first operation] in *The Lancet*. I remember Douglas Robb came to me with *The Lancet* under his arm, and said, 'You've been beaten to the draw,' which was by only a few weeks." Surprisingly, this did not appear to be a major disappointment for Barratt-Boyes. "I don't remember it so. In those days, I was totally unaware of what we were achieving relative to everyone else. We just went ahead and did our thing."

His first patient was a 14-year-old girl who later married, had three children, and required the valve to be replaced successfully by a second homograft 25 years later.

Like Ross, Barratt-Boyes thought that a natural valve would be better than a mechanical prosthesis. "I was lying in the bath one night, and it suddenly struck me how to do it—invert the valve downwards so we could do the lower suture line first. We used a double suture line technique from the beginning. Ross made the mistake of using a single suture line. His initial results were very bad. A lot of the patients died, and other valves did not function well. In our first hundred cases, we only had four deaths, which was outstanding really. Even today, some people can't match those results. Frankly, if we had not been able to show that this operation could be done with a low mortality, it might not have lasted."

## Deep Hypothermia

The idea of using "deep" hypothermia in infants came to Barratt-Boyes from a Japanese surgeon who was working with him. This approach entailed cooling a baby by means of the heart-lung machine from a normal body temperature of 37°C (98.6°F) to 16 to 22°C (61–72°F) or less. At this low temperature, the brain and other vital organs could survive for approximately one hour without further oxygen. The heart-lung machine could therefore be turned off, the heart stopped, and the blood drained from the body. (If you touch the child's skin during this period, you would swear the child is dead, so cold does he or she feel.) This provided the surgeon with a perfect operating field: a nonbeating heart with no blood to obscure his view. The Japanese group had been using this technique in Kyoto for several years, but not much had been published about it, and they had not used it in young babies.

"The guy who came out first [to Auckland] was the professor in Kyoto, Professor Hitoshi Shirotani," Sir Brian told me. "He had this young guy with him, Atsumi Mori. They came out to learn homograft work. They spent a month or so with us. Then Professor Shirotani decided to send Mori back to us for a year as a registrar. He was a very good surgeon, and he presented their experience using deep hypothermia. I cottoned on to it immediately. It was obviously a damn good idea. We then went into the lab, and did a whole lot of experiments in animals. I modified the technique somewhat and, in particular, the anesthetic. They thought ether was very important, but it wasn't. Dr. Mori helped me with the first operations. Then we rapidly developed it. Our first case [in 1969] was a complete atrioventricular canal defect [a very complicated lesion to repair]. Then we did atrial septal defects, ventricular septal defects, tetralogies, everything."

The Green Lane group was extremely successful in this field, operating on babies only a few days old. Soon they could boast the best results in infant heart surgery in the world. Following this success, for the next few years Barratt-Boyes was at the height of his fame within the cardiac surgical field. Indeed, so good were his surgical results that it sometimes proved difficult to get other surgeons to believe them. "That was one of my problems when I went over to the U.K. as Paul Wood's visitor. [Paul Wood, British by birth but educated in Australia, was the preeminent cardiologist in the United Kingdom at that time.] No one would believe my results. They all thought I was telling a pack of lies because they were just so far behind — behind the U.S., and certainly behind New Zealand by a large margin."

Barratt-Boyes rated his work on infants as an achievement equal to the homograft work, but "it was more exciting. It was an enormous challenge to develop new techniques for these babies, operate on all sorts of conditions, and do some new operations. We did the whole gamut of heart operations in neonates too [infants less than one month old], and that wasn't reintroduced really until the 1990s, but we did them in the 1970s."

At about this time and as a result of the outstandingly good results he was achieving, Barratt-Boyes was approached about leading the heart surgery program at Boston's prestigious Children's Hospital, where Robert Gross had initiated the modern era of heart surgery. The job was offered first to Kirklin, who refused it. Barratt-Boyes also refused it. "In a way, I am rather sorry I did that. The reason I did was because I would only be operating on children, and I didn't want to do that. I wanted to keep my interest in adult work. That was the main reason." But perhaps, as some have suggested, he was worried about his ability, at the age of 52 and with heart disease himself, to adapt to a new environment, a new set of colleagues, and the challenge and stress of all the complicated cases that would face him.

Although he had extremely good results, in those early days deaths were not that uncommon. "They *did* affect me. It was worse with the children than with the adults because of the attachment of the families to their kids. That could be very, very heart-wrenching. It was particularly difficult when a patient had come from overseas — traveled all the way from Europe or wherever it may be — and the operation was not successful. That was shattering. Really."

But he was resilient enough to bounce back, and he never stopped operating even for a day or two.

Pertinent to this topic, in *From the Heart,* a biography of him by Donna Chisholm, Sir Brian is quoted as saying, "I think saving life is one of the more traumatic sides of cardiac surgery, which makes it very wearing emotionally. It is perhaps the most difficult area of medicine, because so much of the time what you do is intimately involved with the possibility that the patient may not survive the operation, and that is rare in other forms of surgery. It is very rare for the general surgeon to have that experience. There is a particular challenge when you have this very close association with life and death. I don't think one particularly relishes it, but clearly if you can save a patient's life you have that much more satisfaction."

## The "Book"

As early as 1966, Barratt-Boyes's family life was deteriorating and, according to his biographer, Donna Chisholm, "aloof and self-absorbed," he had been "a rare sight in his own home." Some of his colleagues believed his intense desire to achieve made him relegate his family life to second place. His work was a major contribution to the breakup of his marriage. He told me, "My wife literally couldn't handle it. It put my five sons off medicine. They wouldn't consider it. It was too hard work. 'Dad' was never at home, working enormous hours. It affected them because I couldn't take the time to spend with them that I would have liked to have done. My relationship with my sons has never been what I would have liked it to be. That goes very deep. It was difficult because my wife had great trouble coping with the children, and the whole thing worked out as a bit of a disaster, really.

"And, of course, it got worse when I began writing the book [*Cardiac Surgery,* a monumental treatise of 1,500 pages] with John Kirklin. That book took eight years to write, and it was very stressful. It wasn't my idea. He asked me if I would collaborate because he was determined to write a textbook. I said, 'I don't know if this will work. This is going to ruin our friendship.' The only reason it did work is because we were so far apart [geographically], but it almost broke up my relationship with him.

"He didn't like being corrected. His stuff was outstanding, but many of our results were better than his, and we had some problems because he didn't want that to be apparent. At one stage, he rang me, and said, 'I'm not going to go on with it. I'm going to take it over myself.' We had gotten about halfway through it. I had contributed a really long chapter. I got legal advice about it. I indicated to him that, if that was the case, then all of my material would be removed, and certain conditions would be put on use of the remainder of it. He backed off.

"We had to work out differences of opinion and make the book uniform. I think in many ways it was an outstanding achievement to be able to do that. Without question, he was the moving force. I got wrapped into it to the extent that it was with me night and day. I got to the stage where I thought, my God, can I ever get rid of it? I used to work on it from about four o'clock in the morning, do my operating, and then work again late at night. At one stage, I gave up operating for six months to get it finished."

Sir Brian admitted that his family problems had not been a major distraction for him in his work, largely because he "put them aside. I didn't leave my wife until after we had got all the children through university education, because I didn't want to leave her with that responsibility."

## Strengths and Weaknesses

I asked Sir Brian to comment on his strengths as a surgeon.

"I was technically very adept, probably one of the best in the world. People would generally acknowledge that. That was a natural gift. You train a whole lot of surgeons, and it's only very seldom that you find one who is a 'natural' surgeon. You can develop your skills, of course, but very few are naturally gifted. You have to pay attention to detail. It also helps to have an ability to run a team. You've got to make everybody feel they are contributing and are an important part of the team. I had that ability to make it work — the ability to make the team work as a team.

"After the initial stages at Green Lane, I got too involved in private practice so that I handed over a lot of the responsibility of the Green Lane service to others. [Many in London would say that this was also an impediment to Donald Ross's academic work.] I began to get distracted from the public service in the late 1970s or early 1980s. It evolved around my own illness, and the fact that I really cut down on call work because I really thought I couldn't do it. It was too stressful to have to do that as well as a full operating program. Then, later, writing the book got in the way. That was a mistake. I have always regretted that I didn't spend more time with the patients. That didn't happen in the earlier days, but it did subsequently. You have to decide what are your priorities; there is only a certain amount that you can do."

I asked Sir Brian whether he felt that his contributions to surgery had been well recognized.

"Yes, I think so. I think the book has contributed to that recognition. John [Kirklin] always used to say, 'If you want to be remembered, you've got to write a textbook. Not just a book—you've got to write a major work.' That was his motivation. And that's why I think it was a great achievement, because it was recognized."

It surprised me how much emphasis Barratt-Boyes placed on *Cardiac Surgery*. From his biography, we learn that he considers it the greatest of all his achievements, and that such a monumental volume was the only way to seal his place in medical history—to prove himself as a great cardiac surgeon. Although it was a major contribution to the training of the next generation of cardiac surgeons, his original contributions to the field would seem to me to greatly outweigh it. My own opinion is that his reputation was already well established before the book was published, and that people would have recognized his contributions anyway. I suggested to him that writing the book doesn't compare with his innovative homograft work or the infant surgery, which were major advances in cardiac surgery. With some hesitation, he agreed.

After lunch, as Sir Brian drove me back to my hotel, I asked him whether he felt the benefits of being in a relatively isolated place, such as New Zealand, at some distance from others doing cardiac surgery, had outweighed the disadvantages. He thought it had actually been an advantage because "we did our own thing, and weren't so influenced by what other people said would or wouldn't work." I found this an interesting attitude, and possibly this was of benefit to Christiaan Barnard also (chapter 12).

What drives men like Barratt-Boyes to work and work to the point that it disrupts their marriage and family life? From his biography, we learn that he believed he inherited from his mother an innate desire to achieve, a singleness of purpose to overcome problems that would cause most people to falter. He is quoted as saying, "Many times I have thought if only I could give it all up. Many times I have wondered why am I doing it; that I can't continue. But you don't give up, despite all the irritations and frustrations, because of that ambition."

Sir Brian was divorced from his first wife and, when I met with him, was living with his second wife on a farm outside of Auckland. He died in 2006, at age 82, from complications following open heart surgery at the Cleveland Clinic in the United States to replace two of his heart valves.

## CHAPTER 11

# The Floodgates Open: Surgery for Coronary Artery Disease

―――――

## VASILII KOLESOV AND RENE FAVALORO

THE OPERATION OF coronary artery bypass grafting (Figure 41), established by Rene Favaloro (Figure 42) in the late 1960s, has become one of the most common operations performed in the Western world. The incidence of coronary artery disease, leading to angina (central chest pain) or a heart attack, is so common that, once an operation was developed to prevent the pain and/or a heart attack, it soon became frequently performed. At one time, more than half a million of these operations were being performed in the United States alone each year.

## Coronary Artery Disease and Anginal Chest Pain

In coronary artery disease, fat deposition in the walls of the arteries (atherosclerosis) narrows them to the point that not enough blood passes down the artery to supply the heart muscle. The needs of the heart for blood and, in particular, for the oxygen that it carries, are considerable. When the blood and oxygen supply is diminished to a certain point because of the obstruction in the coronary artery, then the heart muscle cells will not receive enough oxygen for their needs, and central chest pain results.

This is most likely to occur when more is demanded of the heart, such as during exercise, when the heart rate increases and an increased cardiac output is required, or during emotional stress, which may similarly increase heart rate and blood pressure, or after eating a heavy meal, which places an increased demand on the heart to pump more blood to the gut. The chest pain can be accompanied by a feeling of suffocation, and has been given the name *angina* (literally, "strangling" or "suffocation"). The pain usually subsides when the patient ceases the activity that initiated it. Anginal pain is therefore a warning that one or more coronary arteries are becoming diseased.

The first description of anginal chest pain would appear to have been by the Roman philosopher Lucius Seneca, who recorded his own symptoms in the first century, but it was Edward Jenner, the English physician best known for his work in vaccination for smallpox, who in 1776 concluded that there was an association between angina and disease of the coronary arteries.

If the obstruction in an important coronary artery develops to the point that no blood and oxygen can get to the heart muscle supplied by that artery, then the subject will experience very severe and prolonged pain that does not subside when the subject rests, and he or she will suffer a heart attack. Unless the obstruction is relieved rapidly — within a few hours at most — that area of muscle will be irreparably damaged, and will no longer be able to contribute to the muscular activity of the heart. With death of the muscle cells, the pain will subside, but those cells will never contract again.

For many years, it was believed that the arteriosclerotic narrowing of the coronary arteries was diffuse, i.e., extended over the whole course of the artery. It was not until the early 1960s that this was found not to be necessarily so. The artery can be narrowed in one segment alone, the rest of the artery being relatively spared of disease.

## Arthur Vineberg's Operation

Attempts to surgically treat obstruction of the coronary arteries go back in the experimental laboratory for almost 100 years. In the late 1940s and early 1950s, a Toronto surgeon, Arthur Vineburg, developed an operation by which an artery that supplies some of the chest wall was diverted to supply the heart muscle. Doubt was cast on the efficacy of this technique by many surgeons for several years, but it was eventually determined to be beneficial. Before 1967, several surgeons had made occasional attempts to try to bypass or replace diseased sections of coronary arteries without great or consistent success.

There was no satisfactory form of surgical therapy for the disease in the Western world until Mason Sones, an American physician, and Rene Favaloro, an Argentinian surgeon, working at the Cleveland Clinic, came onto the scene. However, recognition of Favaloro's pioneering surgical role in this field should rightly be shared with that of the little-known Russian surgeon Vasilii Kolesov. His is a remarkable story.

# VASILII I. KOLESOV — THE "UNKNOWN" RUSSIAN

Vasilii Kolesov (Figure 43) was born in 1904 in the small village of Marthianovskaia, in the Vologda province of Russia. He studied medicine in Leningrad (now St. Petersburg), where he graduated from the Leningrad Medical Institute in 1931. From 1934 to 1938, he undertook training in general surgery, and then spent a period of time in research. After German troops invaded the Soviet Union in 1941, Kolesov was given the rank of major in the medical corps of the army and was appointed surgeon-in-chief to one of the municipal hospitals in the heart of the city.

During the siege of the city that lasted for 872 days, almost one million citizens died of cold and starvation, including Kolesov's brother, with whom he shared a room in the basement of the hospital.

Kolesov himself became bedridden but survived. In 1953, he became chairman of the department of surgery at the First Leningrad Medical Institute, which he headed until 1976. He began experimental work in dogs, and, after some discouraging results, used an artery in the chest to bring in a new blood supply to the heart muscle (joining the internal mammary artery to one of the coronary arteries); although this procedure is now in common use worldwide, at that time Kolesov was way ahead of the field.

On February 25, 1964, Kolesov performed the first successful coronary artery bypass graft in a patient. He published his early results and, indeed, an entire book on direct coronary revascularization (in Russian) in 1966, one year before Rene Favaloro published his first results. From February 1964 until May 1967, the department of surgery headed by Kolesov was the only place in the world where coronary artery bypass operations were regularly performed.

What is perhaps equally remarkable is that before Mason Sones developed the technique of coronary arteriography (see below), there was no definitive way of identifying exactly where the obstruction in the coronary artery was situated. How did Kolesov know where to insert his grafts? It appears he made intelligent "guesses" based on changes in the electrocardiogram (EKG) and by feeling the coronary arteries at the operation. With such primitive diagnostic capabilities at his disposal, it is remarkable that his patients did so well.

In the West, virtually all surgery for coronary artery disease in the early era was performed using the heart-lung machine, to enable the heart to be stopped while the operation was completed. Today, there is an increasing trend for the operation to be carried out on a beating heart without the support of the heart-lung machine. Special techniques and devices allow for stabilization of the heart (which continues to beat) and/or the artery while the surgeon sutures the new blood vessel to the obstructed coronary artery. Kolesov was probably the first to advocate the use of "off-pump" coronary artery bypass grafting. In the early 1960s, following careful study, he concluded that while the heart-lung machine was safe and reliable, the deleterious effects were too great to justify its use for coronary artery bypass grafting. Although use of the heart-lung machine was well established in Kolesov's clinic, he performed coronary artery bypass grafting without its help, believing in the superiority of the off-pump technique. Remarkably, between 1964 and 1974, only 18% of his coronary artery operations were performed with the help of the heart-lung machine.

He was also one of the first to advocate the advantages of using an artery, rather than a vein, as a graft for coronary artery bypass grafting. It was only during the mid-1980s that the advantage of arterial grafts in terms of superior long-term patency was first appreciated worldwide.

Vasilii Kolesov died in 1992. Because most of his studies were published in Russian, his work still remains almost unknown and inadequately appreciated by surgeons outside of Eastern Europe. He was a major pioneer in heart surgery, and has not received the requisite credit his innovations deserve.

## MASON SONES AND CORONARY ARTERIOGRAPHY

In 1958, F. Mason Sones Jr., a cardiologist at the Cleveland Clinic, was injecting radio-opaque dye (that would show up on an X-ray) through a catheter that had been passed into the root of the aorta to assess the state of the aortic valve. His main interest was in the aortic valve, not in the coronary arteries, but at the moment he injected the dye the catheter by chance became lodged in one of the two major coronary arteries. When he took the X-ray he found, to his horror, that the dye had traversed down one coronary artery alone. Sones anticipated that the presence of a catheter in a coronary artery, and the injection of dye directly into the artery, would cause a serious rhythm disturbance of the heart (ventricular fibrillation) and result in fatal cardiac arrest. In fact, the heart did temporarily stop beating but, to his great surprise and relief, began again after he thumped the patient's chest. From this chance occurrence developed one of the major medical and surgical advances of the 20th century.

The idea immediately came to Sones that, if a catheter was designed that could be purposely passed into a coronary artery orifice without difficulty, then selective dye injection could be carried out, allowing identification of the state of each coronary artery in turn. He went ahead and developed this radiological technique, which became known as coronary arteriography or coronary angiography.

Mason Sones was a workaholic perfectionist who led a chaotic lifestyle, sometimes reportedly spending the night asleep on the catheterization table in his laboratory. This lifestyle played havoc with his home life, family events frequently being sacrificed. The stresses and strains led to divorce from his first wife, divorce from his second wife, and remarriage to his first wife.

Mason Sones's colleague Rene Favaloro (Figure 42) took full advantage of Sones's ability to identify narrowed (or stenosed) areas in the coronary arteries, and developed surgical techniques for bypassing these narrowed areas. Favaloro initially used a vein taken from the patient's leg (the saphenous vein) to bypass the obstructed area of the coronary artery, just as a ring road may pass around a city to allow traffic to bypass the congested center of the city relatively quickly. Unlike Kolesov, he quickly popularized this form of surgical treatment for coronary artery disease worldwide. When judged by the number of patients who have benefited from the advances he contributed, Favaloro's impact on cardiac surgery has been immense.


## RENE FAVALORO — THE TRAGIC MAN

I had written to Dr. Favaloro in Buenos Aires, where he then lived, in 1991 asking whether he had any plans to visit the United States. He replied, telling me he was attending the annual meeting of the American College of Cardiology in Dallas during April 1992. We met outside the convention center in what appeared to be an old cemetery where there were trees and a statue to the Confederate infantry erected as a memorial by the Daughters of the Confederacy on June 25, 1896. We sat in the sun and talked at length.

I found Dr. Favaloro, who was by this time in his late 60s, to be very pleasant and communicative. He spoke with a fairly heavy South American accent. He was rather taller than I had expected — I would estimate about six feet tall — and he still had a full head of hair, rising fairly low on his forehead and temple and streaked with gray. He had a slightly protuberant stomach but was not grossly over-weight, although he did not look to be in great physical shape. The impression was of one who didn't get a great deal of exercise. He was dressed casually in a light green-blue shirt, blue casual slacks, a light windbreaker, and no tie. He looked very relaxed, as if he were about to take a stroll along a beach.

Rene Favaloro was born in 1923 and brought up in La Plata, a town approximately 30 miles south of Buenos Aires. He spent almost the first 40 years of his life in Argentina before moving to the United States to further his surgical training, in particular, to gain experience in heart surgery.

## Early Days in Buenos Aires

Having read in an article he had previously mailed to me that his father had been a carpenter and his mother a dressmaker, both origi-nally immigrants from Italy, I opened our conversation by mentioning that these sounded like very good occupations for a couple whose son was to become a surgeon.

"You are correct. My old professor at the University of La Plata in Buenos Aires used to say, 'If you want to be a good surgeon, first you will have to become a carpenter.' During my childhood, I worked with my father. Even when I went to college, I worked with him dur-ing vacations. I did a lot of carving, veneer work, and so on. The example of my parents was very important for me, not only because I saw my mother doing all kinds of sewing, but because both of them were really working very hard. We came from a very low-middle-class family, and I learned a lot because they were working all the time. I think it was very important that I grew up in that atmosphere. I always say that if you are born into a rich family, maybe you aren't lucky. This is my theory.

"Elementary school in Argentina has been totally free by law since the end of the last century. That means I went to a common public school. In Argentina you attend elementary school for six years, and then attend for six years in what is known as a college or secondary school. To get into the college school that is connected to the University of La Plata, you take an examination. If you passed through the 'college,' you could choose any place at the university.

"My mother told me that when I was four or five years old I was already certain I was going to medical school. For as long as I can remember, I always thought that I would become a doctor. Maybe the one who influenced me was an uncle — the youngest brother of my father — who was a doctor. He was in practice in a suburb of Buenos Aires. Many times I used to go with him to see patients. I was eight, ten, twelve years old. I think his influence was very important. In secondary school, I hated mathematics, but I loved biology."

At medical school, Favaloro spent as much time as he could in the operating room.

"I shall tell you a true story. The university campus in La Plata is a beautiful place, with acres and acres of trees. One day I was walking in a place where there were oak trees, and I said to myself, 'Look, if you make a little bit more effort, instead of being in the upper third of the class, you could be number one.' I made that decision walking between the trees. I really started working a little bit more, and it was not difficult to be number one. I used to get up very early in the morning, and follow a schedule and work hard."

Favaloro graduated in 1949. He soon left the University Hospital and spent several years in a rural surgical practice; I asked him why he had done this.

"There were several factors. Number one, my family was not well-off. Secondly, my only brother [who was two and a half years younger and was a medical student at the time] was involved in a car accident and lost his left leg. As a consequence, I felt I had much responsibility. And thirdly, the most important one, was the political situation in Argentina. It was during the first years of [President] Perón. It was a dictatorship, no question about it.

"After my graduation, there was an empty post in the hospital working in the emergency room. The director of the hospital called me, and said, 'This place belongs to you because you were number-one in the class, but you have to fill out this paper that you are not against the Peronist ideas.' On the other side of the paper, you required support for your application from somebody who was important in the Peronist party. I thought for about 24 hours, and then I talked to the director again. I said, 'Because of my background and because of my hard work in the hospital, and because I am number one in the class, you told me that I should be nominated for that particular empty place. How come you are telling me that I have to have the support of a political party? I am not a Peronist, and I'm not for the Peronist party. I always believe in freedom.'

"You have to remember that I was a medical student during the Second World War. Many people in our ruling class were in favor of Germany and the Nazi party. The influence of the German military school was very strong in our army; the majority of our army officers had received some instruction in Germany. As a consequence, our government was a typical Fascist government. I'm talking about 1945, 1947, et cetera. The students, on the contrary, were in favor of the Allied Forces. We were fighting inside the country for freedom and liberty. The students were making demonstrations in the street. I went on all those demonstrations, and twice I was in jail for short periods of time. All my life, I believe in freedom and liberty. So I emigrated from the big city, and from the university that I loved so much, to work in a smaller area where nobody was going to look for me. That was maybe the most important reason for my decision to work in a rural area."

## In Surgical Isolation — Jacinto Arauz

Favaloro, later joined by his brother, Juan José, opened a small clinic, where emergency surgery became his main work. (Juan José Favaloro would appear to have been born under a very unlucky star in that, apart from losing a leg as a young man, he died while still young as a result of a second automobile accident, having received less than adequate surgical treatment when in Mexico.) Favaloro remained in Jacinto Arauz for 12 years, performing large numbers of operations and gaining immense surgical experience.

However, he felt a persistent desire to train in the field of thoracic and cardiovascular surgery, and so he decided to move to the United States. "My old professor used to tell me, 'This is not your place. Your capability is much greater.' Then finally, my nephew, who was already in the U.S.A., urged me to come to the U.S.A." Favaloro chose the Cleveland Clinic because he was advised it had one of the best cardiology departments. Like the Mayo Clinic, the Cleveland Clinic is based on the concept of group practice. The excellent reputation of its cardiology department, which persists to this day, was in part associated with the pioneering work of Mason Sones. Favaloro traveled to Cleveland in February 1962, with his wife — without a definite offer of a job.

## The Cleveland Clinic

"I arrived not knowing anything about the examinations I would have to take to practice in the U.S.A. I told myself that in two or three months I will realize what is going on. When I interviewed for a job for the first time, the interviewer told me, 'You don't have the qualifications. You can only be an observer, and we won't pay you for anything.' I said, 'Look, I've saved some money, and I can live on my own money. Don't worry about it.' That surprised him — no question — I could see on his face. I'm sure he thought, 'Here is a guy that doesn't want money. He wants only to learn.'" After that, despite Favaloro's relatively poor English, he took the examinations that all foreign doctors take in the United States and became a junior fellow and then a senior fellow. "Everything went in the right direction. I worked hard. I was living just across the street, and I was at the clinic all the time."

By 1964 he was the chief resident, and by 1966 he was a member of the senior staff. Donald Effler, the chief of cardiothoracic surgery, gave him every freedom in his work. Favaloro and Sones spent many hours together reviewing the coronary arteriograms that Sones had taken.

## The Surgical Treatment of Coronary Artery Disease

Early in 1967, Favaloro thought that the use of the saphenous vein as a bypass graft could solve the problem of an obstructed coronary artery. As in many other centers, there was experience at the Cleveland Clinic in the reconstruction of occluded arteries in the leg and elsewhere with that kind of graft. He reasoned, "Why not at the coronary level?" The plan was to insert a length of vein to carry blood around the obstruction; the graft would need to be connected to the artery above the obstruction and to the same artery below the obstruction.

He discussed the matter with Sones and some other associates. The two criteria for the operation they felt essential were that the patient should have a totally occluded coronary artery, but that the artery should be patent (open) beyond the occlusion so that they could anastomose (join) the vein graft to it satisfactorily. They decided they should begin cautiously by selecting patients with occlusion of only the right coronary artery, since this was a less important vessel than the left coronary artery as it supplies less of the heart, and the operation would therefore be less risky. "At the beginning, we were very conservative," he told me. "We were very careful in our selection of patients. We progressed slowly."

The first operation was performed in May 1967. The postoperative pictures of the vein graft to the coronary artery showed a good result, with good blood flow through it. They soon modified the technique so that the vein graft carried blood from the aorta (rather than from the coronary artery itself) to the coronary artery beyond the obstruction (Figure 41).

Favaloro and his colleagues subsequently developed enough confidence to carry out the operation on the left coronary artery, the first operation for left main coronary artery obstruction being performed in 1968. Left main coronary artery disease is a very serious condition that carries a high risk of sudden death for the patient; indeed it is known among cardiologists and cardiac surgeons as the "widow-maker." This is because the left coronary artery soon divides into two major branches that supply a large part of the heart, particularly the left ventricle, which pumps blood around the entire body with the exception of the lungs. Obstruction of the left coronary artery, therefore, almost always causes the left ventricle to stop beating.

By the end of 1968, the largest series of patients in the world (171 cases) — with the possible exception of Kolesov's series — had been accumulated at the Cleveland Clinic. Favaloro emphasized the need for the surgeon to use magnifying lenses, as they were operating on arteries as small as one millimeter in diameter. (Take a look at a ruler or tape measure, and imagine stitching together two blood vessels of this small size without the help of magnification.) By June 1970, 1,086 coronary artery bypasses had been performed at the Cleveland Clinic, with an overall mortality of only 4%. Hearing of the benefits of these procedures for patients with coronary artery disease, very soon many other groups began to offer these operations to their patients.

After initial experience by others, Favaloro began to divert the internal mammary artery (the artery that normally supplies blood to part of the chest wall) to bring blood to the diseased coronary artery (as advocated earlier by Kolesov). This became preferred to the saphenous vein, since the long-term results were superior when the artery was used as the graft; the vein tended to clog up (become narrowed) with time, but the internal mammary artery did not. At the time of my meeting with Dr. Favaloro, he told me that he used the artery in 98% of his patients.

The impact of Favaloro's innovations on the practice of cardiac surgery, particularly in the United States, was rapid and immense. At one meeting in London in 1970, when Dr. Favaloro arrived an hour early to organize his slides, the room was already packed with doctors filling the seats, sitting on the floor, or standing against the walls. People crushed in through the doors, and they went away only when the chairman assured them that Favaloro would repeat the symposium later that same day.

## Surgical Dexterity

Surgeons who had watched Favaloro in the operating room unfailingly reported that he operated with great ease and skill. "Surgery is complicated," he explained. "It's not only your hands. It's a combination of your head and your hands. The greatest surgeon is the one who has good hands that know how to work but, at the same time, has enough judgment to make the right decision in a difficult moment. I was born right-handed, but I use the left hand many times. I trained myself to use the left hand. There are some parts of the operation that can be done much better with the left hand. You can train your left hand by eating with it, et cetera. Slowly and steadily you will be able to use the left hand. It's not necessary, but I use the left hand.

"I am relaxed [during an operation]. The operation has to be simple and standardized. If you simplify and standardize, anybody can learn, and you can teach. Once in a while you get involved in very difficult problems, and you have to solve them. Anybody can then be tense. But I feel pity for the surgeon who goes to the operating room not relaxed."

Favaloro's emotional response to the death of a patient was similar to that of many surgeons. "Personally, it's always the same. The life of a surgeon is very difficult, and it's difficult to express. We knew that those patients were in a difficult situation. We knew that they could die suddenly. We tried to do *something*. We went ahead with the operation, knowing in advance that many of them would die after the operation. The mortality was never *very* high, but still I suffer with every single death of my patients. I always tell my Uncle Alvareto, 'The day that I don't feel the sensation that I am the guilty one, then I will drop the knife and I won't operate anymore.' I don't mean 'guilty,' but *responsible* for the life of the patient. This is the feeling."

In 1990, Dr. Favaloro wrote, "A surgeon's life means assuming responsibility for the risk that accompanies his decision to operate. The deaths associated with surgery are personal and the surgeon must endure their burden as long as he lives."

## Donald Effler

Despite his undoubted prowess as an operating surgeon, Favaloro had his limitations as a lecturer. In Sir Brian Barratt-Boyes's opinion, "Favaloro was hopeless as a lecturer — too much detail. He got involved in all sorts of stuff, and you just couldn't follow what he was saying. He had a lot of ideas and a lot of knowledge, but he was not a good lecturer."

Possibly because of this fact, Favaloro's titular chief, Donald Effler, often attended international meetings to present their clinical data. "Effler was a very good surgeon," explained Dr. Favaloro, "but he did not play a role in the development of coronary artery surgery. However, he really was a very excellent speaker at the meetings. It was impossible to compare anybody else to him in this respect. He knew how to present our data." The two of them worked well together. "I used to operate on very important people," Dr. Favaloro told me. "I can give you plenty of examples — billionaires, et cetera. When I operated on somebody who was really a VIP, I used to tell Effler to come with me to the room. I presented him as my chief, and said he will do all the social elements. Finally, he would become a very good friend of the patient who I operated on. We never had any problems."

## Return to His Roots

In 1971, Favaloro decided to return to Argentina.

"I knew there was a lack of cardiology and cardiac surgery in Latin America. I had done my job in America, and trained so many people. My job at the Cleveland Clinic was done, and they needed me more in my home country and in Latin America. Everybody says 'patriotism.' I don't know. You cannot deny your roots. They were asking me to come back. Finally, I decided to go back. I sat down and wrote a letter of resignation to Dr. Effler. I confess that, when I left the clinic that day, I was crying all the way home. Dr. Effler called me, and said, 'It is all right. I have the letter.' He finally approved my decision. I sent a copy of my letter to Mason Sones, but he never answered because he thought that I was foolish. He couldn't accept that it cut our professional relationship. I told him, 'Look, the only thing for you to do is to come to Buenos Aires. We can work together in Buenos Aires.'" Dr. Sones did not take up this offer.

Favaloro did not say good-bye to the scrub nurses in the operating rooms, "because I am a very sensitive fellow and I cry very easily. I knew that I wouldn't have been able to say good-bye. Even though people feel I'm very energetic and aggressive, I am a very sensitive fellow. Many times when they gave me an honorary degree and I was supposed to talk, the only thing I could say was 'Thank you very much,' because I was crying. I sent letters [to the nurses] afterwards.

"When the medical profession found out that I was leaving the Cleveland Clinic, I received all kinds of offers to stay in the U.S.A. The maximum one offered me $2 million free of taxes. But my decision was final. It was not a decision related to any problems in Cleveland. I love the place. I wanted to dedicate a lot of time in Argentina to teaching and research, and we have accomplished a lot. The whole of Latin America is full of people trained in our department [at the Favaloro Foundation in Buenos Aires]. Even in very difficult moments in Argentina—with military governments, dictatorships, et cetera, I never regretted it." Dr. Favaloro told me something of the excellent facilities the Fundación Favaloro had established in Buenos Aires. He was clearly very proud of the "higher institute" that had just been built. "The architecture and technology is the best you can get now in the world. There is no question about it."

This was the beginning of the breakup of the Cleveland Clinic team. Sones and Effler had always had personality conflicts, often very bitter, and fell out over many topics, despite Favaloro's efforts to be the peacemaker. With him gone, and in the absence of someone in a position of seniority who could handle the explosive situation between the two men, Sones eventually was fired.

"The Board of Governors fired Mason Sones by a letter," Dr. Favaloro told me, clearly shocked by this decision. "Can you imagine? One day, Mason Sones went to his office and there is a private envelope. He opened the envelope, and he is no more the chief of the department. You cannot do that to a guy like Mason Sones." There were vociferous protests from his cardiological colleagues. In view of the antipathy between Sones and Effler, to redress the situation, the administration decided to demote Effler also.

Favaloro received many honorary degrees and awards in recognition of his contributions to cardiac surgery, but he believed that "the highest reward that you can have in your life, in the silent moment when you are under a tree and alone, is to think that you have done something for your fellow man."

Dr. Favaloro and his wife had no children of their own, but when his brother died tragically, Favaloro took over responsibility for the upbringing of his four children. "When we had lived together in the rural area, his children were living in our house, maybe more than in his house, so we didn't have a problem in taking on his children. The four children of my brother are like our children." The eldest one, Roberto, eventually worked with his uncle as a surgeon in Argentina. Another of Dr. Favaloro's "children" is a cardiologist.

Favaloro had a long-standing interest in Latin American history, mainly of Argentina. He wrote two books on San Martín (considered the founder of Argentina), which became popular in Argentina. He told me he hoped to write more books on history.

## Sad Endings

The three main players in the development of coronary artery surgery at the Cleveland Clinic — Sones, Effler, and Favaloro — have all since departed this world in one way or another.

Sones, a heavy smoker, died of cancer of the lung in 1985. Favaloro and a colleague had operated on him twice. Dr. Favaloro and his wife made a special trip "to say good-bye to him" four weeks before he died. Favaloro later wrote, "Finally we embraced, cried together, and said good-bye for the last time in this world.... I will always thank God for having given me the opportunity to share with Mason many years of common work, understanding, and deep friendship."

In the late 1990s, I tried to contact Dr. Effler but, sadly, by this time he was suffering from Alzheimer's disease and was not able to speak with me. He died in 2004.

In July 2000, a little more than eight years after he and I had met, Rene Favaloro committed suicide — by shooting himself through the heart. He was found locked in his bathroom covered and surrounded by blood. The reason for his suicide was almost certainly the desperate financial status of the Favaloro Foundation that he had set up on his return to Argentina from the United States. The foundation owed money to the construction company that had built its buildings, and to the Siemens company for the expensive state-of-the-art cardiovascular monitoring and investigative equipment it had purchased. The foundation was in debt by an estimated U.S. $50 million, although it claimed that it was owed $18 million by the Argentine government health insurance scheme for services rendered to patients. On the evening of Dr. Favaloro's death, President Fernando de la Rúa of Argentina declared a national mourning with the flag to be flown at half-mast.

In one of the seven letters Dr. Favaloro wrote before his suicide and left to be read after his death, he asked to be cremated and his ashes to be scattered in the rural town of Jacinto Arauz, where he had worked as a general practitioner and surgeon with his brother for 12 years before going to the United States to further his career. In the area of La Plata where he was born and lived throughout his adolescent years, a street now carries his name. A plaque has been positioned in front of his family home, where he had had lunch with his mother every Wednesday until her death.

There were probably warning signs that his mind was disturbed. At the time of his death, a woman who had known him since they were children was quoted as saying, "His decency, honesty, and love for the people were the reasons for his existence, but for some reason these were not enough to continue living; he tried to let them know but nobody listened."

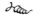

## CHAPTER 12

# The Ultimate Operation: Heart Transplantation

---

## NORMAN SHUMWAY, JAMES HARDY, AND CHRISTIAAN BARNARD

A S WE HAVE seen, the development of open heart surgery in the 1950s was one of the major advances in medicine in the 20th century. Organ transplantation followed as another great medical advance. The first successful heart transplant epitomized both of these great surgical achievements, at least in the public eye, and therefore represents a defining moment in surgery in the 20th century.

The late Keith Reemtsma was a surgeon who helped establish organ transplantation. When chairman of surgery at Columbia-Presbyterian Hospital in New York in the 1980s, he would assist the residents in performing heart transplants. When the donor heart had been successfully stitched in and restarted with an electric shock (defibrillated), it would start to beat. Having been quiescent for several hours after its removal from the donor's chest, it would suddenly burst into life again. Even though he had experienced this phenomenon many times before, Keith would inevitably exclaim, "Another goddamn miracle!" Indeed, heart transplantation is in many ways miraculous.

By the late 1960s, birth defects in the heart could be corrected, diseased valves could be replaced, and narrowed coronary arteries could be bypassed. But little could be done to reverse the heart failure caused by severely damaged or dead heart muscle. Only replacement of the entire heart would correct this problem, and that would require either heart transplantation or the implantation of a mechanical device—a total artificial heart or a ventricular assist device.

By the late 1950s and early 1960s, kidney transplantation was underway, but it was limited to few patients and the results were generally dismal. By the mid-1960s, a patient with kidney failure could be kept alive by frequent use of the artificial kidney (dialysis), and this offered an alternative to kidney transplantation. If the transplanted kidney rejected, it could, of course, be removed and the patient could once again be maintained alive by dialysis. No such alternatives were yet available to patients with advanced heart failure. Despite the poor results hitherto associated with kidney transplantation, a very few groups began to take an interest in the possibilities offered by heart transplantation.

The earliest experimental work on heart transplantation was actually carried out in Moscow by the rather eccentric research surgeon Vladimir Demikhov. Since he was not popular with the Soviet hierarchy, I am told he worked in rather poor conditions. A senior British colleague of mine who visited Demikhov in the 1960s told me the Russian's research laboratory was a converted public lavatory. Nevertheless, he carried out some ingenious transplant operations in dogs, though without long-term success. This was followed by experimental work by Shumway, Hardy, and others, and then the first clinical attempts were made by Hardy and, later, Barnard.

## NORMAN SHUMWAY— "LAID-BACK" PERSISTENCE

Norman Shumway (Figure 44) is recognized as the "father" of heart transplantation. Although James Hardy and Christiaan Barnard performed this operation in patients before Shumway, it was largely through his previous experimental studies that the feasibility of the operation became accepted. His group perfected the operative technique and demonstrated that the immunosuppressive drugs available at the time could prolong graft survival and reverse an acute rejection episode. Furthermore, they demonstrated that an autograft (i.e., a heart that is removed and replaced in the same animal so that rejection would not be a factor) would work well for years, indicating that division of the nerve supply to the heart did not prevent good function.

Before I interviewed Dr. Shumway in 1994 for the purposes of this book, I had known of him for almost 30 years. I'd heard him lecture on many occasions, and had met him informally at meetings of the International Society for Heart and Lung Transplantation, of which he was honorary president. I eventually came to know him, I believe, as a friend.

Neither in appearance nor style did Dr. Shumway give you the impression of being a surgical heavyweight. He was a very "laid-back" character, always seemingly relaxed, unworried, and irreverently, even cynically, humorous. His lighthearted manner and humor gave you the impression that he wasn't a great intellectual, and this may have been so, but he was clearly very intelligent. One did not get the impression of a person who was "driven," as one did with some of the other surgeons whose achievements are discussed in this book. His relaxed, casual manner, however, disguised an immense determination to achieve his goals. If it had not, he would not have achieved the medical advances that he did. And he was no respecter of authority, having frequently gone his own way in opposition to those above him. Possibly only in this way was he able to achieve the breakthroughs that he did.

Examples of Shumway's irreverent humor abound. The most glaring example was perhaps when he was giving a presentation at a meeting in Minneapolis celebrating the pioneering heart surgery of C. Walton Lillehei. Lillehei's troubles with the the Internal Revenue Service were well known to the audience. He had been heavily fined and compelled to do many hours of community service, and was perhaps fortunate to have avoided a prison sentence. To some extent, the meeting had been arranged by Lillehei's admirers as a means of rehabilitating his reputation, which had suffered as a result of his personal problems, not least of which was the IRS trial. In his presentation, Shumway referred to the fact that in the early days of open heart surgery, many patients had died during or soon after undergoing heart surgery performed by Dr. Lillehei. Then, with Lillehei and those who had come to honor him in the audience, Shumway added that, in many ways, Lillehei reminded him of Al Capone. "He killed a lot of people, but the government could only get him on unpaid taxes." That was Norman Shumway.

Several times I had broached the subject of an interview with him for the purposes of this book. On each occasion he expressed interest in the book, but courteously and casually declined my invitation. I wondered why. It could have been humility or shyness, of course, though heart surgeons are not generally noted for a lack of ego or a wish to avoid the limelight. I considered that my close association with Chris Barnard, with whom I had worked for several years, might be the problem. In the eyes of many Americans, including many of Shumway's supporters and protégés, Chris Barnard had "jumped the gun" when he performed the first transplant in a patient. The implication was that if Barnard had been a decent and honorable man, he would have left it to Shumway, who had done so much of the background experimental work.

Whether this rivalry was a factor in Dr. Shumway's early reluctance to discuss his career with me is uncertain. I suspect, however, that it was not a major factor, since he was also reluctant to agree to interviews with several professional authors who were compiling books on heart transplantation.

In September 1994, Dr. Shumway and I were in Cambridge, England, when the opportunity came for me to interview him. At the time, he was aged 71. We met one Sunday morning at 9:00 in my hotel. He had white hair, which was very thin on top and tended to sprout upright in a rather chaotic fashion. He had a receding chin, which was particularly noticeable when he laughed or smiled because his upper teeth were prominent compared with his lower; the receding chin disappeared into a wrinkled neck. Dr. Shumway was dressed very casually.

## Early Years in Kalamazoo

Norman Shumway was born in Kalamazoo, Michigan, in 1923. In high school, he was a good student. "I was the so-called valedictorian; the rest of the class wasn't too bright. [A typical Shumway throwaway remark.] I was very interested in law at that time and so, when I went to college at the University of Michigan, I was a pre-law student. After only about a year, pre-law students went into the service; this was 1943. I started out with infantry basic training in Texas. One day, they sent us to have an IQ test. As nobody knew how long the war would last, everybody with even a relatively modest IQ was put back into college. They wanted us in specialty areas, and so they sent me to engineering school. I was there for only six months, when they put us down for a medical aptitude test because they thought they might be short of doctors. I was sent to premed at Baylor in Waco, Texas. We completed that in nine months. We had only three quarters of premed before they decided to send us to medical school. So I have no bachelor's degree at all. I never finished anything but medical school."

Shumway attended medical school at Vanderbilt in Tennessee. Alfred Blalock had already left to go to the Johns Hopkins Hospital, but his name was still well known there.

"I graduated and moved to Minneapolis in 1949. I had an internship and one year of residency. It was just an unbelievable stroke of luck that I got to Minnesota. The atmosphere in Minneapolis was unbelievable; it was really electric. We used to say there that you had to invent an operation to get on the operating room schedule." It was in Minneapolis that Shumway came under the influence of John Lewis, who he admired considerably.

During the Korean War, Shumway had to go back into the services because he had received so much money from the government — basically his entire education. He joined the air force for two years. He then returned to Minneapolis to finish his residency. "By that time, Lewis had done the first successful open heart operation using hypothermia, in September 1952. Lillehei was still working mainly in the laboratory on the cross-circulation techniques with Cohen and Warden. Almost everybody who was doing anything in cardiac surgery at that time was on the program. It was a very exciting, stimulating program. Everybody who was there will remember it."

Shumway left Minneapolis in late 1957 and entered private practice in Santa Barbara, California. However, it was not to his liking, and soon he joined the staff of Stanford Medical School, which was then based in San Francisco.

"The only way I could get on the faculty there and get any kind of a stipend was to take over the artificial kidney program. The nephrologist was only available at night, and so we would run all of our patients on the old Kolff artificial kidney machine through the night. In the daytime, I would work in the laboratory. We were hoping that we could get heart surgery started."

Stanford Medical School soon relocated to Palo Alto. This was an opportunity for Shumway because none of the recognized cardiac surgeons moved from San Francisco to Palo Alto with Stanford, but "of course, there also weren't very many patients." This gave him plenty of time for research. Richard Lower was the resident assigned to the lab at that time.

## Local Hypothermia — Cooling the Heart

It was during this period that Shumway made his first major contribution to open heart surgery: an investigation of the concept that cooling just the heart would enable the surgeon to operate inside it while it was in a nonbeating, ideal state. While the heart-lung machine pumped oxygenated blood around the body, the blood supply to the heart itself was occluded and the heart was cooled to a very low temperature in order to protect it from the lack of oxygen. The concept was, of course, the same as Bigelow's for cooling the entire patient, but Shumway restricted the cooling to the heart. (Senning had utilized this approach three years earlier.) Reducing the metabolic demands of the heart, since it was no longer beating and was cold, protected the heart from injury and allowed the surgeon to operate on a quiescent heart without the presence of blood impairing his vision.

Richard Lower explained to me, "We demonstrated that you could get up to about an hour of aortic cross-clamping [i.e., discontinuing the blood supply to the heart] with very good recovery of the animals. That really opened things up. The operative mortality of most open heart surgery was around 50% at that time. But we operated on a bunch of dogs with zero mortality. Shumway's approach to myocardial cooling probably saved the lives of many more patients than did transplants."

## The Stimulus of Boredom

Quite remarkably, Shumway's interest in heart transplantation began almost by chance. He explained to me that, in the research laboratory, "We would stand there for an hour with a dog supported by the oxygenator, the aorta clamped, and the heart being cooled. We were both getting bored as the dickens, so I said to Dick, 'We can take the heart out and put it in cold saline,' which we were using for cooling the heart, 'and then we can stitch it back in. It will give us something to do while we're standing here for this hour's time.' Of course, we were trying to improve our surgical skills.

"We started to do that. The problem we had was that we had just silk sutures at that time and there was a lot of bleeding and other problems. Lower said, 'Why don't we get another dog's heart, leave more of the atrial tissue on it so, as we suture, we can semi-bolster the suture line?' [The technique of implanting a donor heart is easier than replacing the native heart.] So that's how we started to do heart transplants. We'd take the heart out of one animal, and put it into another animal. To our amazement, these animals began to live. They would be jumping around the laboratory for awhile. Depending on the degree of tissue compatibility, this might be anywhere from three or four days to almost three weeks, without any immunosuppression. So that was pretty interesting. It wasn't long before it became a project."

The operation proved relatively straightforward for a competent heart surgeon (Figure 45); it was preventing rejection of the organ that was the major hurdle that needed to be surmounted and that proved very difficult to achieve.

Shumway and Lower found that when they gave immunosuppressive drug therapy to prevent rejection of the heart, there was a high incidence of infectious complications. Lower noted changes in the electrocardiogram (EKG) when rejection was occurring, and so, to avoid infection, they gave the immunosuppressive drugs only at the time that EKG abnormalities developed. "That was the only way we were able to get any long-term survivors," said Shumway. "Until then, we were totally unprepared to believe that heart transplantation would be clinically possible. The most important thing we did, I think, was to show that the denervated heart can work very successfully in taking over the circulation."

It is perhaps remarkable that the "father" of heart transplantation began research in this field because he had nothing much else to do.

A group at the University of Mississippi, led by James Hardy, had also carried out considerable research in dogs. By 1964, they felt ready to attempt the procedure in a patient.

## JAMES HARDY—
## TWO UNSUCCESSFUL FIRSTS

James Hardy (Figure 46) has the unique distinction of being the surgeon who performed the world's first lung transplant, in 1963, and the first heart transplant, in 1964. His attempt at heart transplantation in 1964 has largely been forgotten in the wake of the immense publicity that surrounded Christiaan Barnard's transplant in 1967. Furthermore, Chris Barnard can still claim he performed the first human-to-human heart transplant in that year, because James Hardy's attempt utilized a chimpanzee heart.

Both Hardy's lung and heart transplant operations must be viewed as "experimental" surgery in human patients, but then so are nearly all pioneering advances in surgery. The change in attitude toward such experimental surgery that has occurred in the last 40 years can be illustrated by a look at the informed consent form that Hardy used at the time of his first heart transplant (Figure 47). The patient was semi-comatose and not in a position to sign the form himself, and so a member of his family signed on his behalf. The consent form consisted of only one paragraph, whereas today several pages — or even a small book — would probably be necessary to meet medicolegal requirements. Although the consent form indicated that no previous heart transplant had been performed in a human subject, it failed to mention that the "donor" was going to be a chimpanzee, or any other animal, for that matter. I mention this not to be critical of Hardy and his team, but purely to indicate the great change in what is considered "informed consent" — i.e., in medicolegal requirements — that has taken place since that time.

I had met with Dr. Hardy, a bespectacled man of average height with a full head of white hair, on several occasions over a period of 15 years or so and always found him to be a courteous and genuinely friendly person. Indeed, I liked him very much.

## Youth in Alabama

James Hardy was born in Newala, Alabama, in 1918, and had a twin brother. After graduating in medicine from the University of Pennsylvania in 1942, he was called up into the U.S. Army, where he spent three years with the ground forces in Europe. "We were heading for the

Panama Canal to take part in the invasion of Japan," he told me, "when the captain announced the ship was turning back as the atomic bomb had been dropped. That was about the happiest thing I ever heard."

After training in surgery, and three years on the faculty of the University of Tennessee Medical School in Memphis, he was appointed chairman of the department of surgery of a new medical school in Jackson, Mississippi, where he established a team to investigate the possibility of transplantation of the lung and the heart.

The first lung transplant in a human, carried out on June 11, 1963, went well. During the operation, one of Hardy's residents had to leave the operating room to attend to a black civil rights activist, Medgar Evers, who had been shot, and who subsequently died. When Hardy emerged from the operating room, he found the clamor outside was not about the world's first lung transplant, but about the tragic event that had just taken place. On the following morning, the lung transplant, which might well have been considered to be headline news, was relegated to the bottom of the first page in the local newspaper. The patient lived approximately three weeks, dying of kidney failure. Although the public reaction was generally favorable, there was considerable criticism from within the medical profession for what was considered a premature operation. Nevertheless, the initial relative success of the lung transplant encouraged Hardy and his colleagues to go ahead with heart transplantation.

From his experience with kidney transplantation in Mississippi, Hardy realized it would be extremely difficult to persuade a potential donor's family to donate the heart. He began to think of alternatives. In 1963, Keith Reemtsma, then at Tulane University, had transplanted no fewer than 13 chimpanzee kidneys into patients with kidney failure, one of whom was to live for nine months. Hardy visited Reemtsma in New Orleans.

"They had two patients in the hospital at that time, one of whom was a young female schoolteacher who had had a chimpanzee kidney transplant some seven months previously. She was doing surprisingly well, and there was a man there who was also doing pretty well. So I decided that, if they can do this at Tulane, *we* could give it a try. After all, we had nothing else to offer. There was no chronic dialysis then [long-term use of the artificial kidney machine]. We bought four large chimpanzees, and had them available for kidney transplants."

Hardy's selected patient for heart transplantation, 68-year-old Boyd Rush, was by no means an ideal candidate for a heart transplant, even by today's relatively liberal criteria. The report of this historic operation (performed on January 23, 1964) in the *Journal of the American Medical Association* describes the patient as a relatively large man "who was in a stuporous or semi-comatose condition [of uncertain cause] and who responded only to painful stimuli [indicating some brain injury, which would absolutely exclude him from a transplant today]. He had a tracheostomy and was being mechanically ventilated." His left leg had recently been amputated for gangrene. The chimpanzee heart was successfully implanted, but it proved too small to support the circulation of the patient, who died on the operating table.

There was not much criticism locally, but there was nationally, most of it directed toward the use of an animal heart. "I don't think Keith Reemtsma got similar criticism," Dr. Hardy told me. "At least, I didn't hear that much of it. In the first place, to many, the heart was almost the seat of the soul. Certain religious people felt that it just shouldn't have been touched. It was loaded with difficult problems. I think using the chimp was certainly part of it, but doing it at all was so far from what people could imagine and accept that it just took years for it [the concept of heart transplantation] to sink in."

In Norman Shumway's opinion, Dr. Hardy was "an unbelievable enthusiast, but there was absolutely no evidence to suggest the damn thing would succeed. I always thought Jim was a naive, enthusiastic, wonderful guy. I just thought it was kind of foolish. If you'll pardon the expression, we called it a 'foolhardy' procedure."

It so happened that within a week or ten days of the transplant, the Transplantation Society was meeting at the Waldorf Astoria Hotel in New York City, and they called Hardy and asked him to join a hastily organized panel on heart transplantation.

"When I got up to talk," Dr. Hardy recounted, "the chairman, who was Willem Kolff [the inventor of the artificial kidney] [chapter 13], said, 'I want to ask Dr. Hardy a question before he begins. Dr. Hardy, do they keep the blacks in one cage and the chimpanzees in another in the Southern states?' [Kolff was clearly referring to the bitter integration and civil rights struggle then raging in the Southern states of the United States.] That obviously didn't help, you know. [I thought this was something of an understatement by Dr. Hardy.] Anyway, I gave my presentation, reporting exactly what we had done and, at the end of it, there was not one single hand raised in applause. Not one. Afterwards, Kolff came up to me, and said, 'You realize, of course, I was joking.' I replied, 'I didn't think you were joking, and I don't think the worldwide audience thought you were joking either.' It was a bad day."

Subsequently, Hardy thought it best to keep a very low profile. "I just hunkered down and let things pass, and they finally came back to the norm. As the years passed, things got better, but I decided we weren't going to do heart transplants of any sort until Shumway or someone else did something to take the heat off of us. It wasn't that I couldn't take the criticism, but we were living off National Institutes of Health (NIH) grants at the medical school and, at about this time, the NIH became terribly suspicious of any research whatsoever on people. I knew if we did anything else that was to one side of the straight-and-narrow, we might lose our grant support, and we couldn't afford to do so."

Interestingly, in his autobiography, Hardy notes, "When I traveled to Europe, I found our heart transplant was known everywhere, and instead of all the carping and criticism going on in the United States, many surgical scientists in Europe simply wanted to know why we had not gone right ahead with another one."

## Reaction to Barnard's First Transplant

Three years later, in 1967, Hardy heard of Barnard's first heart transplant. "I'll tell you exactly when I heard it. It was at a Christmas party for my department, which we had each year. I came up the stairs at the club where we were holding it, and the surgical resident who had most recently been transplanting hearts with me in the dog lab said, 'Dr. Hardy, I just heard on the radio that somebody in South Africa has transplanted a heart. Dr. Hardy, we should have done that years ago.' He had ruined my night, I'll tell you that. I felt like shooting myself.... We *should* have done it. We should have gone on and done it, and not procrastinated, and said the heck with NIH. But I think that, in the situation in which I found myself after the first heart transplant, I made the right decision. I regret that I had to make that decision. I would like to have gone on and done a transplant that worked."

In his autobiography, Hardy recalls that after Barnard's heart transplant, "the attitude of our national governmental institutions changed overnight. All the transplant teams in the United States, plus outstanding heart surgeons who had not been interested in transplantation, were called by the National Institutes of Health to a meeting at O'Hare Airport [in Chicago] on December 28, barely three weeks after the heart transplant in Cape Town, to plan for the future. Barnard reviewed the details of his case. Once again, I was besieged by reporters and telephone calls asking for a review of our 1964 heart transplant. This time there was none of the adversarial hostility that had characterized such interviews in 1964."

The controversy over the chimpanzee heart transplant clearly did not hinder Hardy's rise in the establishment of American surgery. At one time or another, he became president of most of the major surgical societies in the United States, including the American College of Surgeons. He remained extremely productive, not only running his busy department but producing 24 books, 139 book chapters, 466 surgical papers, and 200 surgical films; he was also invited to 36 visiting professorships at other medical schools.

After a very full life, James Hardy died at the age of 84 in 2003. One of the last comments he made to his daughters was, "I had a good run."

By 1967, Shumway and his colleagues at Stanford, still the leaders in this area of research, announced that they were ready to consider moving on to performing heart transplantation in patients. By this time, Lower had moved to a more senior position in Richmond, Virginia, where the leading kidney transplant surgeon, David Hume, was keen to establish the first heart transplantation program in his department. While there, Lower secretly (because he was afraid of an adverse public reaction) transplanted a couple of human hearts (from deceased donors) into baboons to see how they would function. Although Lower was soon prepared to carry out a transplant in a patient, no suitable human donor appeared. Both Shumway and Lower were suddenly preempted by Christiaan Barnard in Cape Town, who was until then not known to be considering transplantation as a means of treating patients.

## CHRISTIAAN BARNARD — SUPERSTAR STATUS

Chris Barnard (frontispiece), who led the surgical team that stunned the world by performing the first human-to-human heart transplant in December 1967, literally became famous overnight. The daring operation captured the public's imagination as no other before or since, and Barnard became one of the best-known persons in the world. This was in part because heart transplantation had a mystical aura about it, but was equally a response to Barnard's youthful good looks and charismatic personality, which naturally drew people's attention to him. Barnard's name has since been inextricably associated with the first heart transplant and with the stunningly beautiful South African city of Cape Town, where the operation was performed at Groote Schuur Hospital, the academic medical center of the University of Cape Town.

## Youth in South Africa

Barnard was born in 1922 in the small town of Beaufort West, situated in the arid Karoo region of South Africa, about 300 miles, or six hours' drive, inland from Cape Town. His father, though white, was the pastor of a church for the mixed-race residents of the town, and was therefore considered something of an outsider, or even an outcast, by the politically conservative white population. As a boy, one of the young Barnard's duties was to pump the bellows of the church's primitive organ that his mother played during services; years later, he would joke that the heart was not the first organ he had had to deal with in his life. His father's remuneration was small and the family of four sons had no luxuries. There had been a fifth son, who died in childhood from heart disease.

After basic education in the local school, Barnard won a place at the University of Cape Town Medical School. He was not an outstanding student academically, being placed in the middle of the class. He qualified as a doctor in 1946. After junior hospital appointments, Barnard married and went into family practice in a small town in the nearby fruit-growing region of the Cape, where he was happy until personal problems between him and his partners led him to return to Cape Town. He took a junior medical post at the local infectious disease hospital and, during this time, wrote a dissertation on the treatment of patients with tuberculous meningitis. He then began a busy surgical residency at Groote Schuur Hospital, where, through his immense energy and enthusiasm, he also found time to carry out some highly ingenious research on the cause of congenital intestinal obstruction in newborn infants. There are surgeons who believe this was the best research work Barnard ever did. Barnard told me that much of this research was carried out in the evenings or even during the night after he had completed his day's busy clinical duties. It appears he had enough energy to work very long hours; indeed, many years later he told me that, as a young man, he could *never* remember feeling tired.

## Surgical Training in Minneapolis

In 1956, the opportunity arose for him to take up a scholarship at the University of Minnesota, which he accepted, leaving his wife and two young children in Cape Town. Much to Barnard's disappointment, Professor Wangensteen assigned him to the laboratory. It was there that he became fascinated by the studies that involved the heart-lung machine, although these were not part of his personal research project. He therefore requested a move to the clinical heart surgery program, becoming chief resident on Walt Lillehei's service. He worked immensely hard, often moonlighting at night to supplement his income to enable him to send money home to his family. "I can't say that I *enjoyed* it there," he told me. "I would like to have the same medical experience, but I wouldn't like to repeat the personal life. It was really very, very tough."

Barnard spent two highly productive years under the tutelage of Drs. Lillehei and Varco, and had the opportunity to learn the surgical techniques of correction of many congenital heart defects that affect children. He remembered that "the medical side was very exciting. We were in a new era."

Even though offered a faculty position in Minneapolis, Barnard had no doubts he wanted to return to South Africa. He recalled, "I was terribly lonely. I loved the work yet I wanted to go back to South Africa to the medical school where I had trained, where I knew the people, and where I would have opportunities to go ahead with my work. If I had stayed in Minneapolis, I don't think they would have given me the opportunities to really explore my capabilities because I would have been working with Lillehei and Varco and all these people. I would never have done the first heart transplant." Wangensteen very generously arranged with the U.S. government for Barnard to be given a heart-lung machine and money for research in South Africa.

## Return to Cape Town

When Barnard returned to Cape Town, he was given the responsibility of setting up an open heart surgery program. He was greatly helped in this endeavor by the collaboration of the professor of cardiology, Velva Schrire, an outstandingly good physician. Barnard's surgical results were superb for that era, and Groote Schuur Hospital quickly established an excellent reputation in heart surgery, both within South Africa and internationally.

It was probably through learning from Schrire, and the British emphasis on clinical medicine that was emphasized at Groote Schuur Hospital at that time, that Barnard became an excellent diagnostician and clinician, in the mold of Russell Brock and Donald Ross. This excellent training stood him in good stead throughout his career. For example, in 1969, after the first few heart transplants, Barnard was invited to Birmingham, Alabama, to participate with John Kirklin in his famous "Grand Rounds" on a Saturday morning. I was told by Terence English, who was a member of Kirklin's research group at the time, "For days beforehand, the chief resident and the residents were all searching to try and find the most difficult cases imaginable to show to Barnard. They wanted to make him look a fool because they thought he was a 'lightweight' cardiac surgeon. He acquitted himself amazingly well, and showed a depth of clinical skill which I don't think any of them could approach."

Barnard was not a naturally adept technical surgeon, and his frustration in this respect resulted in frequent outbursts of complaint against his assistants in the operating room, rather like Brock. He was almost always assisted by another staff surgeon rather than by a resident, and thus always had the benefit of experienced technical help. However, he provided personal and meticulous postoperative care to his patients, which contributed considerably to his excellent results. "When I had a patient who was sick and about whom I was worried, I couldn't do anything else because that patient was with me the whole day. I couldn't leave the patient in the hands of other people.

"You know, I've stood at patients' beds when they died, and I've been upset with everybody around me. I feel so upset, but I realize what I'm really upset about is that, when I write up my series of operations,

I have one more mortality. It wasn't really the death of the patient — it is the ego that is hurt. I should not have had a death with this particular type of operation; I'm too good for that. When I present my series of cases now, there will be one more death. But in the end, the patient benefits from it [this attitude of the surgeon]. That's why it's not all bad. You kill yourself for your records, but at the same time you kill yourself to save the patient."

Although there is certainly some truth in this explanation by Barnard, which is typical of his disconcerting honesty, it would not be shared by many other surgeons. Personally, a patient's death always distressed me mainly for that simple reason — a patient for whose life I was responsible had died. It was as simple as that. The fact that it was detrimental to my surgical results was very much a secondary consideration.

Barnard had soon developed an excellent reputation among cardiac surgeons, particularly in the United Kingdom. Donald Ross recollects, "The first time I became aware of his potential was at a meeting of the British Cardiac Society. He had already started to shine. I can't remember which year it was. He spoke on the surgical treatment of tetralogy of Fallot, one of the commonest congenital heart defects, and he clearly had the best results in the world at that time, and probably the biggest experience. I think everyone at the meeting was impressed, whether they said so or not. I'm sure I was. He had clearly made his mark."

## The First Human-to-Human Heart Transplant

Barnard's excellent surgical work ultimately led, of course, to the development of the heart transplantation program at Groote Schuur. When we met for the purposes of this book, by which time I had worked with him for a number of years and knew him well, I began by asking him when he first contemplated performing a human heart transplant.

"I can't exactly remember the date [it was probably about 1965], but I remember the reason why I started working on cardiac transplantation. I was asked to give a lecture at the University of Pretoria on the past, present, and future of cardiac surgery. When I started preparing this lecture, I realized that, when there is extensive disease of the heart muscle, the future would be replacement of the heart. In my lecture, I predicted that the future of cardiac surgery would be heart transplantation."

I can personally vouch that Barnard had heart transplantation in his mind as early as 1965, when I visited his unit in Cape Town. He invited me to join him on a ward round visiting his patients, and introduced me to one patient with severe heart failure. When we had moved away from the patient's bedside, Barnard turned to me and said, "What that patient needs, of course, is a new heart." I agreed but, so far in the future did I see this form of treatment, I thought the remark had been made almost as a joke. In retrospect, it seems clear that Barnard was at that time contemplating heart transplantation as a realistic form of treatment for such patients. It was little more than two years later that he stunned the world with the heart transplant performed on his patient, Louis Washkansky.

"We perfected the surgical technique in the laboratory," Barnard explained. "We never tried to get long-term survival. All we were interested in was perfecting the surgical technique. I also had a meeting every Friday lunchtime with people whose interest was in immunology. We would have a little lecture, and I used to provide sandwiches and coffee. There was a guy who is now at the Mayo Clinic who was a very good immunologist. He lectured to us very often. He explained all about cellular immunity and that sort of thing, which I didn't know very much about. I became a good immunologist from those meetings and by reading about it.

"When I was ready to embark on heart transplantation clinically, I decided I would get some experience with immunosuppression [the drugs needed to prevent rejection] and the management of patients who were immunosuppressed. I had been already planning to do the heart transplant for a year or two. I arranged a job with Dave Hume [one of the leading kidney transplant surgeons at the time]. This must have been in 1966. I studied kidney transplantation under him in Richmond, Virginia, for three months. Then I visited Tom Starzl's center [in Denver, Colorado] for two weeks to see the work they were doing. Hume taught me more than anybody else to make a successful transplant. I did exactly like he did.

"During the time I was with Dave Hume, I was working in the laboratory. I was aware that they were doing experimental heart transplants in dogs, but I wasn't interested because I had already done what I wanted to do back home. One day I watched Richard Lower for a maximum of half an hour. He was busy doing a cardiac transplant in a dog. That's the only time I ever spent with Lower. If they say that Lower taught me, I must have been a bloody good scholar to learn everything that I needed to learn in half an hour."

Although Barnard plays down the impact that watching Lower had on his plans, and claims he had long been planning heart transplantation, it may well have provided a major impetus. Donald Ross remembers that Barnard "developed a habit of traveling back and forth from South Africa to the States to attend medical meetings and so on, and would always come through London, where I was working. He would always visit the National Heart Hospital, where I was at that time, and was particularly attracted to it, not necessarily because of me but because of the very pretty nurses we used to have. On one occasion, he came through on his way back from the States, where he had seen some experimental work involving heart transplantation, and said, 'Christ, Donny, I'm going to do that!' I thought nothing more of it until, soon after, his historic operation was announced on the radio.... I know he got the idea there during that visit. As I say, I remember it dramatically. And I'm not taking sides on this issue whatsoever. But he had just seen Shumway or Lower's group transplanting hearts in animals, and he came back determined to do it himself."

In preparation for the heart transplant, Barnard carried out one kidney transplant, which was successful. The patient was certainly still alive 21 years later. As this was the only kidney transplant Barnard ever performed, he would subsequently point out that he was the only surgeon in the world who could claim 100% success in patients with kidney transplants.

Following this success, the professor of cardiology, Schrire, agreed to look for a recipient for a heart transplant. Barnard recollects, "Eventually, he called me and introduced me to Louis Washkansky, who was a 57-year-old diabetic. He was in severe heart failure, and was so sick that he had to remain in the hospital; he was terribly ill.

"Then I discussed with the professor of forensic medicine how we would manage the death of the donor. He thought there was no problem because the law in South Africa at that time said that a patient was considered dead when he was declared dead by a physician. Therefore, because the law did not signify what sort of death you should declare, the forensic expert was quite happy we could use brain death as a criterion for declaring a patient dead.

"We had said that the donor must be young so that we would probably get a normal heart. In addition, we decided our first patient should be white and the donor should also be white so we wouldn't be criticized for 'experimenting' on black people in South Africa. Two weeks before the actual transplant, I got a very suitable donor, a young black man. I didn't take this black donor, even though I was very tempted to do so, but Professor Schrire said, 'Please don't do it.' Two weeks later, on Saturday, December 2, 1967, a young white woman, Denise Darvall, presented as a suitable donor, and her father gave permission for the operation.

"I want to tell you one thing. Before the operation, I thought, 'I'm not terribly religious, but I must pray today. I don't usually pray before an operation, but today I must pray.' I thought, 'What shall I say?' I couldn't say, 'Let me be a brilliant surgeon,' because I'm not a brilliant surgeon, so I said to God, 'Please help me to do this operation as well as I'm capable of doing it.' You know, it's no use to ask God to help you run the mile in under four minutes when you don't have the capability, because it's not within God's power. But it is possible for a higher force to help you do it as well as you can. Sometimes you don't do as well as you can, but I think I did it [the transplant] as well as I could.

"Eventually, we had Washkansky in one operating room and Denise Darvall in the next. I decided I would not take out Denise's heart while it was beating, not even open the chest. I was scared that I would be criticized. Although we had discussed it with the forensic medicine people, and they said there would be no problem, I decided not to do that. When we had Washkansky's chest open and we were ready to connect him to the heart-lung machine, I went to the donor and I disconnected the respirator myself. We waited. She didn't breathe. After about five or six minutes, her heart went into ventricular fibrillation [i.e., it stopped beating]. I then said to my colleagues to open the chest and remove the heart. While they were taking the heart out, I put Washkansky on the heart-lung machine, and excised [took out] his heart."

This story of allowing the donor's heart to stop beating before it was removed from the body was told by Barnard repeatedly for more than 30 years until his death in 2001. However, in a recent book, *Every Second Counts,* journalist Donald McRae quotes Barnard's brother, Marius, a surgeon who was present on that first occasion, as stating that the heart was removed while it was still beating. Presumably, Barnard did not admit to this because he feared criticism or even legal problems for removing a beating heart. If Marius's recollection is correct, it is amazing to me that the group of people in the operating room on that occasion remained so tight-lipped and kept it a secret for so many years.

Although Barnard had carried out about 50 heart transplants in dogs, on the day of this first clinical operation his two assistants had never seen a heart transplant in their lives before. At first, the transplanted heart did not beat well and would not take over the circulation; Barnard was not able to turn off the heart-lung machine since the patient was dependent on it.

"I was horrified," he told me. "You could see the heart was not doing well. But at the third attempt [to turn off the heart-lung machine], the blood pressure kept rising. We were very happy. Then I went out and sat with Marius in the tea room, and I said, 'We had better tell the hospital people that we've done a transplant tonight.' It was then the morning of the third [December 3, 1967], a Sunday. I phoned Dr. Burger, who was the superintendent [of the hospital], and said, 'We've done a heart transplant tonight.' He said, 'Why the hell did you wake me to tell me that you've done a heart transplant? I *know* you've been doing them.' Then I said, 'We didn't do it on a dog tonight. We did it on a human, a patient.' So he said, 'How is the patient doing?' I said, 'Well.' He said, 'Thanks for calling me.' I phoned Jannie Louw, head of the department of surgery, and I told him also. He said, 'Why didn't you call me to tell me you were going to do that?' I said, 'I didn't think it was necessary.'

"I left the hospital at about five or six o'clock in the morning. It was summer, so it was already daylight. There was not one photographer, not one television camera, not one newspaperman in front of that hospital. We hadn't announced it; we didn't tell anybody we were going to do it. I got in my motorcar to drive home and I turned on the radio, and there was a news bulletin. Among the items, they said that a group of doctors at Groote Schuur Hospital in Cape Town had done a human-to-human heart transplant. That was all they said — nothing else. I don't know how they got that information. We didn't let the news out. I got home and I sat down to breakfast. A friend of mine, who guessed I must have been involved, phoned me. He said, 'Chris, I heard that news bulletin and they didn't mention your name. If they don't mention your name, I'm going to write a letter to the newspaper to tell them you did the first heart transplant.' Of course, it was only an hour later when phone calls came from all over the world. I remember Australia was early to phone, and the United States. Sweden was early to phone, and England. Then, of course, the whole world just burst.

"We did not realize this was going to be such a big thing. There were no photographers at the first transplant, not because we wanted to keep them away, but because we honestly didn't think it was a big deal. We considered transplantation to be the introduction of a new surgical technique, not something special."

Initially, while the whole world watched — Christiaan Barnard made the cover pages of *Time* (Figure 48), *Life,* and *Newsweek* — the patient did very well (Figure 49). "The one thing that was fascinating," remembered Barnard, "was that this was the first time that anybody had been able to observe what happened when you transplanted a heart into an animal or a human being in severe heart failure. Transplantation had never been done in animals that had heart failure. And it was the first time that anyone had used a brain-dead donor. Mr. Washkansky poured buckets of urine. His edema [the swelling of his body from the collection of fluid that resulted from heart failure] just disappeared. You could immediately see he was doing *very* well. This was the beauty of it — to realize that this operation had a great future."

But after about 12 days Mr. Washkansky developed pneumonia, which was misdiagnosed by the Cape Town team as being due to rejection. Sadly, he died on the 18th day after the transplant.

Barnard has often been accused of taking away from Shumway the privilege of doing the first human-to-human heart transplant, since it was Shumway's group that had carried out most of the experimental work demonstrating the feasibility of this operation.

"In medical meetings," Barnard told me, "I have heard the Americans say in front of me that I stole the idea from Shumway. As far as that is concerned, after all that these people [Dr. Shumway and his colleagues] had published, I ask, 'Do they publish it so other people can learn from it or is it a secret after they have published it?'" Barnard's implication, of course, was that those, such as himself, who built on the background provided by previous studies should not be criticized for doing so.

After Mr. Washkansky had died, Barnard visited a second patient,

Philip Blaiberg, a local dental surgeon, who had been accepted for a heart transplant. "I said, 'Dr. Blaiberg, you probably heard that Mr. Washkansky died, and I just want to tell you that if you don't want to go ahead with the operation, then I understand.' He said to me, 'No, I want to go ahead with it because, the way I am, it is not worthwhile living. I'd like you to do the operation.'" Dr. Blaiberg underwent heart transplantation on January 2, 1968.

"For two reasons," explained Barnard, "Blaiberg was responsible for other surgeons trying to get involved in transplantation. First, Blaiberg left hospital and was the first patient to show that, after a human heart had been transplanted, you could live a normal life. He was on the beach, he was photographed, he lived for one and a half years. So people saw there was a possibility not only of living a normal life after transplantation, but of surviving longer than just a few weeks or months. He was the one who really got the transplant program going. Immediately, there was an increase in the number of transplants. Then all the patients [around the world] started dying, and that got bad publicity, and everybody [the surgical teams] dropped out again. Eventually, there were only three or four centers continuing with heart transplant work. There was even one year when we didn't do a single transplant in South Africa, but usually we did a few transplants every year.

"I never had any idea of stopping. The reason we only did a few is because no patients were referred to us. It's funny, the cardiologists started not referring patients. The neurologists were the worst; they didn't want to refer donors. At first, they were all on the bandwagon to get better facilities, better postoperative care units, because they were going to be involved in cardiac transplants. But as soon as they got all this stuff, they just fell out. The province [of the Western Cape, the regional government] and the university, however, went out of their way to facilitate matters and to get us better facilities. We had the first international heart transplant meeting in Cape Town, and the province provided the money for it. It was a very successful meeting.

We invited two members, a surgeon and an immunologist, from every unit in the world that was doing transplants."

## THE SPECTER OF CHRIS BARNARD

I asked Dr. Shumway how he viewed Chris Barnard in all of this.

"In Minneapolis, he was smart enough to know that the future of surgery lay in cardiac work. And so he was a smart guy. Later on, he got interested in kidney transplants. He went to Dave Hume's place and there, of course, he encountered Lower. Lower was continuing the same great lab work he was doing with us. There, of course, Barnard saw immediately that kidney transplants were interesting, but heart transplants, my goodness! Lower told me once that the [South African] technician who was with Barnard [in Richmond] said, 'You know, he's going to go back home and do a heart transplant.' Lower thought, 'No, no he wouldn't do that.' Then, of course, he did. So he is a clever guy and could see an opportunity."

Dr. Lower confirmed this story to me. At the time, he told his own technician that Barnard "had no real background in this, so why would he do it?" Lower added to me, "So, big surprise! I'm sure I felt a little disappointment maybe. I thought it was going to be fun whether we [in Richmond] or Stanford did the first one. And it wouldn't have mattered. Of course, I think the biggest surprise was what happened regarding the publicity. The media just went crazy after the Cape Town event. That certainly surprised me. I was kind of relieved not to be in that. That maybe superseded any disappointment. I'm sure there was some disappointment, but I would not have been happy with dealing with that kind of situation."

I asked Dr. Shumway whether he resented Barnard's intrusion into the field.

"No, I don't, because we were having a heck of a time trying to get our people to come around to accept brain death as a diagnosis and confirmation of death. Had it not been for his December 1967 case, I don't think our people would have ever submitted to acceptance of brain death. What it did was open the door to brain death. If Barnard made any contribution, it was in this aspect of it. Within a year of Barnard's case, the Harvard committee came out with the criteria of brain death. That's the contribution I see from Chris that really helped all of us."

I asked Dr. Shumway whether he felt disappointment that somebody else had jumped in.

"No, not really. I'll tell you one thing, we were really surprised. As soon as I heard about Chris's first case, I wrote him. First, I congratulated him, of course, on doing the first case, and then I sent him further information which I think and hope was useful. Since I knew he didn't know anything about the diagnosis of rejection because he had never had an animal live long enough, I sent him a fairly detailed account of how to diagnose rejection from the EKG, which had to be done at least once a day, and I recommended augmented immunosuppression when there was a threat to the heart."

Dr. Lower added one more comment about Barnard. "He came to a meeting in the U.S., probably in 1968, to give the honored address. I felt terribly sorry for Chris because he was smart in a lot of ways, but he was really stupid when it came to this transplant thing. All the early pioneers of heart surgery and heart transplantation were in the audience. Chris could have shown a little humility, and said, 'What we did was this and this, but we have really built on what a lot of you had done.' But he never once acknowledged anybody except himself. Every other word was 'I.' After the lecture was over, I saw him sitting in a corner by himself, and I went over and talked to him. I don't think anybody else talked to him until he went out of the front door of the hotel and was mobbed by the press and the teeny-boppers. I thought, 'Gosh, how stupid he was.' He could have had the whole thing. Besides being so extraordinarily popular with ordinary people — young people and beautiful girls — he could have had the profession too if he had just turned that corner. But he couldn't do it."

Although both Shumway and Lower denied feeling great disappointment when "pipped at the post" by Barnard, I cannot help but believe they must have felt considerable pain at the time.

Shumway began his own heart transplantation program in patients on January 6, 1968. Thereafter, seemingly every leading heart surgeon in the world wanted to get on the bandwagon, and there was enormous enthusiasm for transplantation for a period of about two years. For example, 101 transplants in 26 different countries were performed in 1968. Without adequate preparation and expertise, particularly in regard to the prevention and treatment of rejection, the results of many groups were disastrous or, at least, extremely disappointing. This bad experience might have led to the demise of heart transplantation for a generation or more. In fact, in 1971 only 17 transplants were performed worldwide. However, the persistence of Shumway's group, together with three other groups — those of Barnard in Cape Town, Lower in Richmond, and Christian Cabrol in Paris — led to steadily improving results and eventually consolidated heart transplantation as a realistic treatment.

It is interesting to note that three of these men were trainees of Lillehei, and the fourth, Lower, a trainee of a Lillehei trainee (Shumway). Both Barnard and Cabrol told me that despite the immense excitement of the early days of heart transplantation, the most exciting period of their careers was the time they spent in Minneapolis. Cabrol mentioned that the early work on the heart-lung machine, allowing open heart surgery for the first time, "was more a revelation than transplantation. It worked *immediately.*" If the operation was successful, the patient was cured, whereas "heart transplantation had a more difficult course because of problems of rejection." Open heart surgery, therefore, offered "instant" success, whereas heart transplantation did not.

When I asked Dr. Shumway whether, during the very lean years following 1971, he ever considered abandoning clinical heart transplantation, he replied, "There was always just enough success — just enough gratification, if you will — that you could see that it probably would ultimately work and, if everybody kept working, we might get someplace." Shumway was, therefore, not only the leading figure in the experimental development of heart transplantation but, in the formative years of heart transplantation in patients, his group led the way forward.

Nevertheless, he met considerable opposition, and it required great persistence on his part to continue the program. He recalled, "I had a lot of opposition, including the president of the Board of Trustees and the president of the university. They wanted us to declare a moratorium on heart transplants in the early clinical days, but our patients were beginning to survive, and we just couldn't do that. So we very cautiously continued. We finally worked our way forward. We had the competence because of the animal experiments. Had it not been for that factor, we probably would have folded."

## Legal Concerns

Dr. Shumway told me of a donor, a victim of homicide, from whom he took the heart. "The case later went to court because the lawyers for the murderer said that the donor—or, at least, his brain—was 'okay until those guys came over and took out his heart.' The judge, of course, said it was nonsense, and validated the brain death criteria. That actually was the court decision, the judicial basis for the legislation that followed on brain death in the state of California. Prior to that, we had not really been legally justified in doing heart transplants."

I mentioned to Dr. Shumway that I had heard it rumored in one case—maybe the same case—that a murderer's defense lawyer claimed that brain death [of the victim] was not sufficient—the heart had to stop before the victim could have been considered dead; therefore, it was the transplant surgeons who had murdered the man. The lawyer looked pretty pleased with this specious argument, until the prosecuting counsel pointed out that the heart *was still* beating—in the transplant recipient—and therefore, by this criterion, the homicide victim would still not be considered dead.

(It was not until 1974 that the State of California passed an act that allowed a heart to be removed while it was still beating from a potential donor in whom there was no evidence of brain function. Technically, previous donor hearts had been procured illegally.)

Dr. Lower outlined to me a very similar legal case in which he had become embroiled when a donor's family accused him of wrongful death since the heart had been taken from a brain-dead donor while still beating. "Early in this case, which lasted in court for about ten days, it appeared that the judge agreed with the prosecution and thought we had done wrong. But, after hearing the opinions of several experts, including neurosurgeons, the judge instructed the jury to ignore the usual legal definition of death and accept the definition of brain death. That was the key turning point in the case. I gathered from talking to him afterwards that he studied the evidence long and hard before he made that decision. The evidence was that hearts get stopped and restarted all the time [in various medical conditions]. I was surprised myself to read later some of the legal criticisms subsequently directed towards the judge for his instructions to the jury."

Dr. Shumway mentioned to me that, at one point in this trial, the judge, when calling upon Dr. Lower to rise, had mistakenly said, "Will the guilty please stand up." Dr. Lower's morale plunged to the depths.

## Shumway — Personal Qualities

I asked Dr. Shumway what were his own main qualities that enabled him to put heart transplantation on the map. His response illustrated his generosity and humility.

"I was surrounded by bright young men. Wangensteen used to make the comment that he tried to have an environment that was 'friendly to learn.' I think that's what we tried to do."

His submission that his success was to some extent due to the luck of having good young people around him may well be true, but he clearly had the ability to attract these men and to allow them to fulfill themselves, rather like Wangensteen in Minneapolis.

In *Profiles in Cardiology,* Robert Robbins, a former trainee of Shumway and now the head of the department at Stanford, wrote, "Dr. Shumway provided a relaxed, fun atmosphere in the operating room that allowed each member of the team to perform at maximum capacity. During operations he would frequently say [to the trainee], 'Isn't this fun? Isn't this easy? What could be better? Nothing could be better!' He has been known to say that 'I might not be the best surgeon in the world, but I am the best assistant.'"

There is one aspect of Dr. Shumway's approach that sets him apart from most surgeons who pioneered a new field of surgery. The majority of surgeons who have made significant advances in surgery have forged ahead, dragging their colleagues and juniors behind them. It is they who have remained in the hospital late at night, they who have come in for emergencies, and they who have written the scientific manuscripts in which they have reported their progress. To my great surprise, this was not the case with Shumway. His junior colleagues told me that he was rarely in the hospital after 6 P.M., even more rarely came in after hours for emergency operations, and almost never prepared the first draft of a scientific paper. He trusted — and relied on — his juniors to "hold the fort" after regular working hours, and relied on them to collect the data and prepare the manuscripts, et cetera. Of the 500 to 600 publications he co-authored during his career, I am told that he probably wrote fewer than a half dozen himself. I am not sure whether to admire his ability to delegate so successfully or to criticize what could be interpreted as a lack of drive and energy. Nevertheless, although his approach was certainly different from that of most of his peers, there is no doubting its success.

## BARNARD — AFTERMATH

In the months and years after the first transplant, Barnard was offered many jobs in the United States, often with a huge financial incentive, but he never considered any of these offers very seriously. He told me, "I decided I was not going to leave South Africa. I thought about it this way. I'm not a youngster anymore [he was 45 years old at the time of the transplant], and I'm like a tree who has grown and become mature and is bearing fruit. When you transplant a tree like that, it takes a long time before it gives fruit again because it's got to find its roots again and start growth. Only then will it produce. I didn't have the time. If I had been a young man, I probably would have moved to the U.S.A." It is also possible that, at the back of his mind, Barnard realized that if he moved to the United States, the pressure on him to bring in money to the institution from his professional activities would be considerable, whereas in South Africa he would be more free to pursue his rapidly increasing other interests.

Barnard's team performed only ten heart transplants between 1967 and 1973. The results, although poor by today's standards, were exceptional when one considers the limited number and nature of immunosuppressive drugs available at the time, and the team's lack of experience in diagnosing and treating rejection episodes. For example, after Mr. Washkansky, the next three patients survived for an average of more than a year, which was markedly in excess of those at any other center worldwide. Quite amazingly, the following two patients lived very full lives for almost 13 and 24 years, respectively.

## The Consequences of Fame

The early success of the heart transplant program in Cape Town opened up the world to the 45-year-old surgeon. Barnard was asked to write his autobiography, which he wrote with the help of a professional writer, and later wrote a sequel. Rarely, if ever, has any surgeon been invited to speak so extensively worldwide, both to the medical profession and to the public. Barnard proved an outstanding public speaker who could pitch his talk or presentation to exactly the right level for those listening, be they eminent doctors or schoolchildren. He was both informative and entertaining, serious and humorous, a speaker who could immediately capture his audience's attention and hold it seemingly effortlessly for the next hour. He was equally at ease when interviewed for radio or television or when giving a press interview. Honest and direct, sometimes dangerously so, he was a reporter's dream. His personality came to the fore, and his engaging smile and sense of humor, his charisma, won him many admirers.

His lifestyle rapidly evolved; his suits were handmade for him by an Italian tailor in Rome, he grew his hair trendily long, and he mixed with the fashionable and famous. His penchant for being in the company of beautiful women made him a favorite of the paparazzi. His first marriage, which had given him a daughter and a son, broke up, and he married a beautiful and wealthy 19-year-old, some 29 years his junior; they had two sons before divorcing in 1982. This flamboyant lifestyle led to problems with some of his colleagues.

Barnard explained, "When they see somebody enjoying life — young girls and beautiful women and all that — they are jealous because they want to do the same thing. But they are not capable of doing it. That's the point. That's why they criticize you because they feel they can't do it themselves."

Steadily, Barnard became distracted by his travels and by his increasing social activities. One of his junior colleagues commented that after Barnard's second marriage, he did not keep up with advances in surgery anymore. Gradually, in the 1970s, as Barnard was away from Cape Town so often, his brother, Marius, began to take over the day-to-day running of the cardiac surgical program and was an enormous help to his older brother.

As Barnard's interest in surgery began to wane, so his other interests widened. During the 1970s and later, he wrote a number of books on aspects of health for the lay public, particularly relating to the heart, which were well received. For many years he contributed a weekly column to the leading local newspaper, the *Cape Times,* on any topic of his interest. These were invariably both entertaining and thought-provoking; he had the gift of seemingly always finding an anecdote to illustrate the point he was making, and the knack of stating a fact or opinion in a way that caught the reader's attention. Barnard also developed an interest in creative writing; he wrote, usually with the help of a professional writer, several novels, which, although publication may have been helped by his instant name recognition, are certainly as good as, or better than, many others that are found on the bookstands. Like many novelists, he drew heavily on his own experiences — for example, in medicine — to provide the background for his stories. How much of the writing of all this work for the public was actually penned by Barnard, and how much was written for him by others, remains uncertain. Barnard himself, however, was quite open in admitting that, although the ideas came from him, their translation into actual words was frequently provided by others.

His high profile enabled him to participate in several business ventures, including restaurants in Cape Town and a cattle farm on the south coast of South Africa. He developed a financially profitable, but controversial, link with Clinique La Prairie in Switzerland, where he acted as research advisor. The Clinique's main interest and source of income was in the contentious field of "rejuvenation" therapy, whereby extracts from fetuses of sheep were injected into people who felt they needed to renew their zest for life. His association with the Clinique harmed his reputation in the medical profession.

Barnard's lifestyle distanced him from many of his surgical peers, who no longer considered him a major player. His participation in surgical meetings declined dramatically. Barratt-Boyes told me it was "a pity he spoiled it all with his later life, because he was virtually ostracized [from the surgical world]. The situation was a bit like that of Lillehei, who was ostracized at one stage, and then readmitted, but I don't think Chris was ever really readmitted to the clan."

Barnard acknowledged that his lifestyle stopped him from concentrating on his hospital work and research. "If I had it all over again, I would have limited the amount of traveling I did. I traveled too much. The second regret is that I didn't retire earlier. I should have retired in maybe 1980 or 1981, but not stayed on until 1983. I stayed two years too long." During these last two years, Barnard played an ever-decreasing role in the running of his department.

## Controversial Retirement

At the end of 1983, at the age of 61, Barnard took early retirement, and fully pursued his other interests. He accepted invitations as a guest lecturer on cruise liners, which proved both a way of taking a pleasant vacation and of improving his financial status. He participated in advertisements, which was certainly not something one would have expected of a distinguished member of the medical profession. Perhaps his poorest judgment was shown with his involvement in the advertising campaign for Glycel, a cream purported to help prevent aging of the skin. For this, he was heavily criticized by certain physicians and medical organizations. It tarnished his image further. He perhaps can be looked on, like Lillehei, as a flawed hero in a Greek tragedy who, to some extent, was responsible for his own downfall.

In 1985, Barnard accepted an invitation from Nazih Zuhdi to become scientist-in-residence at the newly formed Oklahoma Transplantation Institute in Oklahoma City, where, for the next two years or so, he spent several months each year advising on the development of a heart transplant program. This greatly improved his financial situation, which he put to good use in his beloved South Africa; he relinquished his cattle farm and took an interest in a large sheep farm in the Karoo, which he later transformed into a game reserve catering largely to wealthy tourists.

At the end of 1988, at the age of 65, Chris Barnard married for the third time, this time to a young fashion model 40 years his junior; they had two children, the youngest born in 1997. Sadly, this marriage also broke up in the year 2000.

Barnard received many academic and public honors, but these did not include honors bestowed by most of the world's most prestigious universities or medical schools — the Harvards and Oxfords. Was this because they did not believe his work was significant? Or was their response influenced by his subsequent flamboyant lifestyle?

Chris Barnard died suddenly during what was reported to be an asthma attack in 2001, at the age of 78.

I once asked him to write some words in my copy of his autobiography, *One Life*. He inscribed the phrase "One life is enough, if well lived." This is surely his own epitaph. He worked immensely hard, at least for the first 60 years of his life, but he played just as hard. He had been a surgeon, researcher, novelist, journalist, restaurateur, rancher, traveler, and celebrity. Can we summarize Chris Barnard? Not very easily, for he was a multifaceted character.

To quote Bob Frater, a onetime surgical colleague, Barnard was a combination of a "rough-at-the-edges poor boy and charming sophisticate, democrat and tyrant, selfless healer and boorish egotist, lover and Don Juan, shrewd parvenu and naïve acceptor of glitterati adulation — but, above all, surgical visionary and simply the most unforgettable character of the second generation of cardiac surgeons."

## SHUMWAY — THE "ADDICTION" OF SURGERY

To many surgeons, work is almost an addiction — to some extent to the detriment of marriage and family. Although not a workaholic in that once he was chairman of his department and surrounded by able younger men, Shumway did not remain in the hospital late in the evening and rarely came in at night, nevertheless surgery held a fascination for him. Eventually, as with so many others, his marriage broke up. I asked him if this was related to the demands of his work.

"I think it was probably related. There are so many factors that go into it. Probably the essence of it is that I have never remarried. That may be a significant point. It may even be a summary of the whole situation. Marriage is just too time-consuming. You can't do it justice. It's very difficult. Surgery, not just heart surgery but all kinds of surgery, is so fascinating, and the responsibility is so acute, that it's a terrible addiction. I was just too consumed by it, and loved surgery so much. And the people who were in it were always so fascinating and humorous. They had such a great philosophy, so different from, say, internists or historians or engineers."

I asked him whether he regretted the way his life had been dominated by his work.

"I suppose you do, but you'd still do it again. It reminds me of what John Lewis would say after a patient's death, when the resident would declare, 'If we had it to do again, we would do it the same way.' Lewis would say, 'What do you mean you would do it the same way? The patient *died!*' So obviously things can always be better. But there's that old saying, 'Things are never so bad they can't be worse.'

"I read recently of a British surgeon [from the early part of the 20th century], Lord Moynihan, who, looking back over his career, said that it was a great fun time and he would love to have it over again. I think that summarizes it for me. The reward, you know, is just being there at the time and looking at these people [the patients]. There's nothing else like that."

At the time of my interview with him, one of Shumway's four children, Sara, was an up-and-coming young heart surgeon on the staff at the University of Minnesota. I asked him whether she had been influenced by him in her choice of career.

"I don't know. I never tried [to influence her]; I think it's important to let your children find their own way without saying you've got to do this or you've got to do that. But she's having a good time with it. Remember this too, she has that faculty position at Minnesota that I always wanted, but never got. So I kind of like that part of it."

Although officially retired, Shumway never really left Stanford Medical Center, being a regular—almost daily—visitor to his old department. He loved the staff, and it remained his "home." He never remarried.

Norman Shumway died in 2006, one day after his 83rd birthday.

Richard Lower retired early and spent many years as a rancher in Montana. He then returned to Richmond, where he did considerable medical charity work as a general practitioner. I asked him whether, if he were a young man again, he would choose heart surgery as a career today.

"I hate to say it, but I think heart surgery has gotten a bit routine, certainly in some areas. We were really fortunate to be in that era. I don't know if there is much else that could match it now. Certainly, doing the clinical transplants was pretty heady stuff, and I don't think I ever got over what a fun thing it was to see the heart start up. Even after about 350 or so transplants, it was still great." (As Keith Reemtsma used to say, "Another goddamn miracle!")

Richard Lower died in 2008 at the age of 78.

THERE IS ONE other story that relates to heart transplantation that was recounted to me during my research into writing this book. For reasons that will be obvious, I shall not report who told me the story or where the event took place.

In the late 1960s, when there was initial great enthusiasm for heart transplantation, groups all over the world were attempting this operation with little or no research experience behind them, and possibly without adequate knowledge of the various aspects of medicine that were required. It was a time of relatively abandoned medical experimentation in this field, and this largely accounts for the lack of success.

Heart surgeons in one region of the world were planning their first heart transplant. A patient was identified who was in heart failure and who it was considered would not survive more than a few days or weeks. He was put on the list to await a donor heart. A suitable "brain-dead" donor was identified, and the operation was planned to be carried out within a few hours. The operating rooms and the surgical teams were alerted and prepared. For reasons that are now lost in obscurity, the operation did not take place.

According to my multiple informants, ten years later the potential *recipient* remained alive and in reasonably good health (which was unlikely to have been the outcome had he undergone heart transplantation in those early pioneering days). It was therefore fortunate for him that the operation was abandoned. Even though the news of his long-term survival came as something of a shock to me, since it had been presumed at the time that he had very few days of life left, it came as even more of a shock when my informants told me that, ten years later, the potential *donor* also remained alive and well. The diagnosis of "brain death" had clearly been wrong.

This story remains a lesson to us all that overenthusiasm toward any new medical or surgical development should not be allowed to cloud an individual physician's judgment.

## CHAPTER 13

# In the Realm of Science Fiction: Mechanical Hearts

———

## WILLEM KOLFF, MICHAEL DEBAKEY, DENTON COOLEY, AND WILLIAM DEVRIES

T HE TOTAL ARTIFICIAL heart and its close cousin, the left ventricular assist device (LVAD) (Figure 50), have captured the public's imagination as being close to science fiction — the bionic man. Progress in the development of the artificial heart has been variable, and a reliable device that can permanently replace the native heart without complications, although close, remains the goal of the future. Nevertheless, mechanical assist devices that augment, rather than totally replace, the heart (such as LVADs) are being implanted in increasing numbers and have achieved good reliability, many functioning well for a year or two.

Willem Kolff (Figure 51), the creator and developer of the dialysis machine (artificial kidney), was among the first to pursue the goal of designing and building an artificial heart. But it was the well-known surgeon Michael DeBakey (Figure 52) who, through his connections and influence in Washington, D.C., did much to ensure funding for this expensive area of bioengineering and surgical research.

The first implantation of a mechanical heart was in Houston in 1969, an event surrounded by great controversy that led to the disruption of the hitherto productive collaboration between DeBakey and his junior colleague, the equally famous Denton Cooley (Figure 54). This operation was planned as a "bridge" to heart transplantation, i.e., the device was implanted with the aim of maintaining the patient's life until a human heart became available for transplantation. It was another 12 years before a second attempt was made — also in Houston — and a further year before attempts were made in Salt Lake City to *permanently* replace a patient's diseased and failing heart with an artificial device, with no plan to subsequently transplant a heart from a deceased human when one became available. This first permanent replacement was carried out in 1982 by Utah surgeon William DeVries (Figure 55), using a device designed by Kolff and his colleague, Robert Jarvik. All of these initial operations in both Houston and Salt Lake City hit the headlines and generated as much public interest as the heart transplants of Barnard and Shumway a few years earlier.

As in every field of surgical endeavor, many have played major roles in the mechanical heart story, but two teams in particular — in Salt Lake City and Houston — were especially pioneering, in part because of the personalities involved. Kolff had already achieved immortality through providing the world with the dialysis machine. DeBakey and Cooley played leading roles in the development of vascular surgery and in the expansion of open heart surgery, and are two of the great characters of 20th-century surgery. Like Barnard, DeVries found himself thrust into the limelight in the media blitz that accompanied the first permanent implantation of an artificial heart.

## WILLEM KOLFF — BIOENGINEERING GENIUS

Willem Kolff (Figure 51), though never a heart surgeon nor even a cardiologist, was one of the most remarkable medical inventors of the 20th century. He is probably most remembered for his development of the first truly functional dialysis machine (artificial kidney), which, remarkably, he developed while working in a small country hospital in German-occupied Netherlands during World War II. Observations he made at that time led him to develop a membrane oxygenator, a new type of oxygenator that would eventually be incorporated into standard heart-lung machines. Furthermore, he was involved in the development of the aortic balloon pump (a device that provides some augmentation to the performance of a failing heart), which has saved literally hundreds of thousands of lives in patients suffering acute heart failure. Finally, he led the team that initiated the development of the artificial heart that became the first to be used in a series of patients. Kolff has also contributed toward the development of artificial eyes and ears. There are, therefore, numerous reasons why he should be remembered in the history of medicine, but he is included here primarily because of his work in developing the artificial heart.

When I met Dr. Kolff in August 2001, I found him to be a moderately tall, white-haired man with an old-fashioned white "Puritan" or "Amish" beard (with no mustache). He was born in Leiden in the Netherlands in 1911, the oldest of five brothers, and studied medicine at Leiden University. In 1939, early in his medical career, one of his patients, a young man, died slowly of kidney failure; it was a miserable death, and it impressed Kolff greatly. He immediately began to experiment to make a dialysis machine.

## The Dialysis Machine

The basis of Kolff's dialysis machine was that toxic waste products in the blood diffused through a membrane into a bath of fluid. The membrane he first used was a commercially available cellophane that was normally used to make sausage skin. A thin film of blood circulated slowly through a long coiled cellophane tube (of sausage skin) lying in a bath of fluid. He found that urea (one of the toxic waste products that the patient's kidneys could no longer excrete) diffused from the blood through the membrane into the surrounding fluid in the bath. The level of this toxin in the blood was therefore steadily reduced.

The Germans then occupied the Netherlands, and Kolff took a position as a physician in the small town of Kampen, where he completed development of the first dialysis machine under very difficult conditions. In order to obtain the supplies he needed from the German occupiers, all kinds of papers had to be falsified, but his Dutch compatriots were willing collaborators. His first brief use of the machine was in 1943. He treated 15 patients before one survived. Ironically, the first to recover from kidney failure and survive was 65-year-old member of the National Socialist (Nazi) party, Maria Schafstade, who had been imprisoned by the Dutch for having collaborated with the Germans. According to Kolff, she was comatose when she went on to dialysis in 1945. After six hours, he bent over her and said, "Can you hear me?" She slowly opened her eyes, and the first words she said were, "I am going to divorce my husband." And she did.

Kolff made four dialysis machines for the specific purpose of sending them abroad, paying for them himself, including the transportation. In 1946, when the war was over, the four machines were shipped to hospitals in London, Montreal, Boston, and New York. These hospitals invited him to show them how to run the machine.

From observations he made while working on the dialysis machine, between 1946 and 1950 he designed several heart-lung machines. Kolff had observed that as blood passed through the "sausage tubing" in the dialysis machine, it could pick up oxygen and thus become pinker. He used this concept to oxygenate blood passing through a heart-lung machine.

"But Kampen was too small a place to develop open heart surgery," he told me. "In 1950, for several reasons, I wrote to the Cleveland Clinic in the U.S.A. and said I would like to work with them there. I used the artificial kidney as a stepping board to come to the Cleveland Clinic, not predicting that nobody there would be interested in heart-lung machines. When I came, they paid for me to bring all the heart-lung machines I had made. Closed heart surgery was underway, and no surgeon in his right mind wanted to fool with any part of my machines. It was a very difficult five years."

During that period, Kolff became friendly with John Gibbon in Philadelphia, who was working on his machine. The first clinical use of Kolff's membrane oxygenator in a heart-lung machine was eventually made at the Cleveland Clinic in early 1956. Membrane oxygenators have now become stamdard in heart-lung machines for open heart surgery, and have long largely replaced the earlier "bubblers" and "filmers."

## The First Artificial Heart

In the spring of 1957, Kolff started work on an artificial heart that could be implanted in the patient. In 1967, he moved to Salt Lake City, where he was able to set up an institute for research into the development of this device.

The basis of the artificial heart that Kolff and his colleagues, particularly Robert Jarvik (with whom he was later to fall out), designed and tested was a two-chambered structure that replaced the patient's ventricles (pumping chambers) and was sutured in place through connections with the two atria (collecting chambers) and the aorta and pulmonary artery (Figures 50 and 56). Within each artificial "ventricle" was a polyurethane diaphragm, which was moved by air pressure pumped in and out from an external pump through drivelines. When the membrane relaxed, the ventricles filled with blood. When air pushed the membrane upward, the blood was ejected. Four metal mechanical valves ensured that the blood traveled only in the correct direction. The drivelines could be connected to a portable power source for periods of time to allow the patient some degree of mobility.

It took some years for Kolff's mechanical heart to be ready for implantation in patients, a topic to which we shall return later. In the meantime, however, Michael DeBakey, working independently in Houston, was testing such a device to support a patient either until the native heart recovered or until a heart transplant could be carried out.

## MICHAEL DEBAKEY — "HELL ON WHEELS"

On a sunny, crisp Saturday morning in November 1990, I entered the lobby of the Methodist Hospital in Houston, Texas. I immediately thought I was in a plush hotel foyer. The lobby was beautifully designed and furnished; the floors were of marble, there was a fountain, numerous plants, and small trees, and the chairs were stylish and comfortable. In a prominent position was a massive bronze bust of Dr. DeBakey, commissioned by King Leopold of Belgium.

The position of honor of this bust in Methodist Hospital is a tribute to the massive contribution DeBakey made to the development of Baylor Medical Center. Indeed, DeBakey must be remembered as one of the most industrious and productive people of the 20th century. He can truthfully be called a "phenomenon" or "hell on wheels," two descriptions used by John Norman, a surgeon-researcher who knew him well. He was also dubbed the "Texas tornado."

When I arrived at his office, I found Dr. DeBakey (Figure 52) to be a relatively small man, wearing a white coat over an operating-room scrub suit and a surgeon's cap; I thought this was a little odd since I suspected that, at the age of 82, he no longer performed any surgery himself — particularly on a Saturday morning. I presumed he wore this type of clothing in order to perpetuate the image of the active surgeon. Dr. DeBakey was not a good-looking man; he had a large, hooked nose, small, slit-like eyes, and a very receding forehead. He wore heavy glasses. He wore black boots with elevated soles and stacked heels that gave him a little extra height; it intrigued me that someone who had achieved so much, was so highly regarded, and had been so honored should feel the need for an extra inch or two.

DeBakey was best known for his work in vascular surgery (the surgery of blood vessels), particularly in the surgery of aortic aneurysms (in which the walls of the main artery in the body become weakened by disease and may tear and rupture). As John Kirklin had said to me, "Mike DeBakey wrote the book on aneurysms." DeBakey is well known for introducing synthetic flexible material grafts to replace or bypass occluded large blood vessels, although Arthur Voorhees was the original pioneer in this field. While DeBakey did not play a primary role in the introduction of open heart surgery, he is usually credited with being one of the developers of a pump commonly incorporated into heart-lung machines, now frequently referred to as the DeBakey roller pump.

Perhaps even more than Willem Kolff, DeBakey was, however, the major driving force in the early development of the artificial heart and the left ventricular assist device. In 1963, he was the first to insert a single pump (an LVAD) to provide temporary support for a failing left ventricle after open heart surgery (with the patient's own heart being left in place); unfortunately, this attempt was unsuccessful. The kudos for carrying out the first total artificial heart implant in a human was snatched from him by his junior colleague, Denton Cooley, a highly controversial event that led to the breakup of their professional partnership and to DeBakey not speaking to Cooley again for more than 40 years — indeed, until the year of his death. The bitter feud that developed between the two men is one of the best known in medicine.

## Childhood and Youth

DeBakey was born in 1908 in Lake Charles, in southwest Louisiana. His parents were born in Lebanon, and came to the United States as children in 1885. Michael was the oldest of five children. By the time of Michael's birth, his father was a successful local businessman. DeBakey found schoolwork easy, and led his class.

"My parents were great believers in education for their children," he told me, "and so we were urged to read a lot. So, in addition to our regular schoolwork, we had to read at least one book from the library every week. One time when I was in the general library, I saw the encyclopedias, and started to browse through them. I was fascinated with them. When I got home, I told my father about it. My siblings and I used to fight to get to the encyclopedias. Before I finished high school, I had read the entire *Encyclopedia Britannica*."

He attended Tulane University in New Orleans, where in two years he had acquired enough credits to get into medical school. As a medical student, he worked as a research technician assistant in the laboratories of some of the medical staff, primarily being involved with experiments on blood circulation. That was when he started working on the roller pump that bears his name.

Subsequently, DeBakey and his surgical chief, Alton Oschner, were among the first to report on the link between smoking and cancer of the lung.

## Early Career

After completing his surgical residency at Tulane, DeBakey spent time in Europe, seeing something of the surgical work going on in France and Germany. During World War II, he was closely involved with administration of the U.S. Army surgical units, drawing up policies, preparing directives to surgical units worldwide, and visiting units in Europe. He played a part in setting up the MASH units. Although still a relatively young man at that time, he gained immense administrative experience. After the war, he returned to a faculty position at Tulane, but in 1949 he moved to Houston as chairman of surgery at Baylor University.

He began working with homograft arteries (taken from deceased humans), like Gross and Hufnagel before him, and developing cloth grafts, like Voorhees, to whom, after some questioning by me, he gave credit for the concept of the use of fabric. According to surgeon George Humphreys, when DeBakey arrived in Houston, he decided that the surgical treatment of aortic aneurysms could be his road to success.

DeBakey first performed operations for aneurysms of the abdominal aorta, beginning in 1952. He recalled, "We started climbing up the aorta, and did the first descending thoracic aneurysm [i.e., in the chest — in 1953], the first arch aneurysm [1954], and the first ascending aortic aneurysm [i.e., of the major artery arising from the heart — in 1954]. In 1955, I did the first successful dissecting aneurysm [i.e., replacement of an aneurysm in which the wall had already split and therefore was very close to rupturing]."

In 1953, Dr. DeBakey was also one of the first surgeons to perform carotid endarterectomy (an operation to remove an arteriosclerotic obstruction from an important artery in the neck through which the brain is supplied with blood).

According to George Humphreys, "DeBakey developed the first production-line surgical service that I had seen. He admitted his aneurysm patients or his cardiac patients to a service where they were worked up [i.e., prepared for the operation]; they then went into the operating room to be operated on, then into the recovery room, which was very well set up to take care of them. As soon as they were able to leave the recovery room, they went to a post-recovery room service, and then to a rehabilitation service, and then out of the hospital. It was a regular production line, very well organized."

## Baylor College of Medicine

When DeBakey first went to Houston in 1948, Baylor was in a pretty poor state. "To be honest with you," he told me, "I turned the job down the first and second times I came to look at it. There was *nothing* here." He almost single-handedly turned things around and built Baylor into a major medical center. When he arrived, he was the only board-certified surgeon in Houston. After his first year, he was generating enough income from his private surgical practice so that Baylor never again had to give him any money to run his department. So immense was his impact that, in 1968, he was asked to take on the deanship of the medical school and, later, the presidency of Baylor College of Medicine.

At the time of my interview with Dr. DeBakey, the Texas Medical Center complex had grown to become one of the largest, if not the largest, in the world. DeBakey confirmed, "The number of employees is 55,000. We have several billion dollars' worth of construction here. The overall annual budget is in the neighborhood of several billion dollars. The growth here has been phenomenal. One of the big factors in this growth was the cardiovascular surgical work that drew attention." He admitted, however, that when he first went to Houston, he did not foresee it would grow to this stature.

DeBakey's relationship with Baylor was perhaps a classic example of Ralph Waldo Emerson's statement that "an institution is the length and shadow of one man." The full story of how DeBakey built up Baylor into a world-famous institution would take too long to tell, but, undoubtedly, Baylor could not have achieved its present stature as a medical school so rapidly without him. He achieved this success by drive and relentlessly hard work, which provided an example to those he appointed to work with him. It was as much his incredible energy and industry as his innovative work in cardiovascular surgery that led to him being featured on the cover of *Time* magazine in 1965 (Figure 53).

According to Bud Frazier, an internationally known heart surgeon who trained under both DeBakey and Cooley, "One thing that was really admirable about Dr. DeBakey was that the staff surgeons he hired — Denton Cooley, Stanley Crawford, and so on — were excellent, outstanding people in their own right. He recruited Dr. Cooley and Dr. Crawford in the early 1950s era, and he may have disliked some of the things they did, but he never told them they couldn't do them, and never tried to stop them. But his drive pushed people like Crawford and Cooley because they knew they could never let up. If someone wanted to beat Dr. DeBakey at something, he would have to try to work as hard as he did. He instilled that drive into everyone."

## Open Heart Surgery and Artificial Hearts

Dr. DeBakey related the story of his interest in devices that would replace the heart: "We became interested in the artificial heart as an extension of the heart-lung machine. As we developed more experience with the heart-lung machine, my feeling was that there were high-risk patients who would only be able to be weaned from the machine if we could continue using it for, say, several hours. My reasoning was that, if you could support them for a longer period of time, perhaps the heart might recover. We began doing some laboratory work, and reviewed what had been done in the past, particularly the work by Kolff."

William DeVries, a colleague of Kolff, confirmed to me DeBakey's important role in the development of the artificial heart. "DeBakey was the man," he said. "The artificial heart was one of the first preempted fundings of the National Institutes of Health (NIH). DeBakey is the one who did all this. He said that if the United States would throw enough money into it, we would get an answer. They threw money into it. At the time when I did the artificial heart implants [see below], $400 million of federal funds had been used to develop it. DeBakey had set this up and was actually working towards some type of schedule for implantation. But all of their ideas came from Kolff."

## The Controversial First Artificial Heart Implantation — The Beginning of the Great Feud

When the first artificial heart was implanted in Houston in 1969, there was great controversy. According to Dr. DeBakey, "The man who was partly responsible for this was working in my laboratory as an assistant technician [referring to Domingo Liotta, later to become a well-known surgeon in South America]. He was Argentinian. To the committee that had to investigate this matter, he said that he felt I would refuse to use our device on human beings, and he was quite correct. I was opposed to using it on humans because we couldn't get survival in our animals for more than a few months. They all died. We couldn't figure out why, or how to prevent that. I didn't feel that ethically we could go to an institutional review board and get approval for the device to be used as an experimental procedure on humans. So, secretly, he went to Dr. Cooley and discussed this with him. I'm not sure yet whether he or Dr. Cooley initiated it, but the fact remains that they got together secretly and agreed they would do it.

"So, one night, he removed the artificial heart from our laboratory and brought it over to Dr. Cooley. They had it all organized. This happened when I was out of town. They had this patient with an aneurysm of the left ventricle [a weakening and dilatation of the ventricle resulting from the presence of dead muscle following a heart attack]. They scheduled it as a resection of ventricular aneurysm, but they knew they were going to use the artificial heart; they had the device there [in the operating room]. They had hardly gotten started with the operation when he [Dr. Cooley] said to remove the patient's heart. So they did. Within three days, the device was replaced with a human heart transplant, but the patient was already dead when they did it. By the time they got it [the heart] going, he was brain-dead. Shumway said that this was 'the first time in medical history that a patient had a heart replacement done from one dead person to another.'"

In other words, although the operation to insert the artificial heart was technically successful, complications developed over the next three days and, by the time a human donor heart became available, the patient had suffered severe brain damage.

"But anyway, it was publicized tremendously," continued DeBakey. "You can't help but wonder how it got so publicized. They had obviously called the press to tell them they were going to do it. I was in Washington, and as I went to bed that night and happened to turn on the television in the hotel, there it was on the news. It was a shock. I was at a meeting at the NIH and so, when I got to the NIH the next morning, they asked me about it. I said, 'I didn't know anything about it.' It created a serious problem because all of our work was supported by the NIH. We had to explain to them how this had been done when it hadn't been approved by them or by the hospital review board.

"So a committee was established. Since I was the principal investigator and the college president then, I turned it over entirely to the chairman of our board. He appointed a special faculty committee to investigate the matter. They prepared a report in which they said it was a violation of ethics and was not standard procedure. So Dr. Cooley was forced to resign. We were able to get the NIH to accept our report.

Of course, the controversy was greatly enhanced by the perception of a feud between Dr. Cooley and me. There never had been a feud in the first place. He was a full-time member of my department until this happened, and he had to resign. There was no reason for me to feud with him before or after that. He initiated the process with this other fellow, who also had to resign. It was just a very unfortunate situation. I have a feeling he miscalculated the consequences of it."

This controversy destroyed Cooley's relationship with DeBakey. Indeed, it initiated one of the greatest and best-known feuds in medicine. Only in the last few months of DeBakey's long life did the two resume speaking to each other. Cooley told Bud Frazier that, at the airport, he had on occasions joined a check-in line in which Dr. DeBakey was also standing, and although he had tried to begin a conversation, Dr. DeBakey would not reply. But, more than 40 years later, the two of them did eventually take steps to honor each other's contributions to surgery.

Many jokes among cardiovascular surgeons have been based on this well-known feud. There is the apocryphal story of DeBakey arriving at the hospital parking lot only to find it completely full. When he pressured the attendant to find him a place, and pointed out that he was Michael DeBakey, the attendant reportedly replied, "I don't care who you are. I couldn't find you a place even if you were Denton Cooley."

## The First Successful Left Ventricular Assist Devices

Returning to my interview with Dr. DeBakey, I asked him of his subsequent work on the artificial heart.

"More and more, I became disillusioned about the total artificial heart and, in 1973, I stopped working on it. I became more interested in some kind of cardiac assistance — the left ventricular assist device [in which the failing native heart is not removed in the hope that it will recover] [Figure 50]. In 1967, I had proved with a clinical case for the first time that this concept was good. We had this girl who we couldn't wean off the heart-lung machine. After ten days of pumping [with an LVAD], we finally weaned her off and she recovered. She lived for six years and led a normal life in every way until she was killed tragically in an automobile accident. Of course, it was not a long step to go from assisting one ventricle to assisting two ventricles."

## Discipline and Perfectionism

DeBakey had a reputation for being a disciplinarian and perfectionist, and I wanted his perspective on this. I cautiously mentioned to him that he had a reputation for being "strict" with his junior staff.

"I think that's true. I also have a reputation for being a perfectionist. Sometimes that's used in a derogatory sense. I think people who have great self-discipline are perfectionists. That's why they have that discipline. They want to be sure everything is correctly done, and sometimes they overdo it. That's why they are difficult to get along with. But I admired those qualities [in others] because I was brought up highly disciplined. My father was a very, very highly disciplined person; he was extremely generous, and so was my mother, but we had to toe the line."

My comment to Dr. DeBakey about his having a reputation for being strict was something of an understatement. Of all the surgeons featured in this book, DeBakey had the most fearsome reputation as someone difficult to work with — far worse than Brock, Harken, Kirklin, or Barnard, for example. Stories of his intensity and of the demands he made on his junior staff are legion.

According to Bud Frazier, "Dr. DeBakey is one of the most interesting people I've ever had to interface with in life in that he is not very like anyone else I've ever been around. I've never been around anyone so intense, so obsessed with details, so observant of every little thing. He would make rounds every morning at six o'clock by the clock. He walked into the intensive care unit at six A.M. and, when I was there, we would see sometimes twenty patients with abdominal aneurysms admitted in a day. He cornered the world market on those. When making rounds with him, you never said anything. If he asked you a question, you would answer it, but you never volunteered anything.

"Dr. DeBakey wouldn't let you leave the hospital. As a resident, you were in the ICU for 90 days at a stretch. You were not allowed out of the hospital at all for 90 days — unless you were fired; that was the only way you could get out. You were not allowed to leave the ICU during this period, not even to go to the hospital cafeteria; food was brought up to you. You slept in the ICU. If you were married, your wife and kids could only see you if they came to the ICU. Actually, I spent a little more than 90 days there because the guy ahead of me got fired, so I had to make up some of his time."

Dr. Frazier recounted a story of his long sojourn in the ICU at Methodist Hospital. He overlapped on this rotation with another resident (who we shall call "Smith") who, on his last day, mentioned to Bud that he would thank Dr. DeBakey for all he had learned in the ICU. Knowing how DeBakey hated "small talk" that distracted from his work, Bud cautioned his colleague about doing this, recommending he say nothing. At the end of DeBakey's round, as he turned to leave the room, Smith could not restrain himself, and stepped forward, saying, "Excuse me, Dr. DeBakey, but today is my last day with you...." DeBakey swung around and, thumping the young man hard on the chest with his knuckles, said, "Yes, I know it is, Smith. When I was getting up this morning, I said to myself, 'What is going to be good about today? It's Smith's last day with me,' I thought. 'That's what's going to be good about today. This gave me tremendous enjoyment, and I looked forward to the day.'" All this was said with great viciousness, without a hint of humor. With that, DeBakey spun on his heel and walked out, leaving a very deflated young resident.

DeBakey's own capacity for hard work was legendary. Bud Frazier again: "Dr. DeBakey always said he went to bed at midnight and got up at four A.M., did his paperwork, and made rounds at six A.M. I think he *did* do that because he was always at the hospital very late at night. Dr. DeBakey would take breaks through the day, go back to his office, and he never came out until he was ready. I always suspected him of taking some catnaps, since I don't know how he could have maintained that intensity of work without getting a little more rest than he supposedly did."

In a 1996 interview in the *American Journal of Cardiology*, DeBakey attributed his phenomenal productivity—for example, the 60,000 operations he estimates he personally performed in his lifetime, and the 1,500 scientific papers he authored or co-authored—to the extra time he had available to him through his ability to exist on less sleep than most of us: "You know that you have a certain time span, whatever God gives you. When you are living, you want to enjoy that. When you are sleeping, you are just dead as far as conscious living is concerned; that's part of your death. So I think you have to set some goals and priorities. I try to use my time as efficiently as I can."

"We, and Dr. DeBakey, were always working," continued Dr. Frazier. "I remember making rounds with him one Saturday. You could see the Rice University stadium from the Methodist Hospital, and Rice was playing a football game. All of us, of course, wanted to go to the football game [particularly Bud Frazier, I suspect, as he had been a player when at college]. Dr. DeBakey looked out, saw all those people watching the football game, and said, 'Isn't it amazing how many people could so foolishly waste their time.' There was probably a little bit of tongue-in-cheek about his comment, but I never heard of him going to a sports event like that. I can't imagine him doing so.

"Any marine drill sergeant would be able to take lessons from Dr. DeBakey. He would absolutely blister. It was vicious. In retrospect, you might joke about it, but at the time, you were horrified with terror. It was an intense experience. Anyone who says they liked Dr. DeBakey after working with him is ridiculous. It's like saying you like your drill sergeant; I can make that as an analogy. The marines say that if you like your drill sergeant, he hasn't done a good job. He doesn't *want* you to like him. He wants you to fear him more than the enemy. Machiavelli said, 'It's nice to be loved, but if you're trying to achieve, it's much better to be feared.' Dr. DeBakey was certainly feared. Nobody liked Dr. DeBakey personally because he wasn't a likeable person. He wasn't a person who would sit and have a few drinks with you."

An example of Dr. DeBakey's unforgivable criticism of his residents was given to me. On his teaching rounds, DeBakey would be followed by a group of residents, medical students, and nurses, often totaling up to 30 people. They would surround each bed while the resident summarized the patient's care and progress. When a resident had done something that DeBakey considered was incorrect — mismanagement, not in the best interests of the patient — he would interrupt the resident and ask, "Now why did you do that? That was a stupid thing to do, wasn't it?" Naturally, the resident tried to avoid responding to this question, but DeBakey would persist. "Why did you do that? Did you do that because you're stupid, or did you do that because you just don't care about this patient?" Usually no reply would be forthcoming; most residents were reluctant to admit they were stupid, particularly in front of a group of 30 medical students and nurses. "I want to know why you did such a stupid thing," DeBakey would repeat. "Did you do it because you're stupid, or because you don't care?" If the resident were to admit that he did not care, he knew he would be fired immediately from DeBakey's service. DeBakey would persevere until he received the reply he wanted — "I did it because I'm stupid, sir." Not satisfied even with this submission, DeBakey would continue his verbal torture. "Yes, you're stupid. Does your mother know you're stupid? What has she done to warrant a child like you?" And so it would go on until the resident had been thoroughly humiliated — all this, too, in front of the patient who had been entrusted to his care!

This type of vicious criticism was not confined to public places; DeBakey could be equally vicious in a private confrontation. Furthermore, this insensitivity to people's self-esteem was not confined solely to junior staff.

However, it seems that DeBakey did have a sense of humor, and occasionally allowed a resident to one-up him. There is an apocryphal story of DeBakey arriving at the hospital one Christmas Day only to find several members of his team absent. He commented on their laziness, to which a brave and perhaps reckless resident responded, "Sir, they are at home celebrating the birth of *another* great man." DeBakey reputedly laughed.

I asked Dr. DeBakey whether he ever worried about his image of being someone who is a very difficult person to work for.

"I don't worry about it. I know it exists, and I sometimes sense a certain amount of antipathy. Fortunately, it doesn't affect me and, in a sense, I've gotten adjusted to the fact that I am not always popular. Don't misunderstand me; I don't want to be unpopular. I don't want to be disliked. But, on the other hand, it doesn't bother me a great deal. In other words, I don't resent it if I am not considered popular. If, for one reason or another, people regard my perfectionism as burdensome to them or they are resentful, then I am sorry about that, but I'm not going to change. I have standards I want to maintain, and there are times when it gets a little difficult and frustrating; then it's more frustration anger than it is resentment anger. As you grow older, you begin to realize you have to be a little tolerant; everybody can't meet those standards."

## Awards and Honors

DeBakey received at least 50 honorary degrees and innumerable other prestigious awards, including the Albert Lasker Award for Clinical Research in 1963. Uniquely in medicine, he received both the National Medal of Science and the Presidential Medal of Freedom. In the last year of his life, he also received the Congressional Gold Medal, which has been awarded to only three other physicians. However, he told me, "It's what's *ahead* of you that interests you, that keeps you going, that is challenging for you, that gives you zest in life."

DeBakey's incredible energy and ability to work long hours continued into his 90s. He died in 2008, at age 99. Ironically, a couple of years before he died, he underwent a major operation for a dissecting aneurysm of the thoracic aorta, an operation he had personally established in the 1950s.

On the same day that I interviewed Dr. DeBakey, I also met (surreptitiously) with the surgeon who could be considered his *bête noire,* Denton Cooley. The contrast between the two men was remarkable.

## DENTON COOLEY —
## THE SAM WALTON OF HEART SURGERY

Denton Cooley (Figure 54) is one of the best known of the early cardiac surgeons, both within the medical profession and by the public. He epitomizes the public's perception of the successful surgeon — or, at least, the media's perception — being tall and good-looking, having a charming manner, and possessing a natural and exquisite gift for surgical dexterity. It is not surprising that he was dubbed "Dr. Wonderful."

He became immensely wealthy through his surgical work and subsequent investments in his hometown of Houston, only to overextend himself financially during the period of the oil boom in the early 1980s and see his business interests collapse when the boom dissolved. At one point, when he filed for bankruptcy, it was reported that his investment company owed $100 million.

Such a financial catastrophe might have permanently damaged a lesser man's self-esteem and confidence but, to his immense credit, Cooley picked himself up and continued working, and his reputation has been little tarnished internationally by this falter in what would otherwise appear to have been a charmed life. Indeed, it took him only a few months to restructure his financial situation; over the next few years, it is reported that he paid off all his creditors.

It is difficult to know where to include him in the list of pioneers. Although he assisted Blalock at the very first operation for blue babies, this was by chance, as he had just begun a surgical residency at Johns Hopkins as a young man. He was not directly involved in the other developments of closed heart surgery nor in the development of the initial heart-lung machines. However, once open heart surgery had been introduced and established by such luminaries as Lillehei and Kirklin, Cooley rapidly became the busiest surgeon in this field, performing more surgical procedures than any other heart surgeon in the world. At one time, according to John Norman, a former colleague of Cooley, fully one-tenth of the open heart surgery in the United States was being carried out by Cooley's group. He therefore was in a position to refine many of the techniques, and has a number of "firsts" to his name. He remained one of the world's leading heart surgeons for more than four decades. Among the many honors bestowed on him has been the Presidential Medal of Freedom, the United States' highest civilian award.

A large part of the reason Cooley could perform so many operations in a single day was his natural surgical dexterity. In this respect, he was among the most gifted of the surgeons profiled in this book. I personally watched him operate, and the procedures always seemed effortless for him. Bob Frater extolled Cooley's technical ability, along with that of a handful of others: "They were just beautiful natural surgeons. They never had to think about a move, always seemed to know where to put the needle, always seemed to know how to hold the needle holder in order to do what they wanted to do. Just smooth. Never seemed to hurry in their operations, and yet took less time. These are unusual people. Most of us have to think about it."

Cooley demonstrated that heart surgery could be "easy" and could be done on a large scale. Indeed, he is quoted as saying that he "always wanted to be known as the Sam Walton of heart surgery," in reference to the founder of Walmart. Cooley's example instilled many lesser surgeons with confidence.

## Equanimity and Charisma

Cooley's good looks, and relaxed and humorous personality — indeed, his charisma — did much to ensure his popularity among colleagues, patients, and public alike. I have met him on several occasions, and he has always been courteous, extremely pleasant, and with an enviable sense of humor.

John Norman, an early researcher into the artificial heart and a long-term colleague of Dr. Cooley, told me that he had *never* seen Cooley in anything but a good mood: "I worked with Cooley for ten years, across the operating table from him every other day. I was with him the day that we ran 44 open heart operations through the Texas Heart Institute. I watched him through a series of patients where we had mortalities in the range of 50%. I watched him when tornadoes came up main street and flooded the building. He *never* lost his composure. I've *never* heard Dr. Cooley curse."

A good example of Cooley's excellent sense of humor was given to me by Chris Barnard. Soon after the first heart transplant in Cape Town, when Barnard was at the height of his worldwide fame, he was visiting the United States. As part of his treatment as a VIP, the U.S. Air Force offered to fly him anywhere he would like within the nation. As he had never visited Cooley, Barnard asked to be flown to Houston. A large jet was placed at his disposal and he was accompanied by several military top brass. When the plane landed, a huge crowd had gathered to greet him, a military band was playing, and a red carpet was laid from the plane to the terminal, where Cooley and several colleagues formed an official greeting party.

As Barnard walked down the red carpet, flanked on either side by senior military officers each literally sparkling with braid and medals, with the band playing and the crowd cheering, he said he felt, momentarily at least, like a "very important person." The walk to the airport building seemed interminable, but eventually, among all this pomp, splendor, and acclaim, he arrived at where Cooley was standing. Barnard recollected, "As Dr. Cooley stepped forward to greet me with outstretched hand — and a twinkle in his eye — he said, disarmingly, 'Hi, boy, what's your name?' If there was any risk of the splendor of my arrival going to my head or giving me any undue sense of self-importance, it was immediately abolished. I burst into laughter, and have never forgotten the incident."

## "Modify, Simplify, and Apply"

Some would question—and indeed some of those interviewed in this book did question—whether Cooley has made any fundamental contributions to cardiac surgery, although most agreed that he, together with DeBakey, contributed immensely to the surgery of aortic aneurysms. For example, when I asked Richard Varco what contributions Drs. DeBakey and Cooley had made to heart surgery, he rather cynically answered, "They did a lot of operations." After discussing with Dr. Cooley and many others the contributions he felt he had made, my conclusion is that he was not one of the key basic innovators, but he was a very important developer; his ability to modify, simplify, and expand cardiac surgery made an immense impact, and contributed significantly to its rapid dissemination and proliferation.

During our conversation for this book, Dr. Cooley reminded me that the motto of the Cooley Surgical Society (founded by his former trainees) is "Modify, simplify, and apply." I mentally noted that this does not include any term that might suggest innovation, but aptly indicates his major contributions to the development of open heart surgery, namely modifying the techniques that others had introduced, particularly by simplifying them and then applying them to the treatment of a large number of patients.

According to Bud Frazier, "Dr. Cooley did for cardiac surgery what Dr. DeBakey did for aneurysms. He made it doable and reproducible by approaching it not as a hardship, but as something that was relatively easy." Cooley's technical dexterity in the operating room stimulated Dwight Harken to describe him as a surgeon who "operates with Woolworth volume and Tiffany quality."

Nevertheless, some would suggest that Cooley to some extent sacrificed quality for quantity. When operating on so many patients each and every day, it was impossible for him to pay the same meticulous attention to postoperative care as, for example, Barnard did. This would be left to others.

Sir Brian Barratt-Boyes, although readily recognizing that Cooley "would have to be included as one of the major contributors to heart surgery," was critical of the work being carried out under Cooley's direction in the early days, commenting, "He did this large bulk of surgery, but his results were not good, and never comparable to those of the Mayo Clinic. A lot of people don't realize that."

## Formative Years

Denton Cooley was born in Houston, Texas, in 1920. He grew up in Houston, attending the public school, and then the University of Texas in Austin, where he majored in biology and zoology, and was an outstanding basketball player, good enough to be on the varsity team. He then attended medical school in Galveston, part of the University of Texas system, but transferred to the Johns Hopkins Medical School, where he graduated in medicine in 1944. He graduated with highest honors from both undergraduate school and medical school. Although the results were not officially announced, it is believed he was top of his class at Hopkins — no mean achievement. He then received an internship in surgery at the Johns Hopkins Hospital under Alfred Blalock.

Dr. Cooley told me, "It was a fortunate circumstance for me to be involved with the first operation for tetralogy of Fallot in November 1944. I can recall that operation very well. Dr. Blalock was the surgeon, and Dr. William Longmire was his first assistant. Dr. Helen Taussig was at Blalock's elbow, along with the black man, Mr. Vivien Thomas, who had gained fame by doing so much of the preclinical work in the Hunterian Laboratory with Dr. Blalock. So from that day forward, I guess, I've been a cardiac surgeon. I consider that operation possibly the dawn of modern cardiac surgery as we know it today, and so I have been privileged to be both witness and participant in the entire history of cardiac surgery."

After his internship, Cooley spent two years in military service between 1946 and 1948 in Linz, Austria (the birthplace of Adolf Hitler). "I was a very poorly equipped surgeon to take over the job as chief of surgery in a 750-bed hospital, which was rapidly reduced to a 250-bed unit, but I enjoyed my two years in Austria. [After completing his residency at the Hopkins] I then decided to take a year with Russell Brock, who was the most notable chest surgeon in the United Kingdom at the time. I spent a year as senior registrar at the Royal Brompton Hospital in London."

Ben Milstein, who was later to become a leading cardiothoracic surgeon in the United Kingdom, worked closely with Cooley during his year at the Royal Brompton Hospital in London. His recollection of Cooley is that he "was great fun to work with. He is *still* great fun to be with. He seemed to have no limitations. He could cope with anything. He came really knowing nothing about thoracic [chest] surgery, but he took to it like a duck to water. He had this fantastic operative technique from the word 'go.' His hands worked like an efficient machine. He was very good from a clinical perspective too [i.e., in diagnosis and the other non-operative aspects of medicine]. I found that rather surprising because, as far as I was aware, he hadn't had the sort of training that would have given him that. He was an exceptional person, and very, very hardworking."

## Return to Houston

Dr. Cooley continued: "In 1951, I joined Michael DeBakey at Baylor University College of Medicine, which was the educational medical school at the growing Texas Medical Center. I was on the full-time faculty at Baylor for eighteen years. My first opportunity to make some sort of a notable achievement was in operating on aneurysms of the thoracic aorta. At the time, the direct treatment of aortic aneurysms had not been introduced. In fact, I think I was the one who stimulated interest in this. My first really important paper on vascular disease was on the definitive treatment of aortic aneurysms. Dr. DeBakey and

I were collaborators on it. He was the chief and I was a young man on the service."

For some time, Cooley and DeBakey operated together on aortic aneurysms, setting a new standard in operative speed and efficiency. John Norman quotes a visitor to Houston at that time who reported back to his institution that "there's a young fellow down there operating with Dr. DeBakey, and they operate like the building is burning down around them." There is a story that, when DeBakey and Cooley were in Stockholm demonstrating an operation for replacement of a large abdominal aortic aneurysm, as they were about to cut the skin, Clarence Crafoord mentioned that he was going to his office for just a few minutes to open his mail. By the time he returned half an hour later, they were closing the abdomen, having completed the operation, much to Crafoord's shock. Viking Bjork, who watched this operation, reported to me that "the two had such synchronicity in their work, it was wonderful to see." Another early heart surgeon who observed them operating together described it "like watching an octopus operate. There were hands everywhere."

Cooley, however, was keen to get into the field of open heart surgery that was just developing. On a visit to Minneapolis to study their heart-lung machine, for the first time he was shown the inside of a beating human heart by Lillehei; he later reminisced that "it was like looking through the gates of heaven."

Cooley continued relating his personal story to me: "Our first meaningful open heart procedure in Houston was in April of 1956. By then, we had our DeWall/Lillehei heart-lung machine pretty much tested in our laboratory. I must say that the results in our animal experiments, particularly with canine, were very disappointing. We never got a real good survival, but I thought the procedure would work in the proper environment of the operating room." By the end of the year, Cooley had operated on 49 patients using the heart-lung machine.

"Once we had this device [the heart-lung machine] available, I didn't take a summer vacation. I stayed right with it, and pushed it as hard as I could. At first, I didn't have a lot of support, I don't think, but I didn't have resistance either. I took the opportunity and got some people to work with me who were willing to push ahead.

"Dr. DeBakey had most of his interest, I always thought, in vascular surgery, rather than cardiac. While I saw him following through with the aneurysm surgery, I rather decided that, since I had all this training and so forth, I would try to keep the cardiac thing to me and my group. It may have been selfish on my part but, nevertheless, I was ambitious. I don't think Dr. DeBakey was really in the professional group who gained great reputation as a cardiac surgeon. Certainly there is no question he has gained a large reputation in vascular surgery.

"We were certainly handicapped by this issue of priming the extracorporeal circuit [i.e., the heart-lung machine] with blood. I saw that as a real handicap. We were so dependent on the blood bank. But then I was challenged and interested in some work that was being done by others [presumably referring to Nazih Zuhdi, although he mentioned no names], and we began studying the use of blood substitutes to prime the system [i.e., to fill the heart-lung machine with dextrose, a sugar solution, rather than blood, before the beginning of the operation]. Our animals did far better if we didn't prime with blood. I began using this hemodilution [i.e., blood dilution] technique in patients with some trepidation. That made it possible to perform even larger numbers of operations. We went on to show that open heart surgery could be done on a much larger scale than previously considered possible."

Without the need to use blood for every operation, Cooley and his colleagues were able to steadily increase the number of heart operations they could perform, and were soon doing more than 1,000 each year. In an interview in the *American Journal of Cardiology*, Cooley stated, "Even though Zuhdi and some others had shown that non-blood prime was possible, they had not really pushed to make it an accepted method. I think we convinced the world that non-blood prime was a practical solution to the demand that open heart surgery was putting on blood-banking facilities." As a by-product of this experience, Cooley almost "cornered the market" in performing open heart surgery on Jehovah's Witnesses, who refuse blood transfusions of any sort. He and his group have operated on 1,200 people of this faith.

Like DeBakey, Cooley had to be highly organized and hard-working to perform operations in the numbers he did — an estimated 45,000 heart operations in his lifetime — and to write the large number of surgical papers that he did — almost 1,200.

He told me, "I don't want to overlook my contribution in aortic aneurysm surgery — indeed, I first recommended an aggressive treatment of aortic disease — but in the field of pure cardiac surgery, my demonstration that we could do open heart surgery without a lot of blood by the use of blood substitutes has been one of my strong points. I had the opportunity to carry out some new techniques for the first time. There is a lot of personal satisfaction in doing things for the first time. The public likes to recognize that. The first man to walk on the moon was probably remembered longer than the second. That's just human nature."

## The Controversial First Use of the Total Artificial Heart

"In 1968, it was evident to me that it was time to try the total artificial heart. We were having a number of frustrations in watching people die who could have been saved with a heart transplant. One of my colleagues was a fellow by the name of Dr. Domingo Liotta, who had spent a lot of time trying to develop an artificial heart. He came to me rather frustrated, saying Dr. DeBakey was apparently not interested in going forward with its clinical application [i.e., its use in a patient]. Dr. Liotta and I decided we would try to develop it in animals and see if we could implant it as a temporary measure in preparing a patient for cardiac transplantation. I knew that if I went to Dr. DeBakey to get permission from our department of surgery, we would get only delay and further negative response. So I decided that the time had come to take a bold step. The opportunity arose to go ahead and do it, and suffer any repercussions that might follow. We did just that.

"We had the ideal candidate who was dying and needed a cardiac transplant, a gentleman named Haskell Karp. We were just interested in seeing if you could sustain a human life with an artificial device. Sure enough, that proved to be the case. The patient did very well with the total artificial heart, but unfortunately he died following his transplant because of an infection. I have no regrets at all for having taken that step. The only regret I have is that the repercussions were such that they delayed further clinical application of the total artificial heart. I think that came about mostly because of Dr. DeBakey's obvious reaction to our operation."

Although Dr. Cooley mentioned that the patient did well after insertion of the artificial heart, this is somewhat debatable. The device certainly maintained his life, but (as mentioned above) there were significant early complications. The widow of the patient eventually sued her husband's medical advisors, and the case came to court.

For an independent opinion on this saga, William DeVries's view may be illuminating: "I studied that to some degree from the court records and talked with some of the people at the time. Basically, Liotta believed that DeBakey had cooled off on the idea [of using the device in a patient]. I've talked with Liotta, who said that Cooley was always sniffing around the lab. Cooley was a visionary-type person and saw where it was going. He wanted to get into the clinical arena as fast as he could. Cooley believed that if you put it into people and it fails, what's going to happen? Great interest is going to come, more funding, more people who want to try it again. He saw what DeBakey didn't see — that people want to live. Given the choice of life and death, people will take life, even if it's an uncomfortable one.

"I'm sure that Cooley waited until DeBakey was out of town, and then did it. I understand exactly why DeBakey was angry. Cooley is the type of person who sees something he wants to do, and does it. I'm sure he knew he was going to have trouble with DeBakey on this.

I'm sure he was upset that it didn't work out the way he thought it would. When it got to court, the widow said it [the insertion of the artificial heart] wasn't ready to be done. It was clear that DeBakey [who was asked to provide opinion] bailed out Cooley in the end. I think the reason he threw himself on that sword was that he saw a lot of [research] work going down the toilet. DeBakey supported it because he realized that, if he didn't support it, it would quell artificial hearts forever. DeBakey did the gentleman thing. When they looked at each other, DeBakey blinked first. I don't think Cooley would have done what he did if he didn't have some antagonism towards DeBakey. This was the nail that sealed the coffin."

There is one other factor that some feel may have been an influence on Cooley's actions at that time. Dr. Cooley was reputedly making approximately $20 million per year doing heart surgery, but he had to give about 50% of it to the institution (Baylor). If he got himself fired or had to resign, he could then transfer to St. Luke's Hospital, where he would be able to keep all of his income. I find this explanation for Cooley's actions difficult to believe, but there may be an element of truth in it, as he is reputed to be rather money-minded.

DeBakey and Cooley—two names inextricably bound together whether they like it or not, two outstanding men who directed the eyes of the medical world, and to some extent the public, on an oil town in Texas—so entwined, and yet so very different. Bud Frazier provided insight into their differences:

"I have a great respect and love for Dr. Cooley as a man and as a physician and surgeon. I have a great respect for Dr. DeBakey. It's a little different feeling, but I don't think it's fair to deny either of them their due. Dr. Cooley and Dr. DeBakey are so different in their approaches and personality. Of course, Dr. Cooley is a very disciplined, driven man. He's always maintained an ability to deal with people in a human way. And yet it's a paradox. I'll never forget when I was a medical student on Dr. Cooley's service, he was operating on three children. Before 10 A.M., all three of these children were dead. He went out and talked to the families, and came back. He came in at six P.M. to make rounds, and said, 'Well, today was a bad day, but maybe tomorrow will be better. Let's go see the patients.' He always had this positivity about him. He felt he was doing the best he could, and that's all he could do. A lot of nurses thought Dr. Cooley was very cold because he could keep on going, seemingly unconcerned about these children who were dying all around him. I don't think it's true. It was one of the qualities that allowed him to accomplish so much as a technical surgeon.

"When Dr. DeBakey would have someone die on the operating table, he would go into his room and close the door and sit in there. We would just wait until he came out. Sometimes he would be so upset that he would cancel the remaining cases for the day. He was always kind to the patient and to the family, particularly if he lost someone. He talked to the family and wrote to them personally. I was always impressed by that. Dr. DeBakey was visibly shaken when he lost a patient. You could tell it affected him. When Dr. Cooley lost a patient, he kept working. I don't know what to imply about that. I think I read in one of my military history books that you never want a general who cries. I guess that's true.

"Dr. DeBakey and Dr. Cooley were so different in their style. Dr. Cooley did a lot of things with ease that Dr. DeBakey did with great intensity. Dr. Cooley was so smooth and always seemed to do everything right. Technically, he was a master, and didn't struggle with anything. Sometimes Dr. DeBakey would have to struggle. He was in his fifties when he started doing vascular surgery with any degree at all, whereas Dr. Cooley grew up with it. The act of surgery was hard for Dr. DeBakey, and doing the surgery was very stressful to him. The only way he could overcome this was by the amazing drive and stamina that he had. In contrast, Dr. Cooley had a gift — technically very gifted. He would do 12 or 14 complex, tough cases in a day, finishing at four or five P.M. and making rounds at six P.M. Dr. Cooley, in a sense, was doing something that he loved to do. He whistled, joked, and laughed through the most difficult cases. You cannot compare

Dr. Cooley and Dr. DeBakey as far as surgical gift. Much of the difference in style stemmed from that.

"Dr. Cooley worked very hard, but he didn't have all the lateral motion that Dr. DeBakey did. He never really tried to undertake all the massive jobs that Dr. DeBakey undertook outside of surgery — the research protocols, dealing with the NIH and with the federal government. If you had to credit any single person for our whole heritage at NIH, it would be Dr. DeBakey, and his personal relationship with President Johnson. That's when the NIH became powerful. I don't think Dr. Cooley could have taken Baylor — a 'nothing' medical school in 1948 — and made it one of the best medical schools in the country by 1968. Their accomplishments, although they were both based on surgery, were in a sense in different arenas."

My own personal impression supports Bud Frazier's comments. Having talked with both men on the same morning, I came away with the feeling that, although Dr. Cooley had made an immense contribution to the development of both vascular and cardiac surgery, the scope of work undertaken by Dr. DeBakey in his lifetime was just so extraordinary that it may never be matched.

John Norman summed up the relationship of the two men: "They have competed with one another forever, and everybody has benefited from it.... Their competition has been for the greater good of the entire Houston as well as for the cardiovascular surgical community."

In Norman Shumway's opinion, "DeBakey had this prodigious capacity for just incredible work, and Cooley is really no different. That's why they had so much trouble with each other — they're the same."

And so, based on Kolff's original work, DeBakey and Cooley laid the groundwork for the use of both the LVAD and the total artificial heart in patients as a means of temporary support for a failing heart until either the patient's native heart recovered or heart transplantation could be performed. It remained for Kolff's young surgical colleague, William DeVries, to attempt to use the artificial heart to replace a failing heart on a permanent basis.

# WILLIAM DEVRIES—
# SURGEON IN THE SPOTLIGHT

William DeVries (Figure 55) was the surgeon who carried out the first real clinical trial using an artificial heart—the "heart" made by Kolff and Jarvik. Having worked with Willem Kolff in the laboratory for some years when he was a medical student, he returned to the University of Utah after his surgical residency and, with Kolff and his associates, decided it was time to go ahead with the implantation of one of their mechanical hearts in a patient. He went on to carry out four such implants, which did much to initiate the drive to use artificial hearts and ventricular assist devices to maintain life in patients with terminal heart disease. Having devoted himself to this program for several years, he dropped out of academic and innovative heart surgery, but remained a busy cardiac surgeon in private practice for the next 20 years.

William DeVries is very tall—six feet five inches. I presume that, as he was a former champion high jumper, originally he was slim, but by the time I met with him, when he was age 60, he had filled out a bit and I would guess weighed more than 230 pounds. He proved an introspective and loquacious person, with whom I found it easy to talk.

## Early Days in Utah

His father, a Dutch immigrant who became a naval surgeon, was killed in World War II when William, who was born in 1943, was only six months old. The boy was raised by his Mormon mother and grandmother in Ogden, Utah, until the age of five, when his mother remarried, after which the family was steadily enlarged by no fewer than eight half-brothers and -sisters. The family was poor, and William worked throughout high school to help out. He attended public high school in Ogden, where he was an outstanding athlete, being a member of the basketball and track teams. He won the Utah state finals in high jumping, and went to the University of Utah on a track scholarship, high jumping and running hurdles. He married during his last year in college, and by the time he finished medical school (also at the University of Utah), he had four children. He held down three or four jobs at any one time throughout medical school, yet graduated top of his class and received the award for the most outstanding graduate.

"All through medical school I got more and more involved in the artificial heart," he explained. "I started helping them in surgery. None of the surgeons at the medical school wanted to be involved with Kolff. We had to use [research] fellows from Holland. These guys would do the surgery, and I'd assist them. One of the other jobs I'd get paid for was to watch the animals overnight. I could study late at night there. I did that for four years. That was my first introduction into the actual animal and surgical world. By that time, I decided I really wanted to be a surgeon.

"After three years as a medical student, I went to Keith Reemtsma [who had moved from Tulane to become chairman of the department of surgery] and said, 'I want to be a heart surgeon.' Reemtsma said, 'You know, Bill, I'd love to have you here. It would be the best thing in the world. You're a smart guy. But really, in all fairness to you, you need to get out of here. You need to go to either the Mass General or Hopkins or Duke, or maybe Alabama. If you want to come back here, I'll make every way we can to get you.' Reemtsma always shot straight with me. He was a good guy, charismatic, and fun to talk to."

This advice sat well with DeVries, who had a great desire to get out of Salt Lake City because "I really wanted to feel my wings. I wanted to know if I was any good or not. So I thought the residency was a great opportunity for me to go east." With a slight smile, he then added, "After all, that was where the center of all knowledge and learning was. As you got progressively more towards the East Coast, you got more and more refined. I really wanted to go up against the best and see if I was going to make it."

The first visit the young DeVries made to the East Coast was somewhat unsettling. He went for a series of interviews at the Massachusetts General Hospital in Boston. "As I was going to the hospital that morning," he recounted, "a guy stabbed someone right in front of me, and ran down the street. All these people were crying. We got the victim to the emergency room, which was about two blocks away. The cops came. I had blood all over my hands and over my jacket. I went in and washed my hands. I started going to these competitive interviews. It was amazing. I went all the way to the top.

"The last interview was in an office overlooking the skyline. They would bring you first into one room, then another, and then another. I didn't understand exactly what was happening, but I remember going into this last room, and all of these guys were the most impressive-looking people in the world. I noticed this podium at the end of this huge table, with all these professors sitting there. Then I went to the other end of the table, and there was a metal folding chair from which part of the legs had been sawn off [he indicated several inches]. I sat in the chair, and the table was like this on me (indicating that the table was at the height of his neck.) I realized that this was some type of game. When I left there, I said to myself, 'I'm not sure I want to be involved in someplace where my family could get killed, and also where I have to deal with this power-play stuff.'

"The next place I went to was Johns Hopkins, which was in the middle of the slums [of Baltimore]. I stayed with a married couple who lived across the street. The man had to have an armed guard to go back and forth to the hospital. I decided that wasn't for me."

DeVries finally chose Duke University in North Carolina, which he described as "a nice, quiet, smokey Southern place .... I felt this was the best place; it was safe. I was kind of watching out for my family."

At the end of his nine-year surgical residency, DeVries found he was expected to return to Salt Lake City, which he did.

## Planning the First Artificial Heart Implant

"I had left Utah when Cooley did his first artificial heart implant [in a patient] in Houston in 1969. At that time, we were working with the artificial heart, and thought we had a pretty damn good one. Our animals [calves] were living like 50 hours. Cooley just went ahead and did it.

"When I went back to the University of Utah in 1979, calves with implanted artificial hearts were living for six, seven, eight months. I said, 'It doesn't take a bright person to see where this work is going.' Jarvik was young and I was young, and we said this could be done. I went around the surgical community trying to get some senior heart surgeon interested. They weren't interested at all. They thought this was just a pipe dream. At that time, I was probably 35 years old and just out of my residency. I said, 'Let me go ahead and do this.' All of a sudden, I realized we were going to do it, and I started going through the Food and Drug Administration (FDA). I started long-term animal experiments. I had the time to do it. It was amazing how it all had to fit together in those early days.

"I learned really, really fast that Kolff was a special type of person and had some real strengths. There were some weaknesses — they were small, but he had some weaknesses. Jarvik was a great inventor. He had ideas. We would design a heart, put it in, and he would change the design three or four times by the time the animal was seven months old. The heart would be entirely different. I was no good at suggesting new ideas for the artificial heart.

"Finally, after two years of animal experimentation, we tried getting the NIH and the FDA to give approval. At that time, it was a matter of interest at the university, but nobody paid much attention to what was going on. They all thought that Kolff was going to make a lot of noise, but nothing would come of it. But then, as it got approval and started getting news coverage, the dean started getting interested."

The NIH also became interested. Their representative pointed out that the NIH had not approved the implementation of a clinical trial. DeVries told them, "I don't need your permission. We have a device not made with NIH funds and I'm not getting paid by you at all. You have no influence on me. I'm a surgeon here at the heart center, and I have no NIH grants."

"Of course," he explained to me, "Kolff, Don Olsen, and Jarvik were all funded by the NIH. The NIH guy left very upset, and threatened to cut off all NIH funding to the university if I did this. Timing is important in these things. If he would have come about two months earlier, I would have probably listened to him but, at this point, I was in it. I looked at it as a religious cause. This was the way it was going to be. I was going to do it. I was not impressed with the NIH at all during this first period."

DeVries explained that Kolff's group would initially do NIH-funded research to develop the device but, toward the end of the research, when Kolff was considering a clinical trial, "he would start a corporation or company. The company would employ the same people who designed these things [with NIH grants], but on 'off' hours. They would implant the device [in some patients], and develop it for a couple of years, and then somebody [a larger company] would buy it. That's how Kolff would do it. This was a recurring theme.

"If you were to ask me what my part in this whole thing was, I was the one who really pushed it. The reason I pushed it was that I believed in it. I believed in it in every fiber of my being. I was going to do it regardless of where it took me or what it did to me because this was the right thing to do. People were dying, and there was a way of doing it [helping them]. It might not have been perfect the first time, but the only way you would get there was by doing it. The more I got involved in it, the more of an 'evangelist' I became. So I started looking for patients with end-stage heart disease who were over fifty years of age [which was the approximate upper age limit for heart transplantation at that time, although it is much higher today]."

## The First Patient — Barney Clark

A dental surgeon named Barney Clark agreed to be the first patient. His wife later told DeVries that Barney had said, "I've been kept alive by medications that other people have died to give me. Now it's my turn to pay them back." DeVries found managing a device in a sick patient more difficult than in a healthy animal. A few days after the operation, which was carried out in 1982, "I turned the pump up to about 140 beats per minute. His [blood] pressure went up briefly to about 150, and he had a little bit of a seizure. So I took him back down, and he got better. I think I was probably overperfusing him. He wasn't used to that."

One of the researchers called DeVries. He said, 'Turn him off.' I said, 'Excuse me, *turn him off?*' He said, 'Yeah, we can't have a complication like this at this particular time. The NIH is going to give us increased funding, and we cannot have a complication. Turn him off.' I was in shock. I remember sitting back and just saying, 'Jeez, I must be on Saturn or something.' He maintained that that was really important. 'You've had it successful so far. The guy's been alive for a couple of days, he's talked, and everything like that. Just bail out.' I said, 'This is a patient. This isn't an experiment. This is a *patient.*'

"I realized then that the feelings of some of these researchers were quite different. I realized at that point that I was the only one standing up for that particular patient. I was the physician and, by God, that's where I should be. That's where I was, and where I was going to be. That's the difference between basic scientists, innovators, and the guy taking care of the patient. That's the way it ought to be. I do a procedure on a patient, and I'm responsible. The patient is unconscious, and I'm the only one who can watch out for his needs. That is the typical surgical mentality, and that's why I was able to do it."

Barney Clark and the surgical team caring for him were thrust into the spotlight. The media were everywhere. DeVries, still early out of his surgical residency, described it as being "like Christiaan Barnard. It was crazy. It was absolutely crazy. That was an interesting time.

"Then we started getting into the issue of money. How were we going to pay for this? [Figure 56] Medical insurance can't pay for it. They said, 'Barney, you're going to have to pay for it,' which was crazy. The guy had to pay for an experiment on himself?"

Barney Clark sold the rights to his story to a newspaper for

$1 million, which meant that the newspaper had access to all of his medical charts. DeVries described the situation he found himself in as "real bizarre."

Mr. Clark lived for 112 days, but his life was plagued by complications. He was never well enough to leave the hospital, and, naturally, at times he became depressed and frustrated. On one occasion he asked for the artificial heart to be switched off, though he soon changed his mind. According to DeVries, "He realized he was in this thing and there was no way out, except to die. I continued in my mind thinking that this is an experiment, but the center part of this whole thing is this patient. I wanted him to live.

"We had the entire world breathing down our necks. These guys were coming out of the woodwork and criticizing. I was a little too sensitive about it those first few days, and I had to learn how to be thick-skinned. I realized that the best thing for me to do was not to read the newspapers, because I got hurt by what I read. It really hurt me what people were saying.

"About the same time, I started getting all kinds of legal things. The Attorney General's office started asking questions. 'How do you turn the patient's artificial heart off?' 'Who has the right to be assisted in suicide?' Am I a murderer? Things like that came up. The state of Utah was a very conservative state, and I realized the implications of this. Those were really hard issues. Am I prolonging death or prolonging misery, or am I accomplishing something? Those were the issues I dealt with daily.

"After Barney Clark died, the institution became very tempered, very lukewarm about the whole thing. I was ready to do another one. 'We've got to keep this ball going. We've got it started, let's keep it going.' Barney Clark had given his life for this. Everything we had was tied up in this work. It was a very successful first experiment in the history of medicine. It needed to go on, but I had a very hard time getting anybody interested in it. You realize that you're the only one in the world who's going to push this thing. I became absolutely evangelical about doing it again. Once I could get the second, third, and fourth done, I could step back because by then the ball would have started rolling.

"I was told that I had to raise at least a half million bucks. I ended up trying to raise funds with no help at all, and I wasn't good at it; I hated it. At that time, really strange things happened. There were Middle Eastern guys who wanted to put money into it, but I had to promise I would be around to put the heart into any of them if they ever died—really weird stuff."

It was then that DeVries received an offer from Wendell Cherry of the Humana Inc. (a major health care company) to relocate to Louisville, Kentucky; Cherry offered to pay for the next 100 implants!

## Move to Louisville, Kentucky

"So I left the University of Utah, and went to Louisville. I did it for one reason, and that was that I *had* to do it. The Humana people were very honest about it, and said, 'We're doing this because we want the notoriety and the reputation of being on the cutting edge of research, and we're going to pay for it.' The first day after we did Bill Schroeder [the second patient], Wendell Cherry said, 'Our name is now on every single newspaper in the world. This is the type of advertisement that you cannot buy. As far as I'm concerned, you've made your money for the next hundred patients.' I realized what this was all about, but it was okay because it was for advancement.

"When people saw Schroeder standing up and saying to the president of the United States, 'I want my social security,' people realized that these guys are pretty normal. They don't all have strokes. It was acceptable. That's when the 'bridge-to-transplant' people took it all in, and said, 'Bridge-to-transplant' [implying that although the artificial heart might not yet be ideal as a permanent replacement for a failing heart, it could be used for temporary support until heart transplantation could be carried out]. That acted as a catalyst to left ventricular assist devices [LVADs]. That really changed things.

That's something I'm really proud of. You provide the stimulus for it and, all of a sudden, boom — it takes off. That experience was the crystallizing agent for mechanical heart support. That's what the real value of it was."

Over a period of about two years, DeVries implanted two more artificial hearts, and consistently had one or two patients with an artificial heart in his facility. Mr. Schroeder lived almost two years with the artificial heart. The next patient, Murray Haden, lived about a year and a half, but the fourth patient, Jack Burton, lived only ten days. Then Mr. Schroeder had a "stroke" (a brain injury due to a clot of blood from the artificial heart), and, according to DeVries, "the pendulum for good, positive things was starting to turn back, and Humana started getting a little bit edgy about it; they didn't particularly like it."

## Jarvik versus Kolff

According to DeVries, "At that time, Jarvik and Kolff were going into battle. I had to stay far away from that. Fortunately, I was in a different town, which was very good. Dr. Kolff told me he and Jarvik had a very funny relationship together — father and son — with the son rebelling against the father. They went to 'marriage counseling' sessions on a Friday. The counselor would say, 'Now, Rob, I know you're upset with Dr. Kolff, but you've got to start talking. You've got to learn how to communicate back and forth.' That's the only way they got along.

"Jarvik, by the way, liked to be in the jet set. He married 'the world's smartest person,' Marilyn vos Savant [of *Parade* magazine fame]. He saw her in the newspaper, went after her, and met her in Hawaii. I was at their wedding in the Palm Court in New York. Isaac Asimov [known best as a science-fiction writer] was his best man. I said to him, 'How do you know Rob?' He said, 'I've never met him before. Marilyn asked me if I would do it. People like us help each other. One supports the other.' That's how they did it.

"Jarvik and Kolff's difficulties really intensified in the period after Barney Clark's operation. Dr. Kolff's idea for the company [set up to make the artificial heart] was to sell it, and let somebody else do the development. Rob's idea was different. He wanted to keep and build the company, and get other companies to put money into it. They clashed about that. There were rumors that Jarvik would have a meeting of the company's board, and lock Kolff out when he would go to the bathroom. They were going in entirely different directions. I was kind of caught in the middle. The business dealings just broke them apart.

"The first thing that Jarvik did when Kolff Medical was dissolved was to engineer Kolff's exit. The first thing he did after Kolff left was to change the name from Kolff Medical to Jarvik Inc. Suddenly, the Utah heart became the Jarvik heart. Kolff continued to maintain, and I think Kolff was right, that the Jarvik heart was a natural progression of many, many models. Anyway, Kolff was finally moved out, and Jarvik moved to the top. But his support from Wall Street was backing off. That became a real issue. I realized the company wasn't quite as strong, and then I realized they weren't reporting their data. In 1988, the NIH said, 'We are not going to do this anymore.' They withdrew their support. That was the death knell. I realized at that time that the company was more interested in selling the device than in reporting to the FDA. They got dumped big-time.

"The worst day in my life was the day that the FDA told me I had to disable all ten of the mechanical hearts in the Humana inventory. In front of the administrator of the hospital, I took a scalpel and perforated the diaphragms [of the devices]. I was able to save one because we had a patient in the hospital being 'bridged' to transplant."

## Impact of the Media on Lifestyle

The artificial heart saga had changed DeVries's life. His marriage collapsed, which affected his six children.

"I ended up flying all over the world—exactly the same scenario as Christiaan Barnard did. I had been sheltered and, all of a sudden, here I am with President Reagan and King Hussain. You're on television. You realize that this is more than you did back in Utah. Your life is fast; it was just going, going, going. You get into that type of fast behavior. You live in pretty heady air too. You go home, for example, and you've got Bryant Gumbel or Katie Couric wanting to come and talk with you. They want a piece of you. They want you to fly to Washington. You're doing this and this and this, and going back and forth. First of all, it takes time, and you have to be mentally sharp. I knew that all I needed to do was to crash out on something like this, and it would stop. So personally, you have to be attuned and ready to go. You can't come in unsharp. I realized that people would use me.

"The other thing is choices. I grew up in a very religious family. I never smoked a cigarette. I never drank alcohol. You have your first glass of champagne in a crystal glass, with all these exciting people. A normal person who's never been in that situation doesn't understand. All of a sudden you're meeting people who are exciting, whether they are men or women, and they're drawn to you and you're drawn to them. You have choices you never had before. Christiaan Barnard mentioned that to me. It eats you. It can totally consume you. In that type of environment, you can't survive.

"When I was on the cover of *Time* magazine, I went out and bought a copy of the magazine for each of my kids. About six months later, I was in my daughter's room and she had ripped out the page and put on crayon marks; I had horns out of my head and a beard. She had made disparaging remarks on it. She would have been about thirteen or fourteen at the time. When I saw that, I realized, 'Hey, this is not without a price.'" (When Dr. DeVries raised the topic with her, she was so upset he had invaded her privacy by entering her room that they never got to talk about the real issue.)

"The other thing that was difficult was that, in the particular world and environment I was in, it was not appropriate to be a media doctor. You can lose the thing that is most important to you, and that is the respect of your colleagues. The media will say, 'You're famous,' but a lot of times it takes more out of you than it gives you back. These people will come out and suck the life out of you, and then they're gone back to New York, and you're back with the people here [in Utah or Kentucky]. I felt that my colleagues, the guys who were sending me my patients, were not happy with the fact that I was on television all the time. They made fun of people like that. That was before professional advertising came in. You can offend a lot of doctors, and they will cut you off.

"At times, when I'd get on the news, read the newspaper, or watch a TV program, with all the controversy, the best thing I could do was to walk into a patient's room and talk with him. Just say, 'Hey, what's up?' You develop a special relationship."

When the artificial heart and the left ventricular assist device were established in supporting (or "bridging") a patient until a donor heart could be transplanted, DeVries felt his contribution had been made. He was mentally exhausted and drained by the immense effort it had taken. "It had been a tremendously intense time. I realized that I'd accomplished what I thought I should do.... I thought, 'Do I keep fighting this battle?' It had changed every aspect of my life in one way or another. I had had enough of this stuff, and wanted to take care of patients, not worry about the funding, not worry about the ethical considerations of the artificial heart and the termination of the device, and just do what I wanted to do — heart surgery."

He settled into private practice, married again, and for the next 20 years was busy as a cardiothoracic surgeon. Since he retired from surgical practice, he has been active in mentoring trainee surgeons in the U.S. Army.

WILLEM KOLFF RECEIVED many awards for his pioneering work, particularly for the development of the dialysis machine, which has saved hundreds of thousands, if not millions, of lives. These included the prestigious Japan Prize, the Lasker Award, and the $500,000 Albany Medical Prize, but the Nobel Prize, which many in medicine feel he should have been awarded, eluded him. He died in 2009, just three days before his 98th birthday.

## CHAPTER 14

# The Right Stuff:
# Those Magnificent Men with
# Their Heart-Lung Machines

A ND SO OUR STORY has unfolded from the first small step of tying off a ductus to the surreal attempts to replace the heart entirely with a mechanical device. In addition to those highlighted in this book who played major roles in the development of heart surgery, there are many other surgeons and scientists, of course, who contributed significantly, but to mention them all would have made the book unreadable. To them I offer my apologies.

The men who contributed to these developments — and, with the exception of Helen Taussig, they were all men, to some extent reflecting the discrimination against women entering medical school in those days — were outstanding individuals. As Tom Starzl said, "They were all very ambitious, courageous, and skillful. They were incredibly smart people. They had the right stuff." They were the medical equivalent of the first astronauts, all exceptionally bright people and yet so very different from each other in so many ways.

To date, open heart surgery has had far more relevance to the average citizen's everyday life than has the landing of men on the moon. The importance of the development of heart surgery, particularly of open heart surgery, was emphasized by Nobel Laureate U.S.

physician-researcher Joseph Goldstein. Writing in the leading scientific journal *Nature Medicine* of the 50-year anniversaries of important medical breakthroughs celebrated in the year 2003, which included the discovery of the chemical structure of DNA (the double helix), Goldstein wrote, "During this year's celebratory events.... there has been no mention, surprisingly, of one other scientific breakthrough that also turned 50 this year, a breakthrough with ramifications that have had as profound an influence on medicine as the double helix. On May 6, 1953, John H. Gibbon, Jr., used his newly created heart-lung machine to perform the first successful open-heart operation on a human being.... His invention has saved the lives of tens of millions of people over the last 50 years.... Last year alone, more than 700,000 open-heart operations were carried out in the United States, including 610,000 coronary bypass procedures, 90,000 valve replacements and 2,500 heart transplants."

## The Stimulus of Cardiac Surgery

It was very largely the surgeons, not the physicians or basic scientists, who led the advances we have reviewed in this book. Michael DeBakey told me, "If you look at developments in the cardiovascular area, it was the surgeons who moved the whole development forward, including the medical development. It was the surgeons who were pressing for the development of angiography and other diagnostic procedures. When you go back and look at that period up to 1949 and the early 1950s, what was going on in medicine? *Nothing* was going on. It was the surgeons who stimulated the cardiologists to do something; they were doing *nothing*."

Bob Frater confirmed this opinion. The introduction of heart surgery "changed cardiology dramatically. Everything that has happened in cardiology started with cardiac surgery. The notion of intensive care, the notion of monitoring, the notion of measuring cardiac output as a way of monitoring patients who were acutely ill. All of these things were applied first by cardiac surgeons."

Indeed, the fact that internists and cardiologists had little to offer their patients in the form of treatment was a major factor driving several of the young medical graduates in this book to choose surgery as a career, since surgery offered them the opportunity of doing more than just diagnosing the patient's condition. They did not want to be therapeutically "impotent"; they were the "movers and shakers" of their classes.

## The Light Moves Westward

The development of heart surgery represents perhaps one of the earliest shifts of medical and surgical advance from the Old World to the New World. Until the beginning of the 20th century, the Old World had largely dominated medical advances, but during the first 50 years of the 1900s, with discoveries such as that of insulin and heparin, superiority in this respect was moving westward to the New World. It is perhaps relevant that for those surgeons training before World War II, it was still considered highly beneficial, if not mandatory, to spend a period of postgraduate study in Europe. Since World War II, the direction of travel has been reversed, with a large number of trainee physicians and surgeons in Europe traveling "across the pond" to gain clinical or, increasingly, research experience in the United States or, to a lesser extent, Canada.

One should remember that in the early part of the 20th century, academic American medicine was concentrated largely in a dozen or so centers clustered on the eastern seaboard. Although these centers remained heavily involved, the development of heart surgery reflected a move away from this geographic region. Centers such as Minneapolis and Houston began to show their clout as never before. Nevertheless, the East Coast establishments still played major roles, either directly or in the training of those who were later involved in these developments.

## Who Were These Men? Similarities and Differences

Although surgery in the "closed" heart era, before the development of the heart-lung machine, maintained to some extent the reign of the individual surgeon, "open" heart surgery could not be carried out without a team of highly skilled colleagues. In *Cold Hearts,* Bill Bigelow wrote, "Interdepartmental teams are not new, but I believe that there has never been an occasion in the history of clinical medicine when men and women of a variety of disciplines had been required to work so closely and be so dependent on each other's special knowledge, judgment, and talents."

Those in the "closed" heart surgery era tended to be individualists, such as Gross, Brock, Bailey, and Harken, whereas those who came to prominence in the open heart era were forced to be team players, although this did not necessarily mean they were democratic; they sometimes headed the team fairly dictatorially, as exemplified perhaps best by Kirklin, Barnard, and DeBakey.

Many, although not all, of those featured in this book were academically very gifted. However, academic success does not necessarily indicate an innovative mind, nor does a lack of such success preclude such innovation. Charles Darwin, one of the greatest innovative thinkers of all time, was perplexed as to what made a man an innovator. In 1871, he wrote to one of his sons, "Many men who are very clever — much cleverer than the discoverers — never originate anything."

A few of these surgical pioneers were very competent, sometimes outstanding, athletes, notably Cooley in basketball and tennis, DeVries in track and field, and Blalock, Swan, and Hufnagel in tennis. (Indeed, there are several similarities between the surgical team and a sports team — uniforms, locker rooms, an arena, et cetera.)

Several were flamboyant personalities, and others, although perhaps not flamboyant, were not averse to some publicity for themselves or their work. Yet some could certainly not be described in any way as flamboyant. There were, of course, several feuds among these men, but that is not particularly uncommon in any field of endeavor. Even though he was personally involved in one, Harken has labeled such acrimonious personal struggles as "horrible feuds between wonderful men."

It is interesting to note the number who believed they suffered from dyslexia, making learning from books difficult. Once freed from the library, however, and able to learn from actual patients and real medical situations, their difficulties largely evaporated.

Several had direct military experience of World War II. The impact of the surgical experience these young men gained under war conditions cannot be underestimated. Despite this interruption to their careers, many of them were remarkably young when they carried out their major surgical advances — the majority being in their 30s.

Perhaps surprisingly for such gifted individuals, a number of them later went through career crises in which they either resigned from their institution under something of a cloud or were actually forced to leave, disrupting a highly productive career; in some cases, the career could not be resuscitated. A significant number of them went through a divorce or separation, in some cases almost certainly related to the intensity of their work or to the distraction that work caused to their marriage and family.

As one might expect, several were sons of doctors, and others the sons of dentists. Several had sons or daughters who went into medicine, a few of whom followed their fathers into cardiac surgery. Several others, however, admitted that the example of their busy and stressful lifestyle had been a factor in dissuading their children from following medicine as a career.

Both John Kirklin and Walt Lillehei had sons who followed them into surgery. One very nice story involves their training at the Massachusetts General Hospital. At one time, they were both working in the department of cardiac surgery under the then director, Mortimer Buckley, who, to his great credit, tells this story about himself. He was, in his own right, a significant contributor to cardiac surgery, particularly in the field of the aortic balloon pump. The story Buckley tells is that he was standing near the notice board on which the operating list for the day had been pinned. He was to be assisted in his heart operation by John Kirklin's son, James, and Walt Lillehei's son, Craig.

The operating list therefore listed the surgeons as "Buckley, Kirklin, and Lillehei." Buckley overheard two anesthesiologists perusing the list, with one saying to the other, "I've heard of Kirklin and Lillehei, but who the hell is this guy Buckley?"

## Surgical Research — Then and Now

Many of those I interviewed for this book commented on the ease with which experimental laboratory research could be carried out in their day — in the 1940s, 1950s, and even the 1960s. There were virtually no regulations to hold them back. Today, any animal experimentation in the United States, even if it involves only a lowly mouse, is required to be reviewed by a local committee, a process that may take some weeks. The process is, if anything, even more rigorous in the United Kingdom. Similar stringent regulations govern surgical research in most Western countries.

Some mentioned to me that, in the 1950s, if the experiment was even modestly successful in a dog, the next week they would try it in a patient. Although this was something of an exaggeration, there was a considerable amount of truth in it. Today, there would unquestionably be a much greater requirement for extensive laboratory work and a much greater delay in ensuring the safety of a procedure before any clinical trial could be undertaken. Today's restrictions may to some extent impede progress in medicine and surgery. Several of the pioneers I interviewed made this point to me most emphatically. For example, John Osborn told me, "I am convinced that a lot more patients would have died if the Food and Drug Aministration (FDA) had been functioning then as it functions now, because we could not have carried out the crucial experiments which made the whole technology advance."

The novel surgical approaches described in this book could be tested in patients as freely as they were, of course, only because the medicolegal system at the time was so relatively primitive. Today, with lawyers breathing down the medical profession's neck, a surgeon would indeed be foolhardy to undertake unregulated and non–peer-reviewed experimental clinical surgery as did his or her predecessors. The medico-legal impediments have become almost overwhelming, and it is perhaps surprising that surgical advances are still being made. Some balance is required in the scales between the inevitable risks involved in genuine efforts to save a patient's life and to advance medical knowledge, and those associated with reckless or incompetent surgical management.

One excellent example of the changes that have taken place during the past four or five decades is provided by the nature of obtaining the consent of the patient to any surgical procedure, particularly if it is of an experimental nature. Today, great emphasis is placed on obtaining truly "informed" consent from the patient. The informed consent form that the patient is requested to sign provides a detailed account of the potential benefits and, particularly, the risks, and takes on an important medicolegal status.

How different this is from not too many years ago! Look again at the consent form signed by a family member on behalf of James Hardy's (comatose) first patient to undergo a heart transplant in 1964 (Figure 47). This one-paragraph document fails to mention that an animal, rather than a human, donor heart might be used and would be totally unacceptable today, either ethically or legally, but was the norm for the time.

Surgical research frequently necessitates demonstrating that a new procedure is *consistently* successful, or at least more successful than the current method of surgical treatment. One will therefore frequently read a scientific report indicating the results of a new operation or therapy in 10 or 20 animals. If success is not consistent in this group, then doubt is cast upon the new approach. In this respect, there is an apocryphal story (told to me during the preparation of this book) of a young surgical research fellow who did not want to spend a long time on his project since he was absolutely convinced it would constitute a major medical advance. He was particularly concerned about the cost and time of performing a whole series of animal experiments, and wanted desperately to do the minimum necessary to prove his point. Yet, at the same time, he wanted his scientific report to be both acceptable to peer review and strictly honest. He therefore named one of his experimental animals "Ten dogs." When he achieved success in this one dog, he could honestly report, "Ten dogs underwent a successful operation." This saved him the inconvenience of having to operate on a further nine!

## The Nobel Prize

It has always amazed and disappointed me that none of the surgeons who are profiled in this book won a Nobel Prize for his contributions to medicine. The Nobel Prize for Medicine or Physiology is awarded each year by the Nobel Foundation, the recipients being selected by the faculty of the Karolinska Institute in Stockholm. Up to three people can share the prize, but it is never awarded posthumously.

I particularly had in mind recognition for the development of open heart surgery, which really was a quantum leap in surgical technique since it involved not just a new operation, but a dramatic new concept — the development of a machine that would support life while the heart was stopped.

Perhaps a majority of those with whom I discussed this topic believed that the prize should have been shared between Gibbon, for his early and prolonged studies demonstrating that a heart-lung machine was feasible, and Lillehei, who, with his several colleagues, established that open heart surgery could be performed using the cross-circulation technique and subsequently greatly simplified the heart-lung machine so that it was available to surgeons worldwide. Several would have added the name of Kirklin, who was the first (with Lillehei) to demonstrate that a heart-lung machine could be used successfully on a consistent basis, and who subsequently did so much to provide open heart surgery with a scientific foundation. There would seem little controversy if these three had shared the prize. However, the Swedish group, particularly Crafoord and Senning, could certainly claim to be included for consideration.

On a lighter note, Chris Barnard tells the story that a journalist once advised him that his flamboyant lifestyle, in particular his being seen with a stream of beautiful young women, had alienated the Nobel committee. If it had not been for this flaw, he might have been awarded the prize for carrying out the first heart transplant. If he had his life again, the journalist asked, would he follow the same social path? Barnard thought carefully for a few moments. If the journalist were correct, he replied, and if it truly came down to a choice between the Nobel Prize and the company of beautiful young women, then he had to admit that, if he had his life to live again, he would still choose the women.

This is the same Chris Barnard who, when 65 years old, was asked by a journalist whether there might be a health risk in his marrying a 25-year-old girl. "That might be so," he replied, "but she will just have to accept the risks."

## Patients' Deaths

All the surgeons portrayed in this book experienced death at close hand. In contrast to physicians, and indeed most other surgeons, heart surgeons are exposed to death much more frequently. In cardiac surgery, the association between the operation and the death of a patient is frequently clear-cut. The surgeon has to live with the fact that the death of the patient was intimately related to his or her performance of the operation. Of course, surgeons can frequently justify their intervention by reminding themselves that the patient was slowly (or rapidly) dying anyway, but it is difficult to shake off the emotional impact of this obvious cause and effect. The pioneer heart surgeons responded to death in different ways. From my personal experience as a heart surgeon, I know most or all of them would agree with Henry Bahnson, a trainee of Blalock, who, when I asked him how he coped with a patient's death in those early days, replied, "We felt guilty."

Sadly, a small number of patients still die on the operating table, or soon after, today. But contemporary surgeons do not experience the number of deaths faced by the pioneers. One leading contemporary surgeon recently commented, "Can you imagine going to work and having somebody die on you every third day? I think it takes a very extraordinary person who can withstand that and make something positive of it."

One of my early mentors, Bill Cleland, was the first surgeon to perform open heart surgery in the United Kingdom (using the heart-lung machine developed by Dennis Melrose). In the 1970s, I was assisting him during an operation when a cardiologist came to the operating room and asked him if he would consult on a patient later that day. The cardiologist mentioned that the patient had a condition with which he thought Mr. Cleland "had great experience." "What is it?" asked Cleland. "Death?" This slightly cynical remark would not have been in his mind had he not faced its stark reality on many occasions.

One very experienced and internationally recognized Texas vascular surgeon was once asked by a junior colleague how he obtained such good surgical results. "By having good judgment," he replied. But how did he develop such good judgment, asked his junior. "By experience," came the reply. But how did he obtain such experience, persisted the junior. "By having bad judgment," was the surgeon's response.

Making errors of judgment, facing death on the operating table, and agonizing over whether you have performed a surgical procedure adequately can all be very painful forms of "hell" to the surgeon. The lesson that heart surgeons quickly learn is, as Winston Churchill said, "If you are going through hell, keep going." Heart surgery is not a career for someone who lacks courage, persistence, and tenacity.

There is a Native American proverb that is relevant here: "It is not enough for a man to know how to ride — he must also know how to fall." The early heart surgeons had to learn this immensely difficult task — how to accept failure as well as success.

## Life Again

One other point that struck me was the comment by several surgeons that, if they were young men today, they would *not* choose to go into heart surgery. The reason given was that the excitement is over. Most of the problems have been resolved, and there is little or nothing more to develop. Indeed, the so-called invasive cardiologists — cardiologists who carry out catheterization procedures on the patient — are gradually developing techniques that enable them to correct abnormalities and diseased states that were originally the province of the surgeon. Balloon angioplasty for coronary artery disease is perhaps the prime example, but some congenital heart defects, such as ductus, coarctation, atrial septal defect, pulmonary valve stenosis, and some valve conditions, formerly amenable only to the techniques of the heart surgeon, can now be treated by a physician using a catheter. Cardiac surgery has therefore become less enticing for those with an inquiring and ambitious mind who wish to push the barriers of medicine forward. Furthermore, the incidences of common heart diseases, such as coronary artery disease and rheumatic heart disease, are steadily declining, at least in the developed world, as preventative measures take effect.

Today, the real medical pioneer directs his or her attention to other fields, such as immunology, genetics, neuroscience, virology, and other areas where large questions are still being asked, and major answers are still required. James Watson, the co-discoverer with Francis Crick, Maurice Wilkins, and Rosalind Franklin of the helical structure of DNA, advised young scientists "not to bother with small questions, for such pursuits are likely to produce small answers."

## The Moment

The pioneer sees medicine through the eyes of dramatist George Bernard Shaw, who put these words into the mouth of one of his characters: "You see things; and you say 'why?' But I dream things that never were; and I say 'why not?'" But the fulfillment of this dream — to see one's aim achieved — comes to few of us in medical research, or in any other field of endeavor, for that matter. And for those select and immensely lucky few, their achievement is often a "one-off," and rarely sustained.

Nazih Zuhdi's opinion was, "Every man has a moment in life when God permits him to touch the sky." Unfortunately, this is not true. Most of us *never* "touch the sky." But if we do, Zuhdi was correct in stating that it is only for "a moment." Those few who do "touch the sky" are rarely able to sustain this period of innovation for long. For many in this book, the sky was touched only fleetingly. They are remembered for the introduction of a single innovation, or even a single event, though in some cases this epochal event may have followed months or even years of research. But then their contribution, large as it may have been, was over. Their star waned, often rapidly.

Many of the major steps forward in heart surgery garnered much publicity and public attention, not surprisingly given the dramatic nature of the surgical procedures that were undertaken. Most of the surgeons experienced at least Andy Warhol's "15 minutes of fame," sometimes much longer. The impact that heart surgery had on the public is perhaps illustrated by a list of "famous names" drawn up in the 1970s on the basis of public familiarity. Although only six 20th-century "medical men" were included — Albert Schweitzer, Jonas Salk, Paul Dudley White, Michael DeBakey, Denton Cooley, and Christiaan Barnard — three of the six were involved in the development of heart surgery.

Walt Lillehei once said, "Science is an endless frontier." There will always be new challenges to surmount, new knowledge to gain, new concepts to put forward. The contributions to medicine made by those in this book will be enjoyed by a multitude of patients for many years to come, but eventually their discoveries and advances will be forgotten — absorbed into the past — since, in the words of British Nobel Laureate Sir Peter Medawar, "In science, the future devours the past." Indeed, many of the crucial advances highlighted in this book were already outdated within a few years, and yet they were critical to the overall development of heart surgery.

Nevertheless, the names of these men — these magnificent men with their heart-lung machines — will be remembered far into the future. There is another Native American proverb that says, "A man is not dead until the last person who remembers him dies." If that is the case, the men who played major roles in the development of heart surgery, even though they may no longer actually be with us in this world, will remain alive for many, many years.

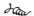

# ACKNOWLEDGMENTS

I THANK THE FOLLOWING surgeons, physicians, and biographers who I interviewed either in person or by telephone in the course of the preparation of this book:

Henry Bahnson, Charles Bailey, Christiaan Barnard, Sir Brian Barratt-Boyes, Robert Bartlett, Erik Berglund, Wilfred Bigelow, Viking Bjork, Christian Cabrol, Sir Roy Calne, Aldo Castañeda, Morley Cohen, Herbert Cohn, Denton Cooley, Michael DeBakey, Clarence Dennis, William DeVries, Richard DeWall, Anthony Dobell, Sir Terence English, Rene Favaloro, Robert Finley, Robert Frater, O. Howard Frazier, Allan L. Friedlich, Harold Goldberg, Vincent Gott, James Hardy, Alden Harken, Dwight Harken, Hardy Hendren, Charles Hufnagel, George Humphreys, John Kirklin, Willem Kolff, F. John Lewis, C. Walton Lillehei, Richard Lower, Dennis Melrose, Bernard Miller, G. Wayne Miller, Ben Milstein, Francis Moore, William Myerly, John Najarian, John Norman, John Osborn, Philip Oyer, Robert Pontius, Keith Reemtsma, Bruce Reitz, Donald Ross, Ake Senning, Norman Shumway, Albert Starr, Thomas Starzl, Henry Swan, Mansur Taufic, John Templeton III, Frank Thomas, Luis Toledo-Peyrera, Richard Varco, Arthur Voorhees, Herbert Warden, Watts Webb, William Weirich, John Wright, and Nazih Zuhdi.

Apart from those quoted in the text, I thank the following surgeons and physicians for providing help or information in the preparation of this book: William Baumgartner, Randall "Chip" Bolman, Leo Buhler, Carl-Gustav Groth, Mark Hardy, Arthur Hollman, Elizier Katz, Christoph Knosalla, Igor Konstantinov, Robert Lanza, Dai Nghiem, Juan Sanchez, Shigeki Taniguchi, Joe Tector, and Tom Treasure.

I also thank Bill Patrick for his expert professional advice on the preparation of this book; my literary agent, Glen Hartley, for his support and guidance; Don Fehr and Katherine Lopaze of Kaplan Publishing, for their editorial expertise; Crystal Taylor and John Schurer for skilled secretarial assistance; and Kameo Muneo for preparing the drawings that illustrate the text.

Certain figures are reproduced by permission of the New York Academy of Medicine Library, the Indiana University Press, the University of Minnesota Archives, or Time, Inc.

# SELECTED BIBLIOGRAPHY

THE FOLLOWING BOOKS and articles have provided valuable sources of information or opinion, and I gratefully and readily acknowledge the information they have provided, some of which has been used in the preparation of this text.

Barnard, Christiaan N. *The Second Life*. Cape Town: Vlaeberg, 1993.

Barnard, Christiaan N., and Curtis B. Pepper. *One Life*. London: Harrap, 1970.

Barr, Brooks. *The Life of Nazih Zuhdi: Uncharted Voyage of the Heart*. Oklahoma City: Oklahoma Heritage Association, 2005.

Bigelow, Wilfred G. *Cold Hearts: The Story of Hypothermia and the Cardiac Pacemaker*. Toronto: McClelland and Stewart, 1984.

Bigelow, Wilfred G. *Mysterious Heparin: The Key to Open Heart Surgery*. Toronto: McGraw-Hill, Ryeson, 1990.

Bing, Richard J., ed. *Cardiology: The Evolution of the Science and the Art*. Chur, Switzerland: Harwood Academic, 1992.

Bjork, Viking O. Fifty years of cardiac and pulmonary surgery 1942–1993. *Scandinavian Journal of Thoracic and Cardiovascular Surgery,* S42, 1994.

Chisholm, Donna. *From the Heart*. Auckland, New Zealand: Reed Methuen, 1987.

Cooley, Denton A. *Reflections and Observations: Essays of Denton A. Cooley,* collected by Marianne Kneipp. Austin: Eakin Press, 1984.

Cooper, David K. C. *Chris Barnard — By Those Who Know Him*. Cape Town: Vlaeberg, 1992.

Derloshon, Gerald B. *One for the Heart: The Story of the Professor Viking O. Bjork, M.D.* Irvine, CA: Shiley, Inc., 1983.

Fenster, Julie M. *Ether Day: The Strange Tale of America's Greatest Medical Discovery and the Haunted Men Who Made It.* New York: HarperCollins, 2001.

Greatbatch, Wilson. *The Making of the Pacemaker: Celebrating a Lifesaving Invention.* Amherst, NY: Prometheus Books, 2000.

Haeger, Knut. *The Illustrated History of Surgery.* New York: Bell Publishing Co., 1988.

Hardy, James D. *The Academic Surgeon: An Autobiography.* Mobile, AL: Magnolia Mansions Press, 2002.

Hardy, James D. *The World of Surgery 1945–1985: Memoirs of One Participant.* Philadelphia: University of Pennsylvania Press, 1986.

Hawthorne, Peter. *The Transplanted Heart.* Johannesburg: Hugh Keartland, 1968.

Hellman, Hal. *Great Feuds in Medicine.* New York: John Wiley, 2001.

Hurst, J. Willis, C. Richard Conti, and W. Bruce Fye. *Profiles in Cardiology.* Mahwah, NJ: Foundation for Advances in Medicine and Surgery, Inc., 2003.

Hurt, Raymond. *The History of Cardiothoracic Surgery from Early Times.* Pearl River, NY: Parthenon, 1996.

Johnson, Stephen L. *The History of Cardiac Surgery 1896–1955.* Baltimore: The Johns Hopkins Press, 1970.

Konstantinov, Igor E. Vasilii I. Kolesov: a surgeon to remember. *Texas Heart Institute Journal,* 2004; 31:349–58.

Lemann, Nicholas. *The Fast Track: Texans and Other Strivers.* New York: W.W. Norton, 1981.

Le Vay, David. *Alexis Carrel: The Perfectibility of Man.* Rockville, MD: Kabel, 1996.

Logan, Chris. *Celebrity Surgeon: Christiaan Barnard—A Life.* Johannesburg and Cape Town: Jonathan Ball, 2003.

Longmire, William, P. Jr. *Alfred Blalock: His Life and Times.* Los Angeles: William Longmire, Jr., 1991.

Lyons, Albert S., and R. Joseph Petrucelli II. *Medicine: An Illustrated History.* New York: Harry N. Abrams, Inc., 1978.

McRae, Donald. *Every Second Counts: The Race to Transplant the First Human Heart.* New York: G. P. Putnam's Sons, 2006.

Miller, G. Wayne. *King of Hearts: The True Story of the Maverick Who Pioneered Open Heart Surgery.* New York: Times Books, 2000.

Miller, G. Wayne. *The Work of Human Hands.* Grantham, NH: Borderlands Press, 1999.

Milstein, Ben B. *The Development of Cardiothoracic Surgery at Papworth Hospital.* Published by the Public Relations Department of Papworth Hospital, Papworth Everard, UK,1997.

Moore, Frances D. *A Miracle and a Privilege: Recounting a Half Century of Surgical Advance.* Washington, DC: Joseph Henry Press, 1995.

Mueller, C. Barber. *Evarts A. Graham: The Life, Lives, and Times of the Surgical Spirit of St. Louis.* Hamilton, ON, Canada: B.C. Decker, 2002.

Naef, Andreas P. *The Story of Thoracic Surgery: Milestones and Pioneers.* Lewiston, NY: Hogrefe and Huber, 1990.

Nose, Yukihiko, and Tadashi Motomura. *Cardiac Prosthesis — Artificial Heart and Assist Circulation — Past, Present and Future.* Houston: ICMT Press, 2003.

Ranier, W. Gerald. *Pioneer Interviews. http://www.ctsnet.org.*

Richardson, Robert G. *The Surgeon's Heart.* London: Heinemann, 1969.

Roberts, William C. David Coston Sabiston, Jr., MD: a conversation with the editor. *American Journal of Cardiology,* 1998; 82:358–72.

Roberts, William C. Denton Arthur Cooley, MD: a conversation with the editor. *American Journal of Cardiology,* 1997; 79:1078–91.

Roberts, William C. John Webster Kirklin, MD: a conversation with the editor. *American Journal of Cardiology,* 1998; 81:1027–44.

Roberts, William C. Michael Ellis DeBakey, MD: a conversation with the editor. *American Journal of Cardiology,* 1997; 79:929–50 and 1078–91.

Romaine-Davis, Aida. *John Gibbon and His Heart-Lung Machine.* Philadelphia: University of Pennsylvania Press, 1991.

Shumacker, Harris B. Jr. *A Dream of the Heart: The Life of John H. Gibbon Jr., Father of the Heart-Lung Machine.* Santa Barbara, CA: Fithian Press, 1999.

Shumacker, Harris B. Jr. *The Evolution of Cardiac Surgery.* Bloomington: Indiana University Press, 1992. (Several figures are reproduced from this book with permission from the Indiana University Press.)

Starzl, Thomas E. *The Puzzle People: Memoirs of a Transplant Surgeon.* Pittsburgh, PA: University of Pittsburgh Press, 1992.

Stoney, William S. *Pioneers of Cardiac Surgery.* Nashville, TN: Vanderbilt University Press, 2008.

Thomas, Vivien T. *Pioneering Research in Surgical Shock and Cardiovascular Surgery: Vivien Thomas and His Work with Alfred Blalock.* Philadelphia: University of Pennsylvania Press, 1985.

Thompson, Thomas. *Hearts: Of Surgeons and Transplants, Miracles and Disasters along the Cardiac Frontier.* New York: McCall, 1971.

Thorwald, Jürgen. *The Patients.* New York: Harcourt Brace Jovanovich, 1971.

Tilney, Nicholas L. *Transplant: From Myth to Reality.* New Haven, CT: Yale University Press, 2003.

Van Noordwijk, Jacob. *Dialyzing for Life: The Development of the Artificial Kidney.* Dordrecht, Netherlands: Kluwer Academic, 2001.

Weisse, Allen B. *Conversations in Medicine.* New York: New York University Press, 1984.

Weisse, Allen B. *Heart to Heart: The Twentieth Century Battle Against Cardiac Disease—An Oral History.* New Brunswick, NJ: Rutgers University Press, 2002.

Wertenbaker, Lael. *To Mend the Heart: The Dramatic Story of Cardiac Surgery and Its Pioneers.* New York: Viking Press, 1980.

Westaby, Stephen, with Cecil Bosher. *Landmarks in Cardiac Surgery.* Oxford, England: Isis Medical Media, 1997.

Wilson, Leonard G. *Medical Revolution in Minnesota: A History of the University of Minnesota Medical School.* St. Paul, MN: Midewiwin Press, 1980. (Several figures are reproduced from this book with permission from the University of Minnesota Archives.)

Wooler, Geoffrey. *Pig in a Suitcase: The Autobiography of a Heart Surgeon.* Otley, U.K.: Smith Settle, 1999.

# INDEX

# ABOUT THE AUTHOR

DAVID K. C. COOPER is a professor of surgery and director of a research group at the Thomas E. Starzl Transplantation Institute at the University of Pittsburgh Medical Center.

Born and raised in London, England, he completed his medical education at Guy's Hospital Medical School of the University of London (now part of King's College London), and then trained in general surgery and heart surgery in the United Kingdom, taking time out for periods of research and teaching at the universities of Harvard, London, and Cambridge (at Magdalene College). In the late 1970s, he was a member of the surgical team that performed the first successful series of heart transplants in the United Kingdom.

In 1980, Dr. Cooper was appointed to the faculty of the University of Cape Town Medical School in South Africa, where he had responsibility for the heart transplant program under Professor Christiaan Barnard at Groote Schuur Hospital. He also directed a program of research into aspects of organ transplantation. In 1987, he moved to Oklahoma City, where he continued his work in heart transplantation and related research. From 1996 to 2004, he held a full-time research appointment at the Massachusetts General Hospital of the Harvard Medical School.

David Cooper holds three doctorate degrees, and is a fellow of both the Royal College of Surgeons of England and the American College of Surgeons. He has published over 600 medical and scientific papers and chapters, and has edited or co-edited six major textbooks, as well as a book of reminiscences on the heart transplant pioneer Chris Barnard. He has also lectured widely on five continents and done innumerable interviews with both print and electronic media. He lives with his wife, Amy, in Pittsburgh, Pennsylvania.